D1570260

GROUP THERAPY FOR
MEDICALLY ILL PATIENTS

Group Therapy for Medically Ill Patients

JAMES L. SPIRA
Editor

THE GUILFORD PRESS
New York   London

© 1997 The Guilford Press
A Division of Guilford Publications, Inc.
72 Spring Street, New York, NY 10012

Printed in the United States of America

This book is printed on acid-free paper.

Last digit is print number: 9 8 7 6 5 4 3 2 1

Library of Congress Cataloging-in-Publication Data

Group therapy for medically ill patients / James L. Spira, editor.
    p.   cm.
    Includes bibliographical references and index.
    ISBN 1-57230-168-6
    1. Group psychotherapy.   2. Clinical health psychology.   3. Sick—
Mental health.   4. Sick—Psychology.   I. Spira, James L.
    [DNLM: 1. Psychotherapy, Group—methods.   2. Acute Disease—
psychology.   3. Catastrophic Illness—psychology.   4. Chronic
Disease—psychology.   5. Critical Illness—psychology.
6. Recurrence. WM 430 G8834 1997]
RC488.G726 1997
616.89'152—dc20
DNLM/DLC
for Library of Congress   96-27736
                                           CIP

Contributors

Mike Antoni, Ph.D., is Professor of Psychology at the University of Miami. He was instrumental in developing and leading the intervention for a gay men's cohort that received coping skills, exercise, and stress management prior to learning their HIV status. Treatment subjects had less disruption on a number of immune measures, both functional and numeric. Recent data on disease progression and survival have demonstrated the effectiveness of this treatment for improving mood and immunity, as well as for reducing disease progression and mortality from AIDS.

Paul Bracke, Ph.D., is a psychologist in private practice in San Francisco, specializing in problems involving chronic stress, self-esteem, Type A behavior, and relationships. As a consultant to the Meyer Friedman Institute in San Francisco, he trains group leaders and conducts groups designed to change Type A behavior. He has conducted research on the role of family in the development of Type A behavior in children and adolescents and was field coordinator for the Recurrent Coronary Prevention Project Update study examining the long-term effectiveness of modifying Type A behavior in postcoronary patients.

Fawzy I. Fawzy, M.D., is Professor, Chief of Consultation–Liaison Psychiatry, Interim Director and Chair of the Department of Psychiatry and Biobehavioral Sciences at the UCLA School of Medicine. He has used group therapy for persons with AIDS and cancer. He is author of several articles demonstrating the effectiveness of short-term group therapy for persons with early-stage malignant melanoma. Treatment patients improved in mood and coping and appear to have less immune disruption. In 1993, he published results of a 5-year survival follow-up revealing reduced disease progression and increased survival for the treatment group.

Nancy W. Fawzy, R.N., D.N.Sc., is Director of Psychosocial Care Programs at the John Wayne Cancer Center in Santa Monica, California, where she coordinates and leads support groups for patients with breast cancer and malignant melanoma.

Carlos M. Grilo, Ph.D., is Assistant Professor of Psychiatry and a clinical psychologist at the School of Medicine, Yale University, where he directed the Eating Disorders Clinic.

Christine S. Hyun, M.P.H., M.B.A., has served as a research assistant for Fawzy I. Fawzy at the UCLA School of Medicine, and is currently Assistant Administrator at Kaiser–Permanente Hospital in San Jose, California.

Robert A. Matano, Ph.D., is Assistant Professor of Psychiatry and Behavioral Sciences at Stanford University and Director of the Stanford Drug and Alcohol Treatment Program.

Judith Rodin, Ph.D., is President of the University of Pennsylvania and Professor of Psychology. She is world renowned as an expert in eating disorders, including physiological, psychological, and epidemiological perspectives. Dr. Rodin is also a clinician, experienced in psychosocial intervention for correcting eating disorders. She serves as director of a MacArthur Foundation Network, exploring the psychoneuroimmunological alterations that occur due to stress.

James L. Spira, Ph.D., M.P.H., is a licensed psychologist, Director of the Institute for Health Psychology in San Diego, and Associate Director of the Scripps Clinic Wellness Programs in La Jolla, California. He has worked with patients with HIV while a graduate student at the University of California at Berkeley, groups for women with recurrent breast cancer and groups for substance abusers while a postdoctoral fellow at Stanford University School of Medicine, and groups of persons with cardiac disease, cancer, arthritis, multiple sclerosis, diabetes, pulmonary disease, Type A, and obesity while serving on the faculty and as Director of the Program in Health Psychology at Duke University School of Medicine. Dr. Spira has written several treatment manuals of group therapy for women with breast cancer, is a consultant with the American Psychological Association group therapy demonstration project for women with breast cancer, and has trained health professionals throughout the United States, Europe, and Asia in utilizing group therapy for medically ill patients.

Carl E. Thoresen, Ph.D., is Professor of Education and Psychology at the School of Education, Stanford University. He directs the graduate program in health psychology education and has collaborated for many years with Meyer Friedman at Mt. Zion Hospital Medical Center of the University of California at San Francisco.

Jennifer G. Wheeler, M.A., has served as a research associate for Fawzy I. Fawzy at the UCLA School of Medicine and is now a doctoral candidate in psychology at the University of Washington, Seattle.

Denise E. Wilfley, Ph.D., a clinical psychologist, is Assistant Professor of Psychology and Director of the Center for Eating and Weight Disorders in the joint San Diego State University/University of California at San Diego clinical psychology program. Dr. Wilfley has conducted research at Stanford University and Yale University Medical Schools on various approaches to group therapy for persons with disordered eating patterns.

Irvin D. Yalom, M.D., is Professor Emeritus of Psychiatry and Behavioral Sciences at Stanford University School of Medicine. He is internationally renowned for his research and teaching in group psychotherapy. He is the author of many now-classic textbooks, including *The Theory and Practice of Group Psychotherapy* and *Existential Psychotherapy*, to name two.

Preface

While at the University of California–Berkeley, Stanford University, and Duke University, I have led medically ill groups that include patients with cancer (early stage, recurrent, mixed), HIV (mixed stage), coronary artery disease, arthritis, multiple sclerosis, pulmonary disease, diabetes, chronic fatigue syndrome, obesity, eating disorders, and substance abuse; families of patients; those concerned with prevention; and Type A persons at risk for cardiovascular disease. I have found group psychotherapy specifically designed for medically ill patients to be without doubt the most effective form of psychotherapy I have encountered for the majority of persons in this population. I must also admit that personally it has been one of the most enriching, maturing, and quite often disturbing activities I have ever engaged in.

My positive experience with groups led me to invite many of the authors in this book to co-present a symposium for the Society of Behavioral Medicine in 1992, entitled "Group Therapy for the Medically Ill." What was unique about this symposium was not only that such a symposium had not previously been held, but that each speaker was involved in the research (and in large part the *only* research on the subject) which had demonstrated that group therapy can improve both quality of life and survival. Moreover, these presenters, all of whom have contributed to this volume, are clinician–researchers in major university settings, and have many years of experience in leading groups for medically ill patients. Rather than staying removed in an "ivory tower," these university faculty members can lead a group as well as describe their methodology with sufficient clarity that other experienced clinicians can understand these methods and begin to incorporate them into their practice or research programs. Such clarity is of special import, because, to date, there have been no books and scant articles specifically devoted to describing group psychotherapy for medically ill patients. That absence of in-depth analysis is of concern because this approach is currently one of the most widely utilized methods of psychosocial support in medical centers throughout the United States, Europe, and Australia.

This book, then, is an initial effort to remedy that concern. As the contributors have researched the effectiveness of their interventions, I have asked them each not only to describe in detail their intervention, but also to present the results demonstrating the efficacy of their research for improving quality of life and physical health of medically ill patients. For, after all, they have been the leaders in demonstrating the positive consequences of psychosocial intervention on health. Although group therapy is doubtless effective for coping with many types of medical illness, these chapters represent areas of health psychology in which group therapy has been shown to affect health outcome. While certainly not exhaustive, these subjects have been chosen to demonstrate a range of effective approaches for a variety of illnesses and health-related behaviors.

The task of understanding what the approaches represented here have in common may at times appear difficult. Throughout my experiences with various groups, I have found that although topics may vary among disease type to some extent, both the groups and the group therapeutic process do have much in common. Patients have similar existential issues (albeit to different levels of motivation, often depending on disease severity). In addition, general principles of facilitating groups, relieving distress, and using the crisis as an opportunity for growth are consistent across all groups. Yet there are also important differences in the approach taken with each disease type and stage of disease which, if appreciated, can lead to maximum benefit to the patients. For this reason, the variety of contributions in this book represents the differing needs of the populations being served, and the correspondingly different approaches.

There is clearly no single approach to psychotherapy that is optimal for all patients. This is partly a result of the range of dysfunctions presented by patients, and also because of the scope of individual differences in the personalities and lifestyles of patients who present for therapy. Such a diversity of patients may help to explain why no single therapeutic system has been able to either universally describe or improve the whole of human functioning or dysfunction. The need for a wide range of therapeutic methods can therefore be appreciated.

At first impression, describing a specific type of health psychology intervention may appear a far less daunting task. After all, most medical patients at least have concern for their health in common and are no more prone to long-standing psychosocial dysfunction than is the general public. Yet, if the variety of psychotherapeutic approaches in existence corresponds to the variety of patients seen, given the scope of the persons who have different illnesses at various stages of development, each with a plethora of responses, and given the fact that there is no single personality factor relating them, developing an interventional method for medically ill patients can be seen as far from a simple matter. Add to this the fact that there are as many approaches to group therapy as there are individual approaches to psychotherapy, and describing group therapy interventions for medically ill patients can pose quite a challenge.

Fortunately, a variety of group formats can serve the variety of special needs that different populations require. The complexity of individual differences that cannot be foreseen in planning for a group can be accommodated by and actually enrich the group. In fact, this is one of its strengths—the variety of members' experiences adds to rather than detracts from the group therapeutic process. Moreover, although it is true that no single group therapy approach is optimal for all medically ill patients, the unique entity which is the therapy "group" can accommodate, and benefit from, a variety of approaches, each tailored to a specific set of outcomes to assist the needs of specific medically ill populations.

With these considerations in mind, the introductory chapter familiarizes practitioners with the range of therapeutic and patient factors needed to select the approach to group therapy that is most appropriate for their medically ill patients. The subsequent chapters describe in detail specific methodologies for particular populations so that clinicians can form such a group (given sufficient background training) and researchers will have confidence in their ability to replicate a methodology reliably.

While most forms of therapy are threatened in a managed care environment, group therapy appears to be the most patient-effective and certainly the most cost-effective form of therapy available. Although clinical researchers have long understood that group therapy as a psychosocial intervention is ideal for intervention research in terms of cost and time, if not effectiveness, managed care is slower to catch on. However, this is bound to change in today's financially austere medical environment. It may well be that the combination of the new managed care environment along with research demonstrating its efficacy will launch group psychotherapy into the forefront of psychotherapeutic methods in the next millennium. The patients are sure to be the beneficiaries.

JAMES L. SPIRA

Acknowledgments

I wish to thank the Society of Behavioral Medicine for sponsoring the symposium that spawned this book, and the contributors who made great efforts to attend that symposium, write and rewrite their chapters, and, finally, wait patiently for this project to come to press. I also wish to thank Irvin Yalom for his mentorship. After years of leading groups geared to training patients in experiential methods of managing pain and stress and conducting exercises to recognize and improve coping strategies, I thought I had learned to present as effective an intervention as was possible for medically ill patients. It took Irv to show me that when one presents, one does not listen, and there is a tremendous amount of experience and maturity to be gained from listening to medically ill patients and drawing out their wisdom.

I also need to thank Janet and Julia for putting up with and permitting endless weekends and evenings buried away in my office. The only more patient person is Seymour Weingarten, Editor-in-Chief of The Guilford Press, who kept faith that this project would eventually come to pass. Finally, I want to thank the patients who have taught me so much and continue to do so in every group I share with them.

JAMES L. SPIRA

Contents

IV. Treating Behaviors that Interfere with Health

PART 1

INTRODUCTION

CHAPTER 1

Understanding and Developing Psychotherapy Groups for Medically Ill Patients

JAMES L. SPIRA

Group psychotherapy specifically designed for persons with medical illness may very well be the most powerful psychosocial intervention available for the vast majority of these patients. Beyond the scope of individual therapy, group therapy can address the major issues facing medically ill patients in a way that members garner the emotional support of persons with similar experiences and use the experiences of others to buffer the fear of future unknowns. For decades, group psychotherapy has been utilized effectively with patients facing a variety of psychosocial issues (Corsini & Rosenberg, 1955; Allen, 1990). Several professional societies and journals have been founded specifically to advance the discipline of group psychotherapy, including the American Group Psychotherapy Association (which publishes the *International Journal of Group Psychotherapy*) and the American Psychological Association, Division of Group Psychology and Group Psychotherapy. However, groups specifically designed for medically ill patients have been utilized, described, and researched far less frequently. This chapter is intended to help reduce that deficiency by providing a clinical framework for health professionals who wish to offer psychosocial support to patients with medically related issues.

Group therapy has been used for almost every type of psychiatric and psychological problem. Although its popularity has waxed and waned over the last several decades (Benezra, 1990), the cost and time-efficient attitudes of the 1990s have brought about a renewed interest in group therapy because group therapy is as cost- and time-efficient as it is effective (Hellman, Budd,

Borsenko, McClelland, & Benson, 1990). This is nowhere as evident as in the application of group psychotherapy for medically ill patients, where this form of therapy is increasingly considered a regular adjunct to usual medical care. Perhaps this emerging attitude is a result of the recent surge in studies linking psychosocial factors to health outcome, or because of several new studies demonstrating health improvement for patients undergoing group psychotherapy treatment. Most likely, such suggestions of clinical effectiveness in combination with renowned cost and time efficiency in this climate of increasingly managed care are responsible for the sudden popularity of this mode of treatment. Whatever the reason, group therapy for the medically ill has seen an unprecedented surge in popularity over the past several years. Yet there has been little written on this application of group therapy and there is no clearly outlined protocol for its implementation. In light of the paucity of literature in this area, this chapter provides a framework for understanding its scope and applications and examines the reasons that group psychotherapy should be considered a viable component of standard medical treatment.

BACKGROUND

Appreciating the styles and applications of traditional group psychotherapy for persons with psychosocial dysfunction as well as other forms of psychosocial support for medically ill patients provides a perspective from which group therapy for persons with medical illness can be better understood.

Group Psychotherapy for Psychosocial Dysfunction

Although group therapy for the medically ill has only recently received considerable attention, as far back as 1905 Joseph Pratt, a Boston internist, reported that group meetings with tuberculosis patients increased their self-confidence and self-esteem. Moreover, those patients also demonstrated clinical improvement (Allen, 1990). Since then, emphasizing interpersonal relationships has been increasingly accepted as a crucial psychotherapeutic tool (Freud, 1921; Adler, 1949; Sullivan, 1953; Bandura & Walters, 1963). Proponents of group psychotherapy have developed a variety of approaches to group therapy (Corsini & Rosenberg, 1955; Moreno, 1966; Minuchin, 1974; Yalom, 1985). With few exceptions, these approaches have been primarily directed at treatment for the psychologically rather than the physically ill. However, because these approaches are usually considered the model for use with medically ill patients, examining them will be helpful.

Why should group psychotherapy be considered over other forms of therapy? First, group therapy can be used along with individual psychotherapy (Berger, 1990) or medical treatments (Morrow, 1984). Yet, at times group therapy should be considered not only an adjunct but also a replacement for individual psychotherapy. Economically, group therapy may be up to four times more affordable for patients and for institutions such as health maintenance organizations (HMOs) (Yalom & Yalom, 1990; Hellman et al., 1990). This approach may enable patients to benefit from additional therapy they could not otherwise afford. Interpersonal problems, behavioral skills, and educational information can often be addressed just as easily in a group setting as in a private tutorial, often with no decrement to the learning process.

Moreover, some aspects of therapy are more appropriately developed in a group than in individual psychotherapy. Just as intrapsychic disturbances that interfere with cognitive or affective functioning may be benefited by individual therapy, difficulties with interpersonal relationships may be more clearly recognized, explored, and worked through during group therapy. Whereas developing a transference relationship to an individual therapist might be of use for working with intrapsychic patterns that have interpersonal ramifications, therapies that use such an approach are often time intensive and not directly focused on extending such insight to behavioral changes outside the therapy session. Group therapy, in contrast, involves learning to recognize interpersonal patterns and to develop interpersonal skills that are more generalizable to interactions in one's life than what can be learned from interaction with only one person (the therapist). Being part of a group also affords patients a sense of community (being understood and understanding others, receiving help from and being able to help others, observing others in such as way as to incorporate their positive attributes into one's own life) in a way that they may have been unable to achieve either in individual therapy or in their lives outside therapy. Thus, a patient can benefit more from interactions with others in a group than he or she usually can in individual therapy. On the other hand, at times personal exploration of long-standing personality patterns may be better addressed in an individual format.

Group therapy can be applied to a wide range of patient problems, including both *intra*personal and *inter*personal disturbances. These applications include working with personality traits that interfere with intrapersonal or interpersonal functioning, helping the patient handle situational stresses, attempting to improve mood, and assisting with interpersonal relationships. Group psychotherapy for persons with psychosocial dysfunction can be conducted with persons with a variety of concerns or groups of persons who all share the same pathology. Types of groups can range from those conducted for persons concerned with relationship difficulties because of early childhood traumas to those with specific anxiety disorders, as well as groups designed to assist such severely dysfunctional populations as schizophrenics (May, 1976).

Styles of Group Psychotherapy for Psychosocial Dysfunction

The therapeutic methods used in group psychotherapy correspond to fundamental principles of group facilitation.

Approaches to Group Facilitation

There are three fundamental approaches to group facilitation, each of which may be suited to a different therapeutic population or structure. The manner with which any topic is discussed can be *deductive*, didactically directed by the therapist, a balanced *interaction* between therapist and patients, or *inductive* facilitation, with patient-generated topics gently facilitated by therapists (see Table 1.1).

   Deductive Process. In situations such as a health education series for prevention or information for the newly diagnosed, the therapist serves as a health educator primarily providing information. The therapist presents topics to be learned, with a goal of patients obtaining information helpful to them now or in the future. At its best, this approach uses sound educational and public health principles, presenting information in the context of patients' lives, world view, and motivational concerns so that each patient can effectively integrate the information into his or her daily life.

   Interactive Process. Therapist facilitation may emphasize interaction with patients around certain topics such as improving communication, dealing with stress, and so on. A structured approach is most commonly used to offer a balanced combination of lecture, experience, and discussion, as per the following example:

   1. Therapists present issues in general, lecturing for 5 to 10 minutes on subject.

TABLE 1.1. Fundamental Styles of Group Therapeutic Facilitation for Medically Ill Patients

Deductive	Interactive	Inductive
Lecture about set topics for educational information or teach specific skills. Patients ask questions for the therapist to answer.	Lecture about set topics. Provide exercise to personalize. Facilitate discussion for integration of topic into patients' lives.	Facilitate discussion of any topic of concern raised by patients to enable authentic expression, stimulate active coping, and provide group support.

2. Participants do an exercise (paper and pencil, dyads, self-hypnosis, etc.) to personalize the exercise for their specific circumstances, lasting about 20 to 30 minutes.
3. Therapists facilitate a general discussion about how these strategies can be implemented in the patient's life, touching on successes and barriers to successful implementation. Or, therapists can ask leading questions about specific topics to structure a group discussion about a topic (e.g., "Let's go around the group and have each person say what his or her biggest stressor is when going for treatment"). The discussion lasts the rest of the 1- to 2-hour meeting.

Inductive Process. Another, more traditional form of group therapy facilitation, occurs when therapists facilitate discussion of any topic that patients raise. Rather than presenting specific topics to be learned or practiced, the focus here is on facilitating the *process* of discussion such that participants are speaking of issues in personal, specific, affective terms, interacting with others to find active coping strategies (Spira, Chapter 5, this volume). In this approach, therapists rarely lecture or give advice to better adjust to new life circumstances. Nor do they give specific exercises to structure the interactions among patients. Instead, therapists facilitate discussion among participants by asking questions as needed to get patients "back on track." When the discussion is going well, there is no need for the therapist to speak at all. This approach can serve as a basis for all types of groups and styles of facilitation during patients' discussion periods.

Therapeutic Methods of Facilitation

Several popular therapeutic methods used by psychotherapists typically correspond to the three approaches to group facilitation discussed earlier, although they can be used in any format. The methods of therapy considered here are educational, cognitive, and interpersonal.

Educationally oriented groups frequently use a brief deductive format to provide information and teach experiential skills to patients in a class-like structure. These groups are popular in addressing such issues as stress in the workplace, anxiety disorders, sexually transmitted diseases, health promotion, and so on—especially for purposes of prevention for those "at risk."

Teaching active coping skills typically utilizes an interactive format, combining some lecture, practice, and discussion to foster healthy alternatives to maladaptive habit behaviors. Cognitive restructuring (Ellis, 1962; Glasser, 1965) focuses on how habitually held beliefs affect cognitions, affect, physiological reactivity, and behaviors in response to particular stressors, both in out of the group. Behavioral medicine methodology teaches specific skills for more appropriately coping with a specific problem (Agras, Taylor, Kraemer,

Southam, & Schneider, 1987). Cognitive-behavioral therapy (Beck, Rush, Shaw, & Emery, 1979) uses a combination of these approaches, as in helping patients to curb their Type A behaviors (Thoresen & Bracke, Chapter 3, this volume). These groups are commonly short term (Fawzy, Fawzy, Hyun, & Wheeler, Chapter 4, this volume; Antoni, Chapter 2, this volume) but can be conducted over extended periods of time (Thoresen, Friedman, Powell, Gill, & Ulmer, 1985).

Interpersonal approaches to psychotherapy most often follow an inductive methodology, where the patient introduces the topics of concern and the therapists focus on facilitating the quality of patients' expressions. This approach emphasizes both interaction between group members and interpersonal relations of patients outside the group. Patients' interpersonal style is seen as stemming from functional relationships learned in childhood (Bowlby, 1958; Buckley, 1986). The interpersonal process in therapy is intended to provide a new model for patients' understanding of relationships and ability to interact in new ways (Adler, 1949; Sullivan, 1953; Yalom, 1985). Traditionally considered a long-term therapy approach, some modern applications of the interpersonal approach are more structured, reducing emphasis on interpersonal relationships within the group in favor of discussing relationships outside the group (Klerman, Weissman, Rounsaville, & Chevron, 1984). Still other modifications of interpersonal therapy emphasize affective support given and received within the group, not for retraining of interpersonal style but rather to make use of the natural support inherent in this type of group for patients experiencing significant distress (Spiegel, Bloom, & Yalom, 1981).

In fact, many psychotherapy groups use some combination of the previous approaches, depending on the type of population seen and the specific goals of the group (Wilfley, Grilo, & Rodin, Chapter 6, this volume; Matano, Yalom, & Schwartz, Chapter 7, this volume). Nonetheless, certain therapeutic goals and techniques appear to work more effectively within certain therapeutic structures (Meyer & Mark, 1995).

Of course, many other formats also exist. Examples of these include maintenance or "holding" groups in an inpatient facility, where economics dictate seeing several severely dysfunctional patients at the same time to (1) check in and (2) help patients control the impulse to be disruptive. In psychodynamic groups (Benezra, 1990), typically composed of patients simultaneously seen in individual counseling, patients use the group as an opportunity to explore how early childhood patterns contribute to their current psychosocial distortions. Family systems counseling (Minuchin, 1974) attempts to reveal family patterns that restrict individual growth and the health of the family system as a whole. Leaderless support groups (used in Alcoholics Anonymous, men's groups, American Cancer Society drop-in support groups, etc.) are also quite popular. Although these types of groups certainly serve a valuable function for reducing social isolation for many patients, they are not generally led by psychotherapists in group therapy for medically ill patients and therefore are not considered here.

Psychotherapy for the Medically Ill

Individual palliative support for patients with medical illness is no doubt as ageless as the capacity to care for others in need. Hippocrates advocated caring for patients' emotional well-being along with their physical well-being, and this caring has extended throughout the history of medicine. However, since the Cartesian separation of mind and body arising in the Renaissance (Starr, 1982), psychological aspects of physical disease have been viewed as either a consequence of the illness or a reason for a lack of diagnosis of "real" disease (Spira, 1991).

Historically, psychological distress was seen as a consequence of medical illness, and efforts to support patient's distress were usually provided by the medical professional or family members. With the rise of psychotherapy as a supportive model in the 1970s, the psychotherapeutic community was able to offer compassionate support as well.

Freud's study of hysterical reactions did much to bridge the mind–body gap, at least in terms of describing how mental processes can mimic physical illness. The field of psychosomatic medicine, which came to prominence in the 1970s, went further in attempting to build a system's model of how such psychological factors as stress or secondary gains could lead to somatizations. Both Freud and these more recent clinicians found that directly addressing issues of psychological neurosis could alleviate the somatic symptoms. In the 1980s, research on psychosocial factors (Type A personality, social support, emotional repression, etc.) affecting morbidity and mortality began to stimulate consideration of the bidirectional interactions between mind and body. By the 1990s, realization of the arbitrariness of the mind–body split led clinicians and researchers not only to consider psychosocial interventions that ameliorated suffering due to illness but to develop psychosocial interventions likely to alter the course of illness.

Today, medical intervention regularly offers relief of psychological distress for medically ill patients, providing palliative support through medication for sleep disturbance, pain, anxiety, and depression. Modern medical systems' approaches offer such psychophysiological support as beta-receptor site-blocking medication for reducing adrenergic responses in patients with cardiac disease, simultaneously reducing central nervous system and visceral organ reactivity.

Modern psychotherapeutic techniques employ a wide range of support for patients with medical illnesses. Many parallel the medical model in offering palliative care to patients, albeit without medication. Such care includes providing supportive counseling to help patients cope emotionally with the illness or teaching behavioral medicine techniques in hopes of reducing psychophysical distress (pain, sleep, nausea). Others go beyond the scope of palliative supportive care, such as the use of cognitive-behavior therapy to improve specific ways of coping with the illness and to improve health-related behaviors, or existential psychotherapy, which views the illness as an opportunity for general growth and enhanced quality of life. This range of psychotherapeutic models is also present in group psychotherapy.

GROUP PSYCHOTHERAPY FOR THE MEDICALLY ILL

Within the background of traditional group psychotherapy and the psychosocial support that has been traditionally offered to patients with medical illness, group psychotherapy for medically ill patients serves the special needs of patients in ways that are distinct from other forms of therapy. This chapter next reviews the specific principles of practice for group psychotherapy serving medically ill patients and ways that this approach serves this population.

Brief History

It has long been known that such behavioral factors as abuse of drugs, alcohol, and tobacco as well as poor eating habits can influence the development of illness. Group clinical interventions of various formats have been developed to assist with modifying these health-related behaviors (Matano et al., Chapter 7, this volume; Wilfley et al., Chapter 6, this volume). However, as has been the case with individual psychotherapy for patients already ill, group psychotherapy was initially palliative in nature, used to help patients adapt to psychosocial sequelae of having contracted a disease (Yalom & Greaves, 1977).

In the 1970s, epidemiological evidence began to accumulate that psychosocial factors themselves could influence survival (Berkman & Syme, 1979; Friedman & Rosenman, 1974). In the mid-1980s, university clinician researchers began to discover that many psychosocial factors appeared to contribute to developing or advancing physical illness. This was first seen with Type A and coronary artery disease (Friedman & Rosenman, 1974), then with emotional suppression and feelings of helplessness in certain types of cancer progression (Greer & Watson, 1985; Stabler et al., 1987; Temoshok et al., 1985) and eventually in illnesses such as human immunodeficiency virus (HIV) (Antoni, Chapter 2, this volume) and other immune-mediated illnesses. Serum immune functions were found to be influenced by psychosocial factors, and psychoneuroimmune (PNI) interactions came to be considered possible mediators of psychosocial factors and health outcome (Solomon, 1981, 1985).

These clinician researchers therefore began to develop interventions intended to modify psychosocial factors thought to be risk factors for disease progression (Antoni, Chapter 2, this volume; Fawzy et al., Chapter 4, this volume; Thoresen & Bracke, Chapter 3, this volume). Although they understood that no single factor always leads to disease incidence or progression, these clinician investigators organized interventions that addressed major psychosocial factors geared toward improving quality of life and, just possibly, physical health as well. For, as these researchers came to appreciate, *the best chance of using psychosocial methods to improve physical health lies in improving quality of life*.

This approach stands in stark contrast to medical interventions that all too frequently reduce the patient's quality of life and sometimes life itself in efforts to reduce the illness. Instead, this approach focuses on improving the host resistance by improving the host.

Comparison with Other Formats

Understanding how group therapy for medically ill patients differs from both individual therapy as well as group psychotherapy for persons with psychosocial disturbance lays a foundation for understanding the power as well as the limits of this treatment.

Group versus Individual Treatment

Although group therapy has tremendous potential to assist most medically ill patients, individual psychotherapy can be of incomparable value for certain persons, especially those with personality characteristics that interfere with social interactions who also have difficulty adjusting to living with their illness and complying or coping with treatment. Yet, whenever possible, group therapy can be considered the "treatment of choice" for most medically ill patients. In contrast to the usual emphasis on examining and modifying personality patterns prevalent in individual therapy, group therapy for the medically ill emphasizes living more fully in each moment and garnering supportive experiences from others regarding ways to handle the stresses faced in coping with life with illness. Certainly individual therapy can assist patients with such adjustments, and group therapy can emphasize recognizing and modifying dysfunctional personality patterns. Still, each is better suited to different therapeutic processes because of its special contextual circumstances. An individual therapist can focus on the complex puzzle that comprises each person's life, whereas a group setting is better suited to utilize the invaluable experience of others in coping with and adjusting to issues com-

mon to most patients facing similar medical concerns. Although a health
professional can suggest a course of action, patients appear to pursue such
recommendations far more readily when they come from someone they know
is personally using this suggestion to help them through a similar situation.
Because of the power of shared experiences, a group format is especially beneficial to medically ill patients.

Persons with Psychosocial Disturbance versus
Persons with Medical Illness

Typically, group psychotherapy is indicated for persons with various types of
interpersonal dysfunction (problems with spouse, women, strangers, authority, etc.), yet members are selected to participate on the basis of similar levels
of ego functioning and cognitive style (e.g., outpatient vs. inpatient, anxious
vs. high functioning). Group therapy for the medically ill is very different,
however. A serious illness can attack anyone at any time. Therefore, these
groups are typically composed of persons with a wide range of past experiences, personal and external resources, and personality styles. Nonetheless,
the patients have much in common. Typical themes discussed in groups of
medical patients include communication with medical professionals; relationships with family, friends, and coworkers; coping with medical treatment
and ill effects of the disease; adjusting to living with a life-threatening diagnosis; and existential issues such as addressing the possibility of dying, examining one's priorities, and shifting self-image (Spira, 1991; Spira & Spiegel,
1993). Although there is much in common among issues addressed by such
patients, the range of personality types in these groups is as varied as those
who can develop an illness—that is, the general population. In this way,
groups with a psychosocial focus differ in both content and style from those
composed of the medically ill (see Table 1.2).

Group therapy for persons with general psychosocial dysfunction most
typically follows an interpersonal format (Yalom, 1985). Group therapy for
medically ill patients can follow a variety of formats, including drop-in meet-

TABLE 1.2. Characteristics of Groups Presenting for Psychosocial versus
Medical Concerns

Group interest	Group characteristics	
	Presenting problem	Cognitive style
Psychopathology	Heterogeneous	Homogeneous
Medical	Homogeneous	Heterogeneous
Behavioral	Homogeneous	Homogeneous

ings with a patient serving as coordinator, educational/didactic class format, teaching and practice of coping skills, Socratic questioning for exploring emotional distress, interpersonal support, and improving coping styles that affect current functioning.

Interestingly, groups for persons with specific behavioral issues potentially affecting health (substance abuse, disordered eating) are more similar to medically ill groups in that these patients present with a specific concern. However, many clinicians believe that there are similar cognitive issues among members of these groups that need to be addressed (impulsivity, dissociative tendencies, etc.). Therefore, although they have similar presenting problems, they also may tend to have somewhat similar ego functioning. Groups for persons with specific behavioral problems have historically emphasized more behavioral interventional styles but in recent years have been as varied as those for medically ill patients (Matano et al., Chapter 7, this volume; Wifley et al., Chapter 6, this volume).

Naturally, the style of facilitating groups depends on group format, patient makeup, stated goals, and therapist training. These issues are examined later.

Topics Discussed in Groups

The group needs to address the most relevant issues immediately facing the patients' quality of life and physical health. Patients' issues, of course, vary depending on the type of illness as well as their stage of illness. Independent of type and stage of illness, however, two perspectives can be followed with regard to what the groups address: (1) scientifically determined risk factors associated with decreasing quality of life and physical health and (2) personal concerns as stated by the patient (Table 1.3). In many cases, these perspectives overlap; however, in many instances they do not.

TABLE 1.3. Examples of Deductive (Therapist-Driven) and Inductive (Patient-Driven) Topics Discussed in Groups

Scientifically determined topics	Patients' personal concerns
Social support/isolation	Psychophysical (pain, nausea, sleeplessness)
Confronting fears/avoidance	Psychological (negative mood, intrusive thoughts)
Emotional expression/suppression	Functional changes (physical fatigue, disability)
Active coping/helplessness	Appearance (cosmetics, prosthesis, reconstruction)
Reprioritizing goals/habitual activities	Communication (doctor, family, friends, coworkers)

Topics most often discussed in groups include both those of concern to the patients and those deemed of value by the therapists. Topics generated by patients stem directly from their immediate needs and concerns, such as coping with pain, nausea, sleeplessness, negative mood, intrusive thoughts, physical fatigue, improving appearance, and improving communication with doctors, family, and friends (Spira, 1991). Addressing these issues early and often goes far in establishing rapport with the patients. As Maslow (1968) so well describes, people must take care of basic functional concerns before they are able to adequately address existential issues.

Topics chosen by the therapists are often emotionally difficult for the patients to pursue at the time, even though they may well feel better afterward. These include issues around establishing meaningful social support, confronting fears, expressing negative emotions, and seeking control over what can be improved while letting go of what cannot be controlled. Although patients may not initiate discussion of death and dying or express negative emotions, such discussions end up being very beneficial and appreciated by the patients. Apparently, discussing these difficult issues in the groups allows patients to focus on living more fully in each moment with less distraction the rest of the week (Horowitz, 1986). Moreover, directly addressing the difficult issues of illness and dying assists patients to reexamine the way they live, with the result of choosing to spend more time in activities that are more meaningful and valuable to them.

Primary Concerns of Persons with Different Illnesses

Despite the range of illnesses and issues facing persons who become ill, all medically ill patients deal with a great number of the same concerns. Yet important differences exist between persons confronting different illnesses as well.

Similarities among Patients with Differing Illnesses

Qualitative analysis of persons with cancer, cardiac disease, arthritis, diabetes, and multiple sclerosis attending group psychotherapy with others with their type of illness reveals group members have many issues in common (Spira, 1991; Spira, 1994a). Patients have similar concerns about their diagnosis, treatment, and recovery. They are concerned with coping with treatment, mood changes, and what to tell others. In addition, patients are concerned with existential issues, albeit at different levels, usually as a function of disease severity. These issues include changes in self-image, reevaluation of priorities in how patients spend their time, and considering life in the face of dying. Of course, the ability to be concerned with these issues assumes that the patient is not so distressed that the distress itself overshadows these considerations. However, with therapeutic group support, these issues can be thoroughly considered and acted on.

Differences between Patients with Differing Illnesses

While patients with life-threatening illnesses have much in common, it is important to consider the special issues that may emerge as most central for patients depending on the nature of their illness. Table 1.4 presents special issues that certainly are common across many illnesses but appear to be of primary concern with specific illnesses. These primary issues of concern have emerged in groups I have led.

TABLE 1.4. Examples of Primary Concerns among Patients with Various Life-Threatening Illnesses

Similar concerns across disease types

Understanding the diagnosis and prognosis
Coping with treatment, side effects, medication
New research and medication for treatments or cures
Adjusting to new lifestyle and level of functioning
Changes in mood, energy levels, and possibly personality
Relationships with family, friends, coworkers, medical personnel
Existential issues: changes in self-image and priorities, living in the face of dying

Different primary concerns between disease types

Cancer: loss of control; unknowns about the disease, treatment efficacy, recurrence
HIV: similar to cancer, but less hope for total recovery; loss of sexual identity, social ostracism
Coronary artery disease: stress, personality characteristics that may predispose, angina, loss of independence for a time, the need to improve lifestyle behaviors
Arthritis: pain, loss of motoric functioning
Multiple sclerosis: loss of energy, motoric and cognitive functioning
Pulmonary: guilt, loss of energy, cognitive and motoric function, lung transplant
Diabetes: motivation to change lifestyle, treatment compliance, progression in distant future
Chronic fatigue syndrome and fibromyalgia: lack of medical and social support, lack of concrete diagnosis variations of the illness, variable course of illness
Obesity: drastically altering lifestyle, passivity and impulsivity, self-image, habitual lifestyle
Eating disorders: cognitive distortions about body, self/other control, influence of social values
Substance abuse: detoxification, secondary gains, resistance, denial, dissociation
Families of patients: coping with distress about loved one, placing one's own distress as secondary, guilt, communicating effectively.
Prevention: avoiding future problems, enhancing current quality of life

STYLES OF GROUP THERAPY FOR MEDICALLY ILL PATIENTS

Understanding the therapeutic intent of the groups and the styles of therapy that best facilitate their goals assists in selecting the most appropriate style of group therapy for a specific patient population.

Therapeutic Intent

Although patients with different illnesses may have different primary concerns, experienced clinicians will recognize the issues listed in Table 1.4 as applying to some extent to most persons who experience life-threatening illness. Because of their universality, given time, most topics emerge at some point during the course of therapy. Exactly what, how, and when topics are discussed vary greatly depending on the special issues faced by each population, as well as the therapeutic goals, methods, and structure. Some forms of group treatment are more inductive in nature whereas others are almost entirely deductive. Different styles lead to differing results and so should be selected with specific goals in mind.

When informational education is the goal, therapists should consider patients' intellectual skills. When active coping skills are being discussed, it is valuable also to discuss the context of the patients' lives within which these skills will be utilized. However, when addressing the emotional distress of patients, therapists must focus on *process*. Rather than *what* is discussed, it is often the therapeutic style that leads patients to examine distress in their lives. When therapists lead patients into exploring difficult realms, they must do so gently lest they meet resistance and lose the trust of the group. Whatever the therapeutic style, the best leader is usually one who can follow the patient, gently introducing new ideas within the context of the patient's relevant experience (Roter et al., 1995).

The style of therapy should therefore depend on the desired outcome. In turn, however, when deciding on the intended goals of therapy, therapists must first consider such patient factors as the type and stage of illness as well as structural considerations including the available resources (therapeutic expertise, time available, costs to deliver, etc.).

Three basic formats can be considered in providing group therapy for the medically ill: informational education, acquisition of active coping strategies, and obtaining emotional and social support. Each of these formats is best served by a different therapeutic style. In general, informational education is best delivered through a deductive presentation, cognitive-behavioral training in coping skills by an interactive therapeutic style, and social and emotional support in an inductive facilitory style. However, each of these formats may benefit at times from partial use of another therapeutic style (see Table 1.5). This next section addresses the different therapeutic styles that best facilitate differing goals of different groups.

TABLE 1.5. Differences in Therapeutic Style by Group Structure and Goals

Goals of groups	Therapeutic style		
	Deductive	Interactive	Inductive
Educational information	X	x	–
Coping skills	x	X	x
Social and emotional support	–	x	X

Note. X indicates primary therapeutic emphasis, x minor emphasis, and – negligible emphasis.

Educational Groups

Education-oriented groups are useful for those concerned with preventing illness and may focus on smoking cessation, breast self-exam, the need for regular screening, the benefits of low-fat diets and exercise, and the like.

Typically brief (one to four meetings), these groups are lecture oriented, with interaction limited to patients merely asking questions of the professional (arguably *not* group therapy in the traditional sense). Educational groups are either information only or information plus simple skill development. An informational focus is commonly offered for those at risk for developing illness or for persons recently diagnosed who wish to learn more information about their disease, what treatments are available, rehabilitative options following surgery (physical therapy, cosmetic surgery, prostheses, etc.), and what, if any, preventive measures they can take for the future (e.g., sun exposure, skin creams, and self-exams for melanoma patients and exercise and diet rehabilitation for cardiac and diabetic patients). Occasionally, experiential skills are also taught, such as relaxation or breast self-exam. In neither informational nor simple skill development is there much interaction between patients. Such groups are frequently coordinated by social workers with clinical nurse specialists as guest speakers and are usually offered as a free service by the institution (Lerman et al., 1995).

There are many examples of the effective use of educational groups. Patients who are newly diagnosed can be given a "health education" prescription along with a medical prescription. These health education groups could meet over four Monday evenings, for 1 hour each meeting. A clinical nurse specialist and a psychotherapist can educate the group about the illness itself, the medications prescribed, compliance with medical protocol, ways to prevent future exacerbations or recurrences through prevention or improving lifestyle, and psychological adjustments to having this illness. Another model is the weekly "drop-in" group on "clinic days" for a particular disease conducted by hospital psychotherapists. Patients and their support persons can attend to learn about a particular topic being presented that day (stress management, prostheses, managing side effects, etc.). Guest lecturers often provide rotating lectures after a brief "check-in" about how members are doing. Rehabilitation psychologists frequently conduct educational groups as part of a rehabilitation program, giving lectures on psychosocial aspects of the pertinent illness followed by discussion and question–answer session. Or, in a preventive model, young women found to be genetically high risk for developing breast cancer can attend a group to find out about options and early detection.

Coping Skills

The most common style of group psychotherapy for medically ill patients teaches active coping strategies focusing on specific and immediate concerns for improving the patient's daily functioning (Fawzy et al., 1995). These concerns include identifiable stressors and stress reactions, communication issues, practicing health behaviors such as diet and exercise, specific self-help techniques for reducing pain and nausea, altering Type A behavior, and so forth. Such groups are usually short term (6 to 10 meetings), run 90 to 120 minutes per session, and most commonly use a cognitive-behavioral therapy orientation.

Cognitive-Behavioral Therapy. Topics are usually deductively selected for presentation, practice, and discussion and focus more on learning skills than on challenging cognitive distortions (Fawzy et al., Chapter 4, this volume; Antoni, Chapter 2, this volume). By actively practicing new strategies of coping in the group, patients will presumably also make these changes at home. Once patients can make such changes in behavior, it is hoped that their cognitive, affective, and physiological distress will be reduced. Typically, a therapist presents a topic for the first few minutes of a group, followed by paper-and-pencil exercises or patient interaction with a partner to practice a strategy. The rest of the session is taken up with discussion on how to implement these active coping strategies in daily life. Many times such groups begin and end with a brief physical relaxation or cognitive meditation training. Most often run by psychologists, social workers, or mental health nurse specialists trained in behavioral medicine techniques, these groups are effective for patients who have specific concerns about a recently diagnosed cancer (Fawzy, Fawzy, & Huan, 1995).

Common examples for teaching functional coping strategies can be found in short-term groups for cancer patients. Each of the six meetings focuses on a different topic. Each meeting introduces the topic in a lecture format, has patients consider how the general topic applies to their specific life through either structured written or small-group exercises, and is followed by a discussion of how this skill will affect their lives and what problems they foresee implementing this new strategy. Common examples of themes presented include managing psychological stress, assertive communication with medical personnel, improving relationships, and managing physical pain and stress.

   Cognitive Restructuring. Occasionally, groups address long-standing personality characteristics of patients that impact negatively on their health. Although also concerned with patients' daily functioning, as in a typical cognitive-behavioral therapy model, these groups often go further by exploring the long-standing beliefs and attitudes that make it difficult for patients to both recognize and change their dysfunctional style of coping. Cognitive restructuring (Ellis, 1962; Glasser, 1965) methods are useful to (1) introduce alternative ways of coping, (2) challenge the beliefs of those clinging to their way of viewing the problem, and (3) explore new strategies, both in the group and at home. The underlying assumption in cognitive restructuring is that one's beliefs about the world, self, and others lead to cognitive, affective, physiological, and behavioral reactions to stressors that affect health. By examining and confronting fixed beliefs that limit health and quality of life, patients can learn to react in healthier ways. For example, if a patient learned in his childhood that the world is a hostile place, he will learn to be more cognitively vigilant, affectively frustrated or angry, sympathetically aroused, and behaviorally aggressive—all characteristics that put patients at risk for increased cardiac disease. These groups can address issues such as Type A behavior for patients with cardiac disease (Thoresen & Bracke, Chapter 3, this volume), impulsivity and low self-esteem for persons with disordered eating (Wilfley et al., Chapter 6, this volume), or denial and externalization in those rehabilitating from substance abuse. Topics to discuss each session may be selected deductively, but substantial opportunity for open discussion about the topic is usually provided because therapists seek opportunities to point out patients' cognitive distortions.

   Formats in which cognitive restructuring approaches are helpful include midlength (12 to 24 months) or long-term groups for Type A cardiac patients, binge eaters with low self-esteem, cancer patients who try not to make too much of a fuss, and so forth. Structured topics and exercises may be introduced into the groups, but long discussions are encouraged so that patients can discuss how the belief was initially formed, ways that this belief helped them at one time but limits them now, and alternative strategies which can be even more effective for them. Therapists are active in guiding the discussions along these lines and challenging the patients to recognize the limitations of their habitual attitudes. Drawing on others in the group to discuss ways they have seen a situation and reacted to it successfully is a component that gives cognitive restructuring-oriented groups more impact than individual sessions. Yet, because therapeutic challenge of deeply held attitudes is an essential aspect of this approach, longer-term therapy with good therapist rapport and group cohesion is usually required.

Social and Emotional Support

Persons with more advanced disease, or those who are having difficulty adjusting to having a life-threatening illness, can benefit from longer-term therapy (3 months to 1 year or longer) focusing on social and emotional support. Because longer-term groups have the opportunity to form intimate bonds of support, patients are able to discuss virtually any issue of personal concern related to living with a major illness. Specific topics rarely need to be introduced by the therapists as patients eventually raise topics important to them. Such groups have the potential to address immediate issues of coping with distress as well as deeper existential considerations of changing priorities, self-image, and directly confronting issues of death and dying. In these groups, the patients are most active, with the therapists typically taking a back seat, only to emerge to keep the patients "on track" and to facilitate interactions. These types of groups are most similar to traditional group psychotherapy, with the modifications made for cancer patients rather than patients with strictly psychosocial dysfunction, as described earlier (Spiegel & Spira, 1991).

Therapists seeking emotional and social support most often use an interpersonal therapy style with emphasis on *authentic expression* of any topic patients feel the need to discuss that day. This means that therapists ask questions that lead patients to discuss their concerns in personal (vs. externalized), specific (vs. abstract), and affective (vs. intellectual avoidance of negative thoughts and feelings) terms. They also ask questions that encourage active coping (vs. passive helplessness) and interaction among group members (vs. solipsistic testimonials), and that focus on patients' distresses (vs. avoidance of negative thoughts and feelings) (Spira, Chapter 5, this volume).

A typical group run along this format might be held for patients with recurrent cancer, cardiomyopathy, or AIDS. Such a group would probably require a commitment of at least 6 months, and would allow members to recommit for an additional committed segments. Therapists might begin and end each group with a few minutes of gentle relaxation or meditation. However, the rest of the group is used to discuss any topics that are of major concern for patients that day, with therapists simply asking questions that keep patients' expressions personal–specific–affective–interactive and seeking active solutions for existential concerns. When discussion is being conducted in this way between group members, therapists remain silent.

Occasionally groups attempt to facilitate adjustment to illness or behavioral change by focusing on the interpersonal context within which the patient lives on a daily basis. These groups, more structured along the lines of a cognitive-behavioral therapy group, focus on relationships outside the therapeutic setting (Klerman et al., 1984). This approach makes for particularly good research and more time-limited therapy constrained by managed care.

These groups are also beneficial for assisting in managing dysfunctional behavior that has health ramifications (Wilfley et al., Chapter 6, this volume).

Although these three styles of therapy represent the main approaches utilized in groups for the medically ill (see Table 1.6), combinations of these approaches, as well as theoretical emphases that guide their use, are quite common as well.

Combinations of Educational, Coping Skills, and Social–Emotional Support

When the group has multiple goals of generally equal importance, group leaders often use combinations of two or three of these major approaches. A health educator may mainly provide a lecture, may then ask participants to practice a skill, and may end by facilitating discussion among the participants. A psychologist in a coping skills class may focus on lecturing about and practice of specific skills or else spend more time in facilitation of discussion, depending on therapeutic orientation or persons in the group.

It is not uncommon to find a typical 12-session group for new breast cancer patients including (1) basic education of prosthesis or reconstructive surgery, (2) relaxation skills and pain management, and (3) discussion on communicating needs and desires to one's spouse. Although certain interventional styles can best facilitate achieving specific group goals, attempting to achieve several therapeutic goals through employing several different therapeutic styles can be problemmatic. Patients in groups find it difficult to change their perception of the therapist as "teacher" to "process" facilitator. When resources permit, different therapists should present different aspects of such mixed-orientation groups.

Additional Stylistic Considerations

Besides distinct styles being suitable for differing goals, several guiding principles are worthy of consideration because they apply across differing styles and populations.

Existential Emphasis

Actually more of a heuristic orientation than an algorithmic method of therapy, existential considerations are useful in guiding therapists' choice of topics and process interventions in groups of patients facing a life-threatening illness. Therapists following this orientation adhere to the belief that although initial buffering of extreme distress may be useful (Reed, Kemeny, Taylor, Wang, & Visscher, 1994), in the long run it is better to (1) acknowledge and express negative thoughts and feelings and (2) use the illness as an

TABLE 1.6. Principles and Methods of Different Group Therapeutic Styles for Medically Ill Patients

Educational

Topics:	Usually selected deductively, based on scientifically determined risk factors.
Assumptions:	Knowledge of information leads to behaviors that can prevent or reduce illness.
Goals:	1. Information about prevention of or living with disease.
	2. Skills to help prevent incidence or recurrence; or to reverse disease.
Format:	1. Lecture/question–answer (what to eat, when to get a checkup, etc.).
	2. Teaching skills (menu planning, self-exam techniques. etc.).

Cognitive

Cognitive restructuring

Topics:	Usually deductively selected, with open discussion of topic, as process of distortion is usually examined.
Assumptions:	Beliefs about the self/others/world lead to cognitive, affective, physiological and behavioral reactions to stressors that affect health.
Goals:	Examining and confronting fixed beliefs that limit health and quality of life.
Format:	Asking questions that challenge distorted beliefs and other alternative solutions

Cognitive-behavioral therapy/behavioral medicine

Topics:	Usually deductively selected for presentation, practice, and discussion—focus more on learning skills than on examining distortions.
Assumptions:	Altering behavior can facilitate changes in cognition, affect, and physiological reactivity.
Goals:	Active healthy coping skills for present and future health-related behaviors
Format:	Lecture, structured exercises, and discussion of applications into one's life

Interpersonal

Long-term

Topics:	Inductively selected, as long as they can be discussed interactively within the group.
Assumptions:	Interacting authentically with others (in personal, specific, affective terms) helps reduce distress and find more optimal ways to cope with existential concerns.
Goals:	Group support for distress, allowing for affect expression, examining existential issues
Format:	Process emphasis—therapists ask questions which draw out authentic expression and interaction among patients.

Short-term

Topics:	Inductively generated, yet constrained to those involving interpersonal interactions.
Assumptions:	Discussing the difficult interpersonal relationships in patient's life in the group helps find alternative methods of interacting which helps improve patient's psychosocial environment.
Goals:	Improved relationships in life help patients reduce psychosocial distress and make active changes within their home environment.
Format:	Discussion of difficult interpersonal relationships in patient's life.

opportunity for growth (Spira & Spiegel, 1993). Of course, existentially oriented therapists are interested in helping patients cope with daily living and reducing excess psychophysical distress. Yet beyond such basic coping, these therapists use the opportunity of the crisis to have patients experience the importance of authentic expression, conscious commitment to meaningful activities, and living as fully as possible in each moment of life (Yalom, 1980).

Typically, existential psychotherapists assist the patient to live in full, open, honest relationships in each moment (Spira, Chapter 5, this volume). This approach assumes that patients' suffering increases when they are unable to suspend their fixed self-image and adapt to changing life-circumstances. Therapists adopt a *hermeneutic* stance with regard to the patient, attempting to understand the patients self-image and expression of meaning from the context of the patient's current and past life experiences. They also pursue a *phenomenological* methodology of helping patients suspend their usual habitual way of looking at themselves and their lives to consider more optimal ways they could be currently spending their time. Such experiential techniques as written exercises or *Buddhist* meditative practices are frequently employed to facilitate this shift from living largely out of habit to living more authentically and consciously in each moment. Topics are usually selected inductively because the focus of discussion is on authentic expression of concerns in personal–specific–affective–interactive ways (Spira, Chapter 5, this volume). However, special exercises might be introduced into the groups to pursue certain concerns raised by patients.

Not a technique in itself, existential therapy can utilize various techniques. Existential therapists use interpersonal therapy to understand and support the patient, cognitive therapy to challenge habit beliefs and to suggest new ways of interacting with stressors, and education through experiential exercises which can more fully address existential concerns (e.g., changing self-image) and facilitate the existential development of patients (e.g., "What would you do differently if you had 2 years to live?"). For patients with life-threatening illnesses, focusing on existential considerations not only honestly addresses issues immediately facing patients but also allows them to adjust better with their changing lives.

Giving Advice during Supportive Group Interactions

When facilitating discussion among patients, therapists must avoid the trap of answering questions with definitive information. Instead, therapists can draw on the knowledge of the group, a superb source of expertise in coping with illness. In educational groups, therapists are teachers relaying information. But in group discussion, therapists' emphasis should be on facilitating the *process*, not providing *content*. Once the therapist becomes the "expert" it is extremely difficult to return to facilitating the process—patients simply will not permit the therapist to "shift gears." Avoiding giving advice may be difficult for a therapist with expertise, yet such restraint is nevertheless very important. The expert therapist should find ways to diffuse the question, such as suggesting that the patient ask his or her medical specialist or that the subject could be discussed after the group. This approach focuses patients on the *group process* rather than allowing the group to become an informational meeting (and correspondingly void of interaction in personal–specific–affective terms).

Table 1.7 compares the therapeutic emphasis of major facilitory styles as to their emphasis on therapeutic intent, advice, and direct experience.

Cautions in Utilizing Coping Skills in Groups with an Existential Focus

As useful as teaching coping skills can be for patients, when conducting long-term groups of patients with serious life-threatening illnesses, over use of these techniques can detract from the interpersonal issues at hand. Patients tend to discuss their use of the techniques rather than the underlying emotional issues at hand. Such exercises can also be inappropriately used as a way of "rescuing" patients who are experiencing negative emotions. Attempting to buffer patients against these difficult emotions unfortunately can also deprive patients of coming to terms with these feelings. Alternatively, such exercises can be used to reduce anxiety to a manageable level, and as a means to

TABLE 1.7. Comparing the Therapeutic Emphasis of Major Facilitative Styles

Facilitative style	Therapeutic emphasis		
	Therapeutic intent	Advice	Direct experience
Deductive (educational)	Informational knowledge	Mostly given	Minimal
Interactive (cognitive-behavioral)	Functional coping skills	Sometimes given	Reflection about problems occurring throughout patient's life; practice specific skills through special exercises
Inductive (process facilitation)	Social/emotional support of existential concerns	Rarely given	Directly experience alternative ways of active coping through naturally arising group interactions

further explore the feelings that arise or exist just below the surface. This latter approach may be instrumental in allowing existing but suppressed negative emotions to surface, yet in a way that allows the patients to better explore and handle what arises. The careful selection and presentation of such structured exercises can serve to circumvent many of the problems discussed here while allowing patients to obtain the benefits such exercises offer.

The Time Course of a Group

First Meetings. Initial introductions are important as they set the tone for the rest of the meetings. Beyond discussing members' names and type of cancer, members can also tell their story about the diagnosis, treatment, and how they are coping with it. This method, used by mental health workers in debriefing disaster victims (Mitchell & Everly, 1993), helps to reduce the stress reaction and possibly future posttraumatic stress reactions (Spira, 1993; Passick & Redd, 1996). It is also an excellent way to set the tone of the group as one of seriousness, openness, and support. In longer-term inductive groups, setting the tone can take several sessions, and a patient's story can stimulate group discussions. In shorter groups, the therapist may need to draw out silent or shy members and manage more verbose members. It is paramount to have each patient's expression met with understanding and compassion, which further allows the other members to feel safer in addressing their own fears. It is important to remember that persons from all walks of life and ways of viewing the world come together in this (for them) unusual setting. They are looking for guidance as to how the group functions, both in terms of *what* is discussed as well as *how* topics are to be discussed. The initial meeting is critical in forming the "group style" that is to continue in future meetings.

Middle Meetings. *Opening* each meeting with some ritual is helpful. When members arrive initially, they generally engage in some light chatting. At some point, it is valuable for the therapist to get up and close the door as a signal that the meeting is formally going to begin. Checking in with everyone (anyone missing?) and showing honest concern for each one helps the group members know that they are cared for, as well as ensuring better compliance with attendance or at least being informed of planned absences. It is useful to begin with a brief (5-minute) meditation or relaxation (Spira, 1994b). Such meditation can serve to settle and focus the mind and the group as a whole. It also serves to teach stress and pain management and self-comforting. The *body of the meetings* consists of presenting information (didactic), discussing the topic to be addressed for the meeting (interactive), or asking whether there are any important issues that need to be discussed (inductive), depending on the format of the group. *Closing each meeting* can sometimes be difficult, especially when emotional issues are being discussed.

Letting the group know that 15 minutes are left can focus the group on essentials and help members begin to summarize important points. It can also be a message that new "hot" topics should not be pursued in much detail at this time but should be picked up again at the next meeting. Finishing on time is important as it offers the security of a much needed structure for the often unexpected feelings that arise. Consistent closure lets the group know that whatever occurs in the group, someone in charge is monitoring the group. Finishing with another 5 to 10 minutes of meditation/relaxation helps to settle down after an arousing session, reinforcing the value of learning to calm the mind and relax the body,. Further, if participants know that they will leave feeling relatively calm and relaxed, they can allow more openness of expression during the meeting itself. It is also possible to lead a "guided meditation" or self-hypnosis as part of the relaxation at the end of a meeting as a way of summarizing the main topic that has been discussed, perhaps helping patients to imagine positive ways of dealing with a negative issue (Spira & Spiegel, 1992).

Final Meetings. The last several meetings can be difficult for members. Bonds that have been formed will be coming to a close, with associated feelings of loss. In groups of 6 months or longer, closure should be discussed for the final month, with emphasis on how members will continue to find social support in their lives as well as what the group has meant to them. Grieving the loss of the group may well prepare them for grieving other aspects of their lives. Shorter groups should also address the ending of the group and what it means to each patient at a final meeting, although such issues may arise with less intensity. In all cases, it is useful to recommend follow-ups to other groups, activities, or therapy, as required by each individual member.

Cautions for the Use of Group Psychotherapy

Any method that has the power to assist also has the potential to disrupt. There are instances in which studies of psychotherapy groups for the medically ill had to be abandoned midtreatment because the treatment subjects were faring worse than the untreated controls. In one instance of patients with HIV disease, unstructured support meetings (where the therapist was mostly a coordinator and observer) were held to discuss issues of mutual concern. After several months, the level of anxiety was so high in the groups that they were considered detrimental to the patients and were stopped. Unstructured meetings of patients with severe illness offer a clear contrast to therapist-led groups, where therapists offer to patients an explicit method of confronting difficult issues and techniques to better handle them. At the other extreme is a therapeutic intervention that was ceased because patients with cancer were progressing in the disease more rapidly than closely matched controls, presumably due to the intense style of therapy. Therapists in this study used a cognitive restructuring approach that directly confronted patients on issues of cognitive denial, emotional repression, and interpersonal assertiveness. Apparently, this confrontational approach was overly challenging, arousing patients without the support needed to adequately handle the fears and worries that arose. Because these studies were abandoned due to therapist concerns for the patients, they remain unpublished. However, they serve as excellent examples of extremes that should be avoided for the medically ill. Instead, establishing an interpersonal approach to emotional and social support for initial rapport, coupled with coping strategies to handle excess arousal, provides a safe and effective way of working with the great majority of persons experiencing distress due to medical illness. From this basis, gentle challenging of dysfunctional beliefs or introduction of existential issues can be highly effective.

Several researchers have investigated the initial phase of an acute crises in a wide range of patients, including initial diagnosis of HIV disease (Reed et al., 1994), newly diagnosed cancer (Levy, Herberman, Lippman, & d'Angelo, 1987; Temoshok, 1987), and rape (Miller, Brody, & Summerton, 1988; Miller, Shoda, & Hurley, 1996). Reports from these investigators and others indicated that initial repression of feelings may very well *help* patients' adjustment whereas later repression hurts. This may be true especially when sufficient psychosocial support is not present to buffer the initial trauma of the illness. However, if psychosocial support is immediately offered to patients, this initial "blunting" phase can be less disruptive to their lives. Early and regular expression of distress allows patients to "get it out" at the group meetings so that they can attend more fully to daily events, with less intrusion of negative thoughts and feelings between meetings. A study by Gellert, Maxwell, and Siegel (1993) found that patients in an "exceptional patient" cancer support group that focused on positive thoughts and feelings without "dwelling" on the negative had no improvement in survival compared to a matched control. Perhaps the difference between this group and the others that did find survival differences lies in the willingness in these other groups to directly address negative thoughts and feelings.

Adjusting Therapeutic Method to Match Patient Needs

Clearly, approaches to group psychotherapy differ in method, goals, and group format. In deciding which therapeutic structures and styles to employ, it is necessary to consider factors associated with the patients being served. These factors include stage of disease, disease type, and the personal characteristics of those who make up the groups.

Stage of Disease

Each stage of illness has its own special issues to which psychotherapists must be sensitive to determine the appropriate therapeutic goals and to select optimal methods and group structures to achieve these goals. The various group structures and therapeutic methods discussed previously can be appropriately utilized to assist persons at various stages of their illness.

Prevention. Persons who are at increased risk for disease incidence or recurrence frequently have education about preventive measures as their goal, although some discussion of stress and its management might be included in such education. The method of education is didactic, which most often occurs in a brief format (between one and six weekly meetings).

Diagnosis. Patients who have recently received a first diagnosis of cancer, HIV, or coronary artery disease (CAD) are naturally distressed over the diagnosis and are no doubt confused about the illness and its etiology, treatment, and prognosis. Goals for this population should include basic education, initial stress management to attend more to the present and cope with immediate decisions regarding treatment, and emotional support. Although some deductive intervention is useful for offering basic information, therapeutic facilitation is primarily interactive for developing active coping skills, with some inductive facilitation for supportive discussion. It is difficult to mix didactic and interactive formats because once they have been lectured to, patients find it difficult to engage in discussion or open emotionally. Therefore, many therapists find it most beneficial to separate the didactic education from the interactive components. Different meetings, different parts of meetings separated by a break, or even different facilitators can help patients get the most out of each type of method.

Treatment. Special issues for persons undergoing treatment may include the need to deal with recovery from surgery, or discomfort from chemotherapy and radiotherapy, which often includes fatigue, nausea, dry or sore mucous membranes, weight changes, flu-like symptoms, and so on. Changes in appearance (weight gain, hair loss, etc.) and daily functioning are also common. With these changes occurring, the urgency of dealing with the initial diagnosis and treatment decisions now largely behind the patient, and the initial shock of diagnosis subsiding, the reality of the illness begins to set in. Patients at this stage are concerned with coping with treatment, adjusting to a lifestyle of being a patient, and receiving emotional support. An interactive therapeutic style that offers emotional support and discussion along with experiential skills is therefore appropriate and can be delivered effectively for most patients in a brief (4 to 12 weeks) group, at least initially.

Recovery. Once initial treatment is completed patients' concerns turn to changes in self-image ("Am I a cardiac patient, or the same person I was but with a diseased heart?"), changes in relationships, questioning and reprioritizing daily activities, wanting more control over their health and course of disease, wondering whether personality or behavior affects their health, and considering the possibility of disease recurrence and death. Therapeutic goals for this stage include training in active coping strategies; offering emotional and social support; reexamining life values, beliefs, and priorities; considering one's optimal future way of living; and learning to live a mentally and physically healthy lifestyle. Utilizing an interactive therapeutic style with a cognitive-behavioral therapy orientation, teaching experiential coping skills, and then switching to an inductive therapeutic style allowing for supportive discussion help achieve these skills, usually in a short-term (8 to 16 weeks) group format.

Recurrence and Dying. Patients who have disease recurrence often experience even greater distress than at the initial diagnosis (Spira, 1993). They face protracted and intensive treatment, greater loss of control, physical discomfort and fatigue, reduced daily functioning and decisions regarding retirement and disability, new ways of relating to family and friends, and also more directly confronting the likelihood of dying. Learning to cope more actively, manage pain and stress, receive emotional support, address existential issues, and live more fully in each moment are extremely beneficial goals to patients at this stage of illness. An inductive approach allowing for supportive discussion and occasional interactive facilitation of experiential skills (relaxation, self-hypnosis) can facilitate these goals in a longer format (24 weeks to ongoing).

Family Members and Bereavement. Families of medically ill patients should not be neglected. Assisting the family members to cope better themselves goes a long way in supporting the patient. Family members to some extent suffer the same issues as does the patient. Therefore, a similar style of therapy is as appropriate for them as for the patient. For earlier stages of illness (patients confronting prevention, diagnosis, and possibly brief groups for coping with treatment), it is valuable to have family members meet in groups alongside patients. However, for longer-term groups (longer than 4 weeks), patients and family members are better served in separate groups so that they each can discuss their own concerns and not worry about distressing the other. Resources permitting, it can be convenient to have patients and family members meet at the same time, in adjacent rooms. Of course, not all patients have family members in the area or family members who can attend such groups, and this lack of support should be addressed in the patient groups.

Family members of patients who have died face considerable emotional distress, existential considerations, and possibly guilt. Offering emotional support to work through distress and help them to live more fully in the moment and plan for the future requires an inductive, interactive format, along with teaching some experiential skills (relaxation, self-hypnosis). Family members who have been involved in family groups while the patient was alive should, of course, be invited to stay on in the group for as long as they like.

Table 1.8 provides a summary of how different patient issues and therapeutic approaches correspond to different stages of illness. For the sake of simplicity, the example of cancer will be used.

Which Therapeutic Style Works Best?

Given that different stages of disease have different issues and goals, which method of group therapy should a therapist choose?

A meta-analysis was performed for all prospective randomized studies examining the effects of *educational, behavioral,* and *counseling* interventions for cancer patients. Not surprisingly, informational/educational approaches were most effective for improving medical knowledge and compliance as well as functional adjustment, behavioral approaches were most effective with managing specific symptoms, and nonbehavioral counseling therapy was superior for assisting with emotional adjustment as well as in more global measures examined. Support groups that lacked psychotherapeutic interventions were not found to be of value for any outcomes examined.

Clearly, therapists should select the style of intervention that will best facilitate the desired outcome. Yet which outcome is most appropriate? Because there is not one single outcome that is optimal for all groups, there can be no one single method of group psychotherapy that is best for all populations potentially seen in a group format. In deciding on a therapeutic style, therapists must consider patients' type and stage of illness as well as the goals of the group. Yet, to a great extent, the therapist's paradigmatic view of illness dictates the type of psychosocial treatment envisioned.

Models for Understanding and Treating Disease in Psychotherapy Groups

The way one understands a problem will lead to possible solutions considered for correcting the problem. This is perhaps nowhere as evident as in diagnosis and treatment for the medically ill (Spira, 1988). There are several possible models for understanding the nature of illness and the selection of subsequent treatments.

TABLE 1.8. Therapeutic Goals, Methods, and Structures Useful for Addressing the Special Issues of Specific Cancer Populations

Stage of illness	Special issues	Goals	Methods	Structure
Prevention	• At increased risk for disease incidence or recurrence	• Education	Deductive • Didactic information	Brief class (1–4 meetings)
Diagnosis	• Distress over diagnosis • Confusion about cancer	• Education • Coping in moment • Emotional support	Interactive • Didactic information • Experiential skills Inductive • Supportive discussion	Brief group (1–6 weeks)
Treatment	• Discomfort: nausea, mucus membranes, fatigue, weight • Reality of illness sets in	• Coping with treatment • Adjusting one's life to having cancer • Emotional support	Interactive • Experiential skills Inductive • Supportive discussion	Brief–short term (4–12 weeks)
Recovery	• Self-image (cancer patient?) • Questioning life activities • Relationships • Sense of control • Possible recurrence or death • Attitudes/behavior affecting health	• Active coping • Emotional/social support • Reexamining life values, beliefs, priorities • Considering one's future • Living a healthy lifestyle	Interactive • Cognitive therapy • Experiential skills Inductive • Supportive discussion	Short-term (8–16 weeks)
Recurrence and dying	• Emotional distress • Death and dying • Coping with treatment • Loss of control • Family and friends • Physical discomfort/fatigue	• Active coping • Pain and stress management • Emotional/social support • Existential issues • Living fully in the moment	Inductive • Supportive discussion Interactive • Experiential skills	Long term (24 weeks–ongoing)
Family support during illness and bereavement	• Emotional distress • Existential issues • Guilt	• Emotional support • Work through distress • Living more in the moment • Planning for the future	Inductive • Supportive discussion Interactive • Experiential skills	As needed • Brief formats, support persons attend with patients • Longer formats, support and bereaved members meet separately

Models of Responsibility. The belief one holds as to responsibility of cause and correction of illness to a great extent determines what psychosocial aspects to focus on in therapy (Parsons, 1951; Fine, 1996). Presumably, if someone's behavior is seen as contributing to the cause of the illness, learning to manage these behaviors should assist in reducing the disease or its chances of recurring. If an individual's behaviors have not been seen as having any role in the disease incidence, such behaviors will not be seen as a target for retraining during intervention.

Unidirectional Models. One simple unidirectional model (see Table 1.9[a]) of illness assumes that genetic and environmental factors contribute to illness, with the result that *physical dysfunction leads to changes in psychosocial functioning* (cognitive adjustment, affect, psychophysical reactivity, and behaviors). A person newly diagnosed with cancer who becomes distressed due to the diagnosis and becomes nauseous when undergoing chemotherapy illustrates this point. Patients are seen as mature and competent normal individuals who just happen to be the victims of a misfortune; they are considered blameless for their condition (Fine, 1996) and are treated by therapists who offer compassionate palliative care. Adherents of this view assist patients to reduce psychological distress, teach methods of coping with treatment, discuss ways to adjust to new lifestyle, and address existential concerns raised by having been diagnosed with a catastrophic illness. Although therapists are the professionals, patients are not seen as "dysfunctional" and the therapeutic relationship is therefore on a more equitable level of discussion than the usual patient–doctor interaction.

A unidirectional view (see Table 1.9[b]) may also consider that genetic and environmental factors contribute to maladaptive behaviors which in turn contribute to disease. Thus, *psychosocial behavior can lead to physical dysfunction.* Early morbidity and mortality can be directly attributable to the use of maladaptive lifestyle behavior that stems from a genetic predisposition or exposure to early childhood dysfunction. Examples can be found in persons with a substance abuse problem who develop hepatic cirrhosis, or a person with anorexia nervosa who develops symptoms of malnutrition. Here, patients are seen to some extent as responsible for having developed their ailments, and although they are offered supportive medical treatment, they are encouraged to take active responsibility for the correction of their problems in the future. Intervention focuses on altering current behaviors and identifying current cognitive–affective patterns that maintain such behaviors, including lifelong beliefs or social attitudes that the patients use to "justify" their injurious actions. Therapists' attitude is usually "compassionate but tough," maintaining a strict doctor–patient relationship.

Bidirectional Models. More complex models incorporate both of the unidirectional models described previously. Whereas illness certainly results

TABLE 1.9. Models of Contributing Factors and Psychosocial Treatments for Medically Ill Patients: Contrast between Treatments for Recurrent Cancer [a], Substance Abuse or Disordered Eating [b], or a Postrecovery Cardiac Patient [c]

Unidirectional views				Treatment considerations

[a] Genetic and environmental factors —*contributes to*→ Disease —*contributes to*→ Psychosocial disturbance —*suggests*→ Palliative care: coping with diagnosis, treatment, and existential concerns

or

[b] Genetic and environmental factors —*contributes to*→ Psychosocial dysfunction —*contributes to*→ Disease —*suggests*→ Cognitive-behavioral retraining: learning to control impulses, maladaptive beliefs, and behaviors

Bidirectional view				Treatment considerations

[c] (= a *and* b)

Multiple factors

Nonpsychosocial
Genetic and physical environment —*contributes to*→

and

Psychosocial
Socioeconomic, lifestyle behaviors, trait characteristics, state coping/mood, social relationships —*contributes to*→

D
I
S
E
A
S
E

—*suggests*→ Palliative care: coping with diagnosis, treatment, and existential concerns

along with

Cognitive-behavioral retraining: learning to control impulses, maladaptive beliefs and behaviors in psychosocial changes, a variety of factors are involved in the incidence and progression of the disease. These exacerbating factors include genetic predisposition, agents in the physical environment, socioeconomic status, educational level, lifestyle behaviors, psychosocial factors such as trait personality and state coping, and social relationships, among others. Moreover, these factors can influence each other. This model is therefore highly interactive, with a variety of psychosocial and nonpsychosocial factors contributing to the disease, the disease contributing in turn to further stimulating this range of factors, and the cycle continuing to interact (see Table 1.9[c]).

A plethora of research has demonstrated that these factors do in fact contribute to disease incidence, progression, and mortality (Spira, 1996b). Of course, group psychotherapy interventions cannot affect some of these factors such as genetics or socioeconomic standing or educational level. However, most other factors, such as exposure to carcinogens or stressors, lifestyle behaviors, trait personality patterns, state coping, and social relationships, have been demonstrated to improve through the provision of group psychotherapy. Therefore, although patients are not held accountable for their actions to this point, every effort is made to (1) ameliorate their current distress and improve their current quality of life, and (2) encourage them to take as much responsibility as possible for improving factors within their control to minimize further exacerbation of the illness. Fortunately, actions to improve current quality of life have been found to be identical with actions intended to minimize further exacerbation of the illness. Such actions include exercise, healthy eating, reducing or eliminating recreational substance use, stress management, active coping, open and honest expression of cognitive and affective concerns, and social support (Sullivan, Cobb, & Spira, 1993). Interestingly, the same therapeutic approach that assists medically ill patients to learn ways to cope with their illness is useful for patients with disordered eating or substance abuse problems to improve their behavioral disorder. For instance, methods common to both cognitive therapy and interpersonal therapy are used extensively in each of these areas, as is evident from the chapters in this volume.

Which Model to Use? Typically, group therapy for persons with cancer have followed a simple, unidirectional model in which patients have no responsibility (as in "blame") for the cause of their illness but can become involved for their personal adjustment in coping with psychosocial disturbance as a result of the illness (e.g., Spiegel et al., 1981). When psychosocial disturbance is seen as the sequelae of physical illness, the reason to focus on improving psychosocial disturbance is to cope with the illness, not to change it. Those working with substance abuse and eating disorders also follow a unidirectional model, although in the other direction, with behavior potentially leading to physical illness. (Of course, genetic and environmental influences are also considered as influencing the behavioral disturbance). When psychosocial disturbance is seen as *causing* a physical disturbance, altering psychosocial behavior improves psychophysical health. However, the role of physical ailments on patients' behaviors is considered to have relatively minor relevance.

Combing both of these simple unidirectional models, many of the contributors to this volume take a more complex bidirectional view of the cause and treatment of disease (Fawzy et al., Chapter 4; Antoni, Chapter 2; Thoresen & Bracke, Chapter 3). These authors are working with disease states in the early stages or those that have potential for many more years of life. Here, patients are not blamed for the cause of their disease but are seen as contributing *to some extent*, along with the other factors mentioned previously, to the future course of their psychosocial adjustment as well as their physical status. In this model, the extent to which patients can contribute to their psychophysical status is the extent to which they are encouraged to actively pursue improvement in their psychophysical behaviors.

Which course of action to follow depends on the therapist's view of the cause of the illness and to what extent the therapist believes that the course of the illness can be altered. If there is no possibility of altering the course of the illness, a simple disease-driven model dictates interventional efforts. If the therapist believes that the course of the illness is completely caused by the patient's behaviors, a behavioral intervention is indicated. If the therapist takes the middle road, believing that the patient's behavior to some extent contributed to the onset of the disease, but also that many other factors outside the patient's control led to the onset of the disease, he or she tends to offer both palliative support as well as cognitive-behavioral retraining (as in the case of coronary artery disease or malignant melanoma).

Stage-Based Model of Intervention. A stage-based treatment model takes into consideration not only the complex factors influencing the course of disease but also the needs of the patients at any given time. If a patient is recently diagnosed and undergoing treatment (e.g., coronary artery bypass graft or radiotherapy), assisting with coping with the distress of diagnosis and handling the treatment is far more urgent than reviewing the patient's beliefs formed in early childhood (e.g., hostile or inhibited emotions). Yet once a patient completes treatment and physically recovers from the illness, turning to such concerns may be of great value. Similarly, patients during drug detoxification or actively purging bulimics need immediate behavioral and emotional support before exploring restrictive personality patterns (see Table 1.10).

TABLE 1.10. Stage-Based Model for Psychosocial Treatment of Medically Ill Patients

Stage of illness	Focus of intervention				
	Medical education	Moderating state mood, pain, stress	Social–emotional support	Coping skills training (psychoeducation)	Exploring and managing personality
Diagnosis (e.g., cancer) or event (e.g., heart attack)	**	**	**	–	–
Treatment (e.g., surgery; radiation)	*	**	**	*	–
In recovery/rehab. program (first 6 months post-acute intervention)	–/*	*	*	**	*
Recovered (posttreatment; e.g., first occurrence cancer; coronary artery disease; sober; controlled eating)	–	*	*	*	**
Chronic–severe (e.g., AIDS; recurrent cancer; cardiomyopathy)	–	**	**	*	–

Note. – indicates rarely appropriate, * somewhat appropriate, and ** highly appropriate.

SPECIAL PROBLEMS IN FACILITATING THE GROUPS

Although the therapeutic methods reviewed here are effective for facilitating most groups, it is also important to consider difficult issues arising in the group and issues in handling difficult patients.

Difficult Issues Arising in the Group

Group issues that are bound to arise in groups in which discursive interaction plays a major role include times when not much is happening, deciding among multiple topics that arise, issues of importance arising in the final minutes of a group, subgroups forming within the group, the mix of single and married patients, and patients receiving bad news regarding their stage of disease.

Downtime

If there is not much happening in the group, it may be possible to get things moving by asking: "If the group was done, and you were on your way home, is there anything you wished you might have said or done in the group that would have made you feel better, or would have made your time here more meaningful?" (I. Yalom, personal communication, 1991). Or, the therapist can ponder out loud how it is odd that a group of persons with this life-threatening disease find it hard to think of difficulties they might be having. If all else fails, this might be a useful time to introduce a specific behavioral technique (e.g., stress or pain management), a specific coping exercise (e.g., assertive communication), or an existential consideration ("If you had one year to live, how would you change your life?"), which is bound to stimulate the conversation afterward (Spira, Chapter 5, this volume).

Multiple Topics

If the therapist believes that several important issues have been raised by one or several patients, the therapist can ask a question concerning one of the points to get the group to explore this area more deeply. The other points can be addressed at a later time. Or, the therapist can simply state that several important points have been raised and they are all important. The group can be asked to decide what topic to address first, giving patients a sense of control over their group.

Late Surges

Frequently, patients attempt to "get everything in" during the final few minutes of a meeting. Too much intensity at the end of a meeting can make the session difficult to end. This is especially true if the intense experience comes from an otherwise introverted patient finally opening to the group. Yet, it is important to give the patient and other group members a chance to wind down and to integrate their feelings and thoughts. One method for handling this situation is to affirm the import of the patient's expression and state that the group will make sure to begin with this concern at the next meeting. If the emotions are very strong in general at the end of the meeting, acknowledging this beneficial expression and then using a relaxation technique to help members settle down before leaving can help them experience firsthand that emotions can be expressed and then allowed to subside.

Recurrence or Death

When a member becomes ill, has a recurrence, or dies, the emotional tone of the group takes a sober turn. It is also a strong stimulus for the group process. This type of event rapidly cuts through denial about the seriousness of patients' illnesses, and helps focus the group on issues they may have been avoiding, such as fears of losing control, death, losing their family, and unaccomplished goals.

Subgroups

Clicks are bound to form within a group. This is to be expected because every member will find a natural affinity with certain other members' views or styles. Such bonds can be useful in establishing social–emotional support. Also, unlike psychotherapy groups, members of cancer groups are encouraged to see each other outside the group meetings to foster supportive relationships. As long as extragroup activities (social events, etc.) are kept out in the open, there should be few problems. However, if one subgroup "gangs up" against another person or subgroup, the therapist must step in to diffuse the situation. This occurs when a group of active problem solvers attempts to help another member "too much," or when there are honest philosophical differences between members (as in the role of "positive thinking," prayer, alternative medicine, etc.). In this case, therapists can point out that different people benefit in different ways from different approaches, how valuable it is to have a wide range of options presented to select among, and how we need to respect this wide range of options.

Being Single

Discussing spouses and family issues when there are single people present should not be avoided. Asking those left out of the discussion how it affects them may uncover feelings of loneliness, regret, or loss, and the need to form new supportive relationships.

Facilitating Difficult Patients

Therapists can interact with the majority of patients in the ways described previously. However, there are bound to be one or more patients in every group who need special management. Several types of difficult patients and ways to interact effectively for them in the group as a whole are described next.

Introverted Patients

Especially quiet, shy, or frightened members can appear to receive benefit from the group by "osmosis." Yet these members can benefit more fully if they are drawn out in a safe way. Other, more expressive members can serve as models, followed by the therapist asking the introverted patient if he or she has similar concerns. In addition, therapists should seek any opportunity to have these patients help others in the group.

Extroverted Patients

Especially verbose, interrupting, or externally focused members need to be managed lest they overtake and redirect the group in ways that may not be optimal. It is useful to allow some expression on their part (they are group members, after all). Yet when they tend to go on too long, it is important for the therapist to interrupt after a few minutes in a polite way and redirect to the group or another group member. One method is to lean forward, raise a finger, and say, "Excuse me. You've said a lot, and I just want to make sure I am following what you've been saying." Then the therapist can summarize in a sentence or two, get an affirmative acknowledgment from the speaker, and finally redirect to the group by saying, "I wonder if anyone else has had this type of experience?" or some such question. Such an approach limits the speaker and yet affirms the value of what he or she has said. At the same time, this approach can be useful in giving feedback to overactive members that they need to limit their expression and allow others to speak. Occasionally, to limit the number of times certain members speak, it may also be useful to say, "We've heard a lot from a few people, but I'd like to give an opportunity to others to discuss their experiences with this situation."

Unusual Patients

Patients that are the most difficult to work with and the most disruptive to the group are those with transient cognitive disturbances and persons with disordered personality function. Patients with significant avoidance can also be problematic for the group as a whole.

Cognitive Deficit and Dissociation. As a result of stroke, primary or metastatic tumors to the brain, or other illness, patients may begin to exhibit unusual patterns of communication and irregular attention. Due to fatigue or medication, other patients may tend to dissociate from current time, place, and logical sequence (Spira, 1996a). It is not unusual to see such patients ramble without a sense of purpose. If the patient is not too disruptive and the therapist decides that he or she can benefit from the group, then managing the patient is important. The best way to manage such a patient is to enter into an interactive dialogue with the patient for a minute or two and then summarize and redirect the group as a whole. This helps the patient stay on track, shows the patient and the group that the therapist cares about what the patient is saying, and eases the worry of the group that this person will go off too far, disrupting the group.

Personality Difficulties. Unlike the progressive or transient dissociative difficulties faced by patients with fatigue or brain involvement, some patients come to the group with long-term personality characteristics that tend to disrupt the group. There are persons who, for example, are interpersonally sensitive (borderline personality in the extreme) or present themselves as continually overwhelmed or especially emotionally demonstrative, crying out for attention (histrionic in the extreme), those who are self-isolating or self-defeating, asking for help and then rejecting it, and those with narcissistic tendencies. In all these cases, it is important first and foremost to form a liaison with the member. Failing to do so sets up an uncomfortable battle within the group. Because such patients are likely to interpret any interaction with them or lack of interaction with them in ways far more complex than the rest of the members, demonstrating an understanding of their feelings and thoughts, without reflection or interpretation, and then asking the group if this discussion has stimulated any thoughts or feelings about their own lives may help to normalize the oversensitivity of these patients and at least to limit their dominance of the group. Still, therapists must be clear that this is not group therapy for persons with personality disorders but, rather, a group that exists to aid adjustment to present circumstances. Therefore, reflecting on the personality characteristics of these patients is rarely of value to the group and may lead to "individual therapy" inside the group or simply results in alienating the patient. If disruption continues, it may be of value to speak with such patients outside the group about their special sensitivities or "insights" and ask for their assistance in allowing others to explore issues in their own way. If all else fails, it may be necessary to suggest to such patients that a group format may not be the best type of support for them and that individual therapy may be of greater assistance.

Distressed Patients

Patients with high levels of distress are to be expected in groups in which a medical condition means loss of function, disruption of basic daily routines, and even the possibility of early mortality. However, when the levels of distress become extreme, patients, and the group as a whole, may not be able to benefit from the planned facilitation.

Mood Disturbance. All patients have some anxiety and depressive attributes. However, when patients have moderate to severe anxiety and depression, it can be difficult to assist them in a group setting. Some patients first need to reduce their general level of arousal before they can address issues raised in the groups. Yet others' personal style is such that they must directly tackle certain issues of vital concern before they are able to relax (Spiegel & Spira, 1991). In either case, when the level of arousal is extremely high, separate groups for these individuals can be very effective in addressing their special needs and individual styles. If simple intake questionnaires can assess level of distress prior to the group's beginning, sufficient numbers of these individuals may be able to be identified to warrant a separate group. At least these persons can be seen individually to obtain additional assistance and to assess their readiness to attend a group. However, the group itself can be extremely distress buffering. If a separate group cannot be developed, then one or two persons in this state may not be disruptive for the group, and the group may likely provide the best possible therapy for them. Certainly, some periods of high distress for most patients in a chronic life-threatening group are to be expected because of the likelihood of disease progression, during which periods the group will serve as a strong source of support.

Cognitive Avoidance or Emotional Repression. Some degree of avoidance and repression may be a buffering against excess distress (Reed et al., 1994). However, when a patient always looks at the bright side of things, always keeps him- or herself busy, and avoids anything to do with the disease, problems may arise. Betty was such a person. She did not want to discuss negative feelings or thoughts in the group and always insisted on telling others that they would be able to beat the cancer as long as they kept a positive attitude and did not let the cancer get them down. Given that this was a group of recurrent cancer patients, initially they wanted to believe her view. But after some weeks, they heard how she would keep herself so busy that she would have no quiet reflective time to let "negative" thoughts arise. In this way, she was so exhausted at the end of the day that she would be able to go to sleep immediately without any negative thoughts intruding. After some time in the group, however, first being able to tolerate others discussing their fears and then being able to tolerate her own expression of fears, Betty was able to be calmer and more comfortably "in the moment," able to better enjoy each day of her remaining life. This was the Betty that other group members grew to respect and learn from.

STRUCTURAL ISSUES IN CHOOSING THE FORMATS OF GROUPS

Finally, it is essential to consider the structural aspects of the group in some detail. Therapists must decide on patients' time commitment, group size, where the groups will be held, the makeup of the groups (e.g., one disease type and stage or mixed), billing for the groups, and whether to use cotherapists.

Open or Closed Groups

"Closed groups" require all patients to join the group at the same time and to remain in the group for a committed duration (e.g., 16 weekly meetings), during which time no other patients can join. "Open groups," in contrast, allow members to join at any time, for any length of time, as is common in American Cancer Society monthly drop-in support groups. Effective groups intending therapeutic improvement are either closed or semiclosed groups (Trijsburg, van Knippenberg, & Rijpma, 1992). "Semiclosed groups" allow members to join when there is an opening in the group (member leaves, dies, or completes commitment), but the patient must make a commitment for a specified duration.

The advantages of closed groups are primarily in the consistency and ease of treatment. The disadvantages of closed groups are found in several areas. If a program has limited resources and has not been able to fill a group, beginning a group with six patients while requiring newly interested patients to wait for months until the present group ends may be impractical. Short-term groups that have a specific agenda to cover may be able to demand a closed group. Yet in a long-term group with recurrent cancer patients, illness and death will reduce the size of the group to a point where it is difficult to continue effectively. Therefore, semiclosed groups, are often used in longer-term formats.

Size of Groups

The number of participants in a group depends on the type of the group and outcomes expected. Educational groups can number in the dozens whereas emotion-focused social–interactive groups do better with about 12 members. Skill-oriented groups lie somewhere in the middle. The more the therapist seeks serious and emotion-based interaction between group members, the smaller the group size needs to be. About a dozen members provide a minimum synergy of diverse experiences and personality styles to keep a group going well. Still, groups as small as 6 or as large as 20 can often be very engaging and productive, assuming that the therapist has the skills to handle such groups.

Choosing the Setting

It is not always possible to choose a pleasant location for group therapy. If psychosocial treatment must be held in a medical center, having the meetings substantially away from the place patients receive treatment can avoid problem associations (e.g., anticipatory nausea for cancer patients). However, if the group leader can only offer the treatment in a medical setting, learning to relax and receive psychosocial support in this setting can aid patients in relaxing and receiving medical support the next time they come for treatment.

Disease Type

In the same way that stages of disease can be broken down to address specific issues, type of disease needs to be considered as well, and not only the system of the disease (e.g., cardiovascular) but the specific type of illness can be important to consider (e.g., hypertension). Cancer patients, no matter what organ is affected, have many issues in common that should be addressed in groups. However, women with breast cancer have some very different concerns than do men with prostate cancer. Members of mixed-gender groups may find it difficult to discuss issues of prosthesis, reconstruction, or sexuality. Lung cancer patients may need to address feelings of guilt and acknowledge the severity of the disease, while Hodgkin's patients typically try to put the disease behind them and learn to move on. Groups for persons with cardiovascular disease may prove less effective than separate groups for persons with stroke, hypertension, or post myocardial infarction.

Demographic Differences

Age, race, income, education, and so on all need to be considered in developing groups. Groups designed specifically to educate poor minority women about the need to receive regular Pap smears and follow-up in case of cervical dysplasia (Miller, Roussi, Altman, Helm, & Steinberg, 1994) are very different than a group of women in a wealthy community who meet to discuss the implications of cervical dysplasia.

Choosing the Makeup of Groups

For the most part, therapists attempt to offer treatment to the most specific population possible. Groups can be organized around disease type or staging, gender, depression, specific issues corresponding to specific organs (e.g., reproductive organs), or any combination of these. Frequently, multiple populations are combined to include any stage of illness, any type of cancer, and any type of individual. There are advantages and disadvantages to homogeneous or heterogeneous groups.

Homogeneous Groups

The more homogeneous the group, the more specific the goals, and the more focused the intervention. Toward this end, it is usually advisable to organize groups with similar disease site and stage, and with age and sex being a factor when possible. For instance, groups of breast cancer patients in treatment who are under 50 years of age would have a more common focus than mixed cancer groups. It is often difficult for patients with earlier-stage disease to discuss issues such as wigs or dating when there are also patients with recurrent disease in the groups discussing their funeral arrangements. Homogeneous groups are certainly the easiest to facilitate.

Heterogeneous Groups

Although more difficult to facilitate, finding sufficient numbers of patients to comprise a homogeneous group often proves difficult, especially with less common types of illness. On the positive side, it can be helpful in confronting their fears of death and dying for early-stage patients to see others at later stages of illness and to see how well these patients handle the later stages of disease. Also, the more varied a group in terms of personality, demographics, gender, and disease type, the more varied are the experiences that members can bring to any given problem.

Often members feel isolated when others in a group do not share some specific factor with which they identify, such as having cancer. (Of course, even in a group of first-occurrence breast cancer patients under 50 years of age, there can be a patient who claims that no one can really understand her because no one else has her specific *subtype* of breast cancer.) One solution is to ask such patients to describe their special issues to help others understand their situation better. This assists the speaker to express and connect and helps others to better appreciate the speaker's concerns.

Assuming that therapists are sufficiently trained to handle the problems that arise from mixed groups, it is better to have a group of mixed cancer patients than no group at all. Some groups that offer an educational format or a coping skills format to large groups of persons with any type or stage of cancer as well as support persons are apparently quite popular and helpful (Gawler, 1987). However, inductive intervention useful for eliciting emotion-focused and supportive interactions among patients is almost certainly sacrificed.

Charging for the Group

Various options exist for justifying a group financially. Institutions that receive grants (research or clinical) to provide such services can offer them free or at very low cost to patients. However, although psychotherapy groups for psychosocially dysfunctional individuals find better compliance and motivation if payment is a factor, groups for patients with life-threatening illness seem to be motivated even without the monetary factor.

Increasingly, hospitals are finding that offering free additional services to medically ill patients (both their own and, if room permits, community patients) increases their reputation as caring for the whole patient, an important factor in competitive medical markets. In addition, hospital administrations evaluating managed care systems are finding that patients who attend therapeutic support groups have improved quality of life, are happier with their care, and tend to utilize the health care system less often for minor ailments. Therefore, many hospitals are finding it well worth their while to hire a psychosocial staff to provide free or inexpensive services for patients.

Fee for service is feasible if there are at least 10 members in the group. Fees commonly run between $20 and $30 per person, typically 50–80% reimbursable by insurance mental health benefits. Typical diagnoses are *316.00— Psychological factors affecting physical condition* (with the disease listed on Axis III of the *Diagnostic and Statistical Manual of Mental Disorders*, 4th edition), *309.xx—Adjustment disorder* (useful for 6 months following a stressor, yet the stressor may be ongoing, as in the case of cancer treatment or cardiac rehabilitation, etc.; to be listed according to Axis IV of DSM-IV), or other relevant diagnoses such as acute stress disorder, posttraumatic stress disorder, major depression, anxiety disorders, and so on. Group psychotherapy (90802) is the procedural code. Managed care companies usually reimburse such groups as long as "medical necessity" is demonstrated. Medical necessity can be shown through the existence of symptoms such as sleeplessness, pain, compliance with medical recommendations, tolerance of medical intervention, and the Axis III disorders as directly affecting their coping with an illness coded on Axis V. Two paid therapists have difficulty justifying their salary from such a group, but one paid therapist and one trainee can work well.

Cotherapists

In a perfectly objective world, practitioners would select the type of group most appropriate for their patients. However, in reality, all practitioners have certain sensitivities and abilities that bias them to select a style or styles with which they work best. Although it is useful for practitioners to stretch their abilities through studying various approaches, they should settle on the style that works best for themselves and then supplement their abilities with a coleader who has complementary talents.

STEPS IN DETERMINING THE TYPE AND STRUCTURE OF GROUPS

A series of steps must be taken to successfully develop a group that is optimally helpful to its intended group members (see Table 1.11). The practitioner must determine the patient population (type and specificity of illness, disease severity, level of patient distress, and gender). Most therapists strive

TABLE 1.11. Steps in Determining the Type and Structure of Groups

1. Determine patient population
   - Type and specificity of illness (cancer, gynecological cancer, ovarian cancer)
   - Disease severity (excellent prognosis, life-threatening, terminal, hospice)
   - Level of patient distress (mild–moderate or moderate–severe mood disturbance)
   - Gender (mixed, single-sex)
   (*Note.* Strive for greatest homogeneity of factors; settle for heterogeneity as necessary to ensure sufficient group size.)

2. Determine goals of therapy
   - Educational information or teaching specific skills
   - Coping skills for living more functionally with one's illness
   - Emotional/social support, addressing existential, emotional, and physical concerns
   - Combinations, and in what proportion

3. Determine style of therapeutic facilitation
   - Deductive/didactic
   - Interactive cognitive-behavioral therapy
   - Inductive Facilitation of Process
   - Combinations (*Note.* Changing between styles is difficult.)

4. Determine structure of therapy
   - Duration of therapy (number of meetings, length of each meeting)
   - Frequency of meetings
   - Family involvement
   - Cotherapists

5. Determine billing for services

6. Train therapists

7. Recruit groups

8. Run groups (debriefing after each group with cotherapist)

9. Evaluate group and modify for future groups

for the greatest homogeneity of factors possible but settle for heterogeneity as necessary to ensure sufficient group size. Next it is important to consider the goals of therapy (educational, coping skills, emotional/social support, or combinations of these). Practitioners need to determine the style of therapeutic facilitation (deductive didactic, interactive cognitive-behavioral therapy, inductive facilitation of patients' emotional concerns, or combinations of these). They must also determine the structure of therapy (duration of therapy, frequency of meetings, family involvement, choice of solo or cotherapists).

Following these critical decisions, it is also important to consider the mechanics of getting the group going, including determining how to bill for services, training of therapists, and recruitment issues. Finally, practitioners must consider debriefing after each group with cotherapists (or getting occasional evaluations from group members if running the group solo). Once the groups have been run, it is valuable to evaluate the experience and modify it for future groups.

CONCLUSION

Group Psychotherapy within a Managed Care Environment

HMO and managed care providers are beginning to see the value of group psychotherapy as being both cost and time efficient as well as highly effective. Studies are now under way that examine reduced health care utilization for patients attending group therapy ("Group Psychotherapy for Women," 1996). In a market competing for patients, it can only serve insurers well to offer services that patients believe help them to adjust and that are inexpensive.

Future Research

There is a need for more exploration of the relative value of different types of groups for different populations. Although the stage-based model presented here describes what is most frequently *used*, is it actually what is *best?* Are heterogeneous groups as effective as homogeneous groups? What level of training and experience is needed for therapists in different types of groups? To what extent is the therapeutic style and focus of the groups what matters, compared to simply giving patients an opportunity to interact? These and other issues need to be more rigorously tested.

Why Group Psychotherapy?

The issues raised in group therapy for the medically ill are in fact of universal concern. Every person must subtly and gradually adjust to interact successfully with a continually changing environment. When medical illness occurs, such subtlety is no longer possible. Modern industrial societies have a way of bracketing illness and death away from the normal experience of most persons. For many, some of the most central issues of their lives, such as self-image, life goals, and the value of their lives in light of their impending death, can be postponed indefinitely. It often takes a crisis before we are able to rally all our resources to deal with our lives as authentically as possible. Yet even in times of crisis, when such matters are bound to arise, they can arouse such distress that related thoughts are avoided and concomitant feelings repressed. Therefore, serious medical illness befalling a person or a loved one has the *potential* to mobilize that person to consider these issues immediately and fully, given the *opportunity* to do so. By providing a safe and supportive environment, group psychotherapy can enable patients to confront these issues, allowing them to live more fully in the face of illness.

Certainly some patients have the ability to handle a crisis well on their own. Some may even discover that they have grown richer from working through the tragedy of illness. Yet those who have difficulty expressing their thoughts and feelings to themselves and others, as well as those who experience anxiety due to their illness, can benefit from the supportive psychotherapy. Individual psychotherapy offers the advantage over group therapy in that individual patterns that lead to or interfere with adjusting to the illness can be examined and potentially modified. However, many persons who become ill do not necessarily have personality disorders that if corrected will cure the illness. Rather, most of the medically ill are psychologically competent yet faced with a situation that would be distressful to anyone.

Group psychotherapy has the advantage of acknowledging every member's intrapersonal as well as interpersonal resources which can help to navigate the crisis of illness. Universal issues that the illness brings forth can be more readily understood and discussed among those who share similar experiences. Group therapy also has the advantage of being able to empower each group member to take responsibility for his or her development rather than facing the long and difficult issue of transference that arises in individual therapy. Moreover, group therapy is more affordable and therefore able to be continued for a longer period for many who cannot afford individual therapy. Certainly, there are instances in which individual psychotherapy is of primary importance for an individual, such as when individual characteristics cannot be sufficiently considered in the group setting. However, group psychotherapy is so effective for persons with medical illness, both from the standpoint of patient and provider, that it is well on its way to being considered a fundamental adjunct to medical care. Although there may be questions as to whether group psychotherapy assists in patients' physical health, there is no doubt that the vast majority of patients receive assistance for improving their quality of life as a direct recult of engaging in this therapy. As the chapters in this volume demonstrate, improving a patient's quality of life offers the best chance for improving physical health as well.

REFERENCES

Adler, A. (1949). *Understanding human nature*. New York: Permabooks.
Agras, W. S., Taylor, C. B., Kraemer, H. C., Southam, M. A., & Schneider, J. A. (1987). Relaxation training for essential hypertension at the worksite: II. The poorly controlled hypertensive. *Psychosomatic Medicine, 49*(3), 264–273.
Allen, M. G. (1990). Group psychotherapy: Past, present, and future. *Psychiatric Annals, 20*(17), 358–361.

Bandura, A., & Walters, R. (1963). *Social learning and personality development*. New York: Holt, Rinehart & Winston.

Beck, A. T., Rush, A. J. Shaw, B. F., & Emery, G. (1979). *Cognitive therapy of depression*. New York: Guilford Press.

Benezra, E. E. (1990). Psychodynamic group therapy: A multiple treatment approach for private practice. *Psychiatric Annals, 20*(17), 375–378.

Berger, M. M. (1990). Combined group therapy: Treating patients with both individual and group therapy. *Psychiatric Annals, 20*(17), 379–384.

Berkman, L. F., & Syme, S. L. (1979). Social networks, host resistance, and mortality: a nine-year follow-up study of Alameda County residents. *American Journal of Epidemiology, 109*, 186–204.

Bowlby, J. (1958). The nature of the child's tie to his mother. *International Journal of Psycho-Analysis, 39*, 350–373.

Buckley, P. (1986). *Essential papers in object relations*. New York: New York University Press.

Corsini, R. J., & Rosenberg, B. (1955). Mechanisms of group psychotherapy processes and dynamics. *Journal of Abnormal and Social Psychology, 51*, 406–411.

Ellis, A. (1962). *Reason and emotion in psychotherapy*. New York: Lyle Stuart and Citadel Press.

Fawzy, F. I., Fawzy, N. W., Arndt, L. A., & Pasnau, R. O. (1995). Critical review of psychosocial interventions in cancer care. *Archives of General Psychiatry, 52*, 100–113.

Fawzy, F. I., Fawzy, N. W., & Huan, C. S. (1995). Short-term psychiatric intervention of patients with malignant melanoma: Effects on psychological state, coping, and the immune system. In C. E. Lewis, C. O'Sullivan, & J. Barraclough (Eds.), *The psychoimmunology of cancer* (pp. 292–319). New York: Oxford University Press.

Fine, C. (1996). Models of responsibility and helping. In J. Spira (Ed.), *Treating dissociative identity disorder* (pp. 81–98). San Francisco: Jossey-Bass.

Friedman, M., & Rosenman, R. (1974). *Type-A behavior and your heart*. New York: Alfred A. Knopf.

Freud, S. (1921). *Group psychology and the analysis of the ego* (J. Strachey, Trans.). New York: Liveright.

Gawler, I. (1987). *Peace of mind*. Melbourne, Australia: Hill of Content.

Gellert, G. A., Maxwell, R. M., & Siegel, B. S. (1993). Survival of breast cancer patients receiving adjunctive psychosocial support therapy: A 10-year follow-up study. *Journal of Clinical Oncology, 11*(1), 66–69.

Glasser, W. (1965). *Reality therapy*. New York: Harper & Row.

Greer, S., & Watson, M. (1985). Toward a psychobiological model of cancer: Psychological considerations. *Social Science Medicine, 20*, 773–777.

Group psychotherapy for women with breast cancer: A joint APA and Blue Cross/Shield of Massachussetts demonstration project. (1996). *APA Monitor, 26*(12), 1.

Hellman, C. J., Budd, M., Borysenko, J., McClelland, D., & Benson, H. (1990). A study of the effectiveness of two group behavioral medicine interventions for patients with psychosomatic complaints. *Behavioral Medicine, 16*(4), 165–173.

Horowitz, M. J. (1986). *Stress response syndromes*. Northvale, NJ: Jason Aronson.

Klerman, J. L., Weissman, M. M., Rounsaville, B. J., & Chevron, E. S. (1984). *Interpersonal psychotherapy of depression*. New York: Basic Books.

Levy, S., Herberman, R., Lippman, M., & d'Angelo, T. (1987). Correlation of stress factors with sustained compression of natural killer cell activity and predicted prognosis in patients with breast cancer. *Journal of Clinical Oncology, 5,* 348–353.

Maslow, A. (1968). *Toward a psychology of being* (2nd ed.). Princeton: Insight Books.

May, P. R. A. (1976). Rational treatment for an irrational disorder: What does the schizophrenic patient need? *American Journal of Psychiatry, 133,* 1008–1012.

Meyer, J., & Mark, M. M. (1995). Effects of psychosocial interventions with adult cancer patients: A meta-analysis of randomized experiments. *Heath Psychology, 14*(2), 101–108.

Miller, S. M., Shoda, Y., & Hurley, K. (1996). Applying cognitive-social theory to health-protective behavior: Breast self-examination in cancer screening. *Psychological Bulletin, 119,* 1–24.

Miller, S., Brody, D., & Summerton, J. (1988). Styles of coping with threat: Implications for health. *Journal of Personality and Social Psychology, 54,* 345–353.

Miller, S. M., Roussi, P., Altman, D., Helm, W., & Steinberg, A. (1994). The effects of coping style on psychological reactions to colposcopy among low-income minority women. *Journal of Reproductive Medicine, 39,* 711–718.

Minuchin, S. (1974). *Families and family therapy*. Cambridge, MA: Harvard University Press.

Mitchell, J., & Everly, G. (1993). *Critical incident stress debriefing: CISD*. Ellicott City, MD: Chevron Publishing.

Moreno, J. L. (Ed.). (1966). *International handbook of group psychotherapy*. New York: Philosophical Library.

Morrow, G. R. (1984). Methodology in behavioral and psychosocial cancer research: The assessment of nausea and vomiting. Post problems, current issues, and suggestions for future research. *Cancer, 53*(10 Suppl.), 267–280.

Parsons, T. (1951). Illness and the role of the physician: A sociological perspective. *American Journal of Orthopsychiatry, 21,* 452–460.

Passick, S., & Redd, W. (1996). PTSD and dissociative disorders. In J. Holland (Ed.), *Textbook of psycho-oncology*. New York: Oxford University Press.

Reed, G. M., Kemeny, M. E., Taylor, S. E., Wang, H-Y. W., & Visscher, B. R. (1994). Realistic acceptance as a predictor of reduced survival time in gay men with AIDS. *Health Psychology, 13,* 299–307.

Solomon, G. F. (1981). Emotional and personality factors in the onset and course of autoimmune disease, particularly rheumatoid arthritis. In R. Ader (Ed.), *Psychoneuroimmunology* (pp. 159–182). New York: Academic Press.

Solomon, G. F. (1985). The emerging field of psychoneuroimmunology. *Advances, 2*(1), 6–19.

Spiegel, D., Bloom, J., & Yalom, I. (1981). Group support for patients with metastatic cancer. *Archives of General Psychiatry, 38,* 527–533.

Spiegel, D., & Spira, J. (1991). *Supportive-expressive group therapy: A treatment manual of psychosocial intervention for women with recurrent breast cancer*. Unpublished manuscript, Department of Psychiatry, Stanford University School of Medicine, Stanford, CA.

Spira, J. (1988). *Understanding paradigms that help and hinder medical advancement*. Paper presented at the symposium Psychoneuroimmunology: Are we ready to proceed with clinical intervention?, Society of Behavioral Medicine, San Francisco, CA.

Spira, J. (1991). *Educational therapy: Existential, educational, and counseling approaches to behavioral medicine intervention*. Doctoral dissertation, University of California, Berkeley.

Spira, J., & Spiegel, D. (1993). Group psychotherapy for the medically ill. In A. Stoudemire & B. Fogel (Eds.), *Psychiatric care of the medical patient* (2nd ed., pp. 31–50). New York: Oxford University Press.

Spira, J., & Spiegel, D. (1992). The use of hypnosis and related techniques for managing pain in terminally ill patients. *Hospice Journal, 8*(1/2), 89–119.

Spira, J. (1993, November). *Dissociation and PTSD in the medically ill*. Paper presented at the meeting of Academy of Psychosomatic Medicine, New Orleans, LA.

Spira, J. (1994a). *Health psychology workbook*. Durham, NC: Duke University Center for Living.

Spira, J. (1994b). *Tai chi chuan and Zen meditation for medically ill patients* [Videotape and manual]. Durham, NC: Duke University Center for living.

Spira, J. (1996a). Understanding and treating dissociative identity disorder. In J. Spira (Ed.), *Treating dissociative identity disorder*. San Francisco: Jossey-Bass.

Spira, J. (1996b). Group psychotherapy for persons with cancer. In J. Holland (Ed.), *Textbook of psycho-oncology*. New York: Oxford University Press.

Stabler, B., Surwit, R. S., Lane, J. D., Morris, M. A., Litton, J., & Feingloss, M. N. (1987). Type A behavior pattern and blood glucose control in diabetic children. *Psychosomatic Medicine, 49*, 313–316.

Starr, P. (1982). *The social transformation of American medicine*. New York: Basic Books.

Sullivan, H. S. (1953). *Interpersonal theory of psychiatry*. New York: Norton.

Sullivan, M. J., Cobb, F. R., & Spira, J. L. (1993). Delaying progression of artherosclerosis: A new frontier in cardiology. *Cardio, 11*(5), 26–30.

Temoshok, L. (1987). Personality, coping style, emotion and cancer: Towards an integrative model. *Cancer Surveys, 6*, 545–567.

Temoshok, L., Heller, B., Sagebiel, R. W., Blois, M. S., Sweet, D. M., & DiClemente, R. J. (1985). The relationship of psychosocial factors to prognostic indicators in cutaneous malignant melanoma. *Journal of Psychosomatic Research, 29*, 139–153.

Thoresen, C. E., Friedman, M., Powell, L., Gill, J., & Ulmer, D. (1985). Altering the Type-A behavior pattern in postinfarction patients. *Journal of Cardiopulmonary Rehabilitation, 5*, 258–266.

Trijsburg, R. W., van Knippenberg, F. C. I., & Rijpma, S. E. (1992). Effects of psychological treatment on cancer patients: a critical review. *Psychosomatic Medicine, 54*, 489–517.

Yalom, I. D. (1980). *Existential psychotherapy*. New York: Basic Books.

Yalom, I. D. (1985). *The theory and practice of group psychotherapy* (3rd ed.). New York: Basic Books.

Yalom, I. D., & Greaves, C. (1977). Group therapy with the terminally ill. *American Journal of Psychiatry, 134*, 396–400.

Yalom, V. J., & Yalom, I. D. (1990). Brief interactive group psychotherapy. *Psychiatric Annals, 20*(17), 362–367.

PART II

PREVENTING ONSET AND RECURRENCE OF ILLNESS

CHAPTER 2

Cognitive-Behavioral Intervention for Persons with HIV

MICHAEL H. ANTONI

Since 1986, the departments of psychology and medicine at the University of Miami have been looking at the influence of psychosocial stressors and stress management interventions on affect, coping, and immune functioning in human immunodeficiency virus—type 1 (HIV-1) seropositive and seronegative gay men. Some of our goals have been to see how these psychosocial factors affect the immune system. In addition, we have used cognitive-behavioral group therapy interventions to manipulate certain psychological variables that may be related to the mental and physical sequelae of the infection. This chapter summarizes our rationale for investigating these psychosocial variables and for using this form of therapeutic intervention with this population.

First I address the question of how stressors and behavioral interventions may influence the immune system by way of the nervous system. In so doing, I build a framework justifying the use of stress management interventions with immunocompromised populations. I summarize the data we have collected with this protocol and discuss, in particular, four findings: (1) how stress management buffers the initial impact of discovering that one is HIV-1 seropositive, (2) how this intervention modulates coping during the immediate adjustment period after people learn their diagnosis, (3) how changes in coping during that adjustment period may predict immune status 1 year later and disease progression 2 years later, and (4) possible mechanisms that we have begun to investigate that might account for how changes in psychological variables may influence the clinical course of the infection. Finally, I describe the steps that went into developing the stress management intervention protocol that we have employed with gay men dealing with a newly learned HIV-1 seropositive diagnosis. Here I describe what happens in the various intervention sessions during the 10-week protocol.

How do behavioral factors influence the nervous system and immune functions? Our group approached this question wanting to put together interventions that followed, to some degree, a psychoneuroimmunological rationale. Specifically, how do stressors, social support, and the way one copes with stressors affect the nervous system and, in turn, the immune system? If we could understand how these variables work together, we felt that we could develop an intervention that could affect both quality of life and some physiological measures believed to be related to health status in HIV-1 infection.

There is now an established animal literature relating experimentally induced stressors such as noise and electric shock (Borysenko & Borysenko, 1982; Shavit & Martin, 1987) to impairments in the immune system. These studies have found that uncontrollable stressors seem to have the largest negative effect on the immune system (for review, see Ader, Cohen, & Felten, 1991). These findings have been discussed in literature since the early 1980s.

Most of the initial studies with humans used stressors such as medical school examinations (e.g., Glaser et al., 1987), which are mild compared to such other naturally occurring major stressors as bereavement (Irwin, Daniels, Bloom, Smith, & Weiner, 1987). On several replications, researchers have reliably found that taking a medical school examination can have an effect on a wide variety of immune system measures, including the ability of lymphocytes to proliferate in response to foreign entities (antigens or the plant equivalent, mitogens). On the other hand, Dr. Michael Irwin has observed that both depression and bereavement are associated with changes in lymphocyte proliferation as well as impairments in the ability of specific lymphocytes—natural killer (NK) cells—to kill tumor targets (Irwin, Daniels, Smith, Bloom, & Weiner, 1987). This latter function, NK cell cytotoxicity (NKCC), is important in protecting against viruses as well as cancer cells.

Several psychological variables associated with chronic stressors, such as perceived loss of control and feelings of helplessness (Rodin, 1988), have also been associated with altered immune functioning in humans. Other studies have revealed that not just stress-related processes but also emotional states (e.g., depressed mood) may, in and of themselves, affect the immune system (Calabrese, Skwerer, & Barna, 1986; Stein, Miller, & Trestman, 1991). Thus, stressors, the way stressors are perceived and responded to, and negative mood states can be related to immunological changes. These phenomena— stressors, appraisals, coping strategies, and depressed mood—are the implicit targets of many interventions used with individuals who are dealing with such chronic medical diseases as cancer, diabetes, and HIV-1 infection, to name but a few.

STRESS MANAGEMENT AND HIV-1 INFECTION

We chose to study the effects of stress management in HIV-1 infection for two major reasons. First, HIV-1 infection presents multiple burdens at the psychological and physical levels. Clearly, HIV-infected individuals are among the groups who might benefit substantially from interventions that teach them to cope with the chronic demands that many of us will never have to face. By learning how these interventions help such people adapt, adjust, and adhere to various lifestyle changes, we may gain insight into ways to facilitate the coping process in other people facing such similar life-threatening conditions as cancer. (For a review, see Antoni, 1991.)

A second major impetus for examining the effects of stress management in this population comes from our conceptualization of HIV-1 infection as a chronic disease whose clinical course may be affected by multiple behavioral and biological factors. As in the case of chronic diseases, such as diabetes mellitus, HIV-1 infection is characterized by a disorder in one or more bodily systems and signs and symptoms of the disorder become manifest across long periods of time as a function of the degree of disorder in the bodily system(s) affected. People with diabetes mellitus or HIV-1 infection die from the "complications" of their chronic disease, not from the disease itself. Diabetics who are unable to maintain their blood sugar levels within a certain range may fall prey to an acute coronary event. HIV-1 infected people who go on to develop acquired immune deficiency syndrome (AIDS) are those whose immune systems have been compromised to the point that they develop complications such as acute life-threatening infections and rapidly progressing cancers.

Because the degree to which the immune system becomes disordered seems to be the strongest predictor of the progression to symptoms and death, much biomedical research has focused on ways to slow either the growth of HIV-1 or the decline of the immune system by modulating the function of its cells. We have been involved in a segment of the research community that examines ways in which psychosocial influences such as cognitive-behavioral stress management (CBSM) can be used to modulate psychosocial and behavioral factors known to affect the immune system. From the point of view of a chronic disease model, *to the extent that CBSM modifies psychosocial factors such as emotional distress, maladaptive coping strategies, and social isolation, might also modulate biological factors such as certain immune system components.* By diminishing the impact of psychosocial and behavioral factors on the immune system, individuals might retard the onset of disease complications by maintaining their immunological status (e.g., T-helper cell counts) within a range necessary to defend against certain pathogens.

Within the subdiscipline known as psychoneuroimmunology (PNI), many studies relate psychosocial and behavioral factors to the immune system. This area is marked by significant agreement and disagreement about the ways in which a wide range of factors affect the immune system in animals and healthy human populations. We and several others have attempted to classify how such things as self-efficacy and sense of control, coping strategies, and social support and such emotional states as depression—all reasonable targets of CBSM—contribute to impairments in the immune system (e.g., Antoni et al., 1990). When we began doing PNI research in HIV-1 infection in 1986, little to nothing was known about how these factors might impair the immune system in infected individuals. However, given prior evidence that experimentally induced and naturally occurring "stressors," perceived loss of control, social isolation, and depression were related to decrements in the numbers and functions of immune cells known to be altered by HIV-1 infection, we reasoned that these psychosocial and behavioral factors might influence immunological status and, possibly, disease course in HIV-1-infected individuals. Similarly, we reasoned that stress management interventions that targeted these factors might provide both psychological and physical benefits for infected people, especially for those who were in the early stages of this chronic disease.

The pieces of the puzzle that were coming together at this point were that several "neurohormones" known to be altered as an function of an individual's appraisal of and coping response to stressful stimuli were also shown to be capable of impairing certain components of the immune system. Some of these hormones, including those produced by the adrenal gland, were also known to be dysregulated in depressed individuals and those reporting significant degrees of loneliness. Because emerging evidence was linking uncontrollable stressors, perceived loss of control (similar to low self-efficacy), and social losses such as divorce and bereavement to alterations in some of these immunomodulatory hormones, we reasoned that the relationships previously observed between psychosocial and behavioral events on the one hand and immunological changes on the other might be mediated, in part, by neurohormonal changes that were linked to an individual's appraisals of and coping responses to environmental burdens. Elsewhere we present a detailed description of the literature supporting the various parts of this model (Antoni et al., 1990). According to this model, stressful events or burdens that are interpreted by individuals as beyond their control might lead to low self-efficacy, avoidance behaviors, social isolation and depression, or distress, which might accompany alterations in some neurohormones and certain aspects of the immune system that may be relevant for the clinical course of HIV-1 infection. Thus, our theoretical model prescribed at least two sets of related targets for intervention: psychosocial experiences and pathophysiological processes involving the immune system.

Psychosocial Targets: Psychosocial Burdens of HIV-1 Infection

We focused our efforts on developing a stress management intervention for HIV-infected gay men because, at the time, this was the group receiving the bulk of energies and resources in HIV-1 research. As such, the psychosocial sequelae of HIV-1 infection had been documented for this population. For some, these include being faced with a wide variety of chronic, uncontrollable, and unpredictable stressors such as changes in health, job status, health insurance, and medical costs. These men may also simultaneously face a loss of social support resources which is triggered by their own withdrawal, the death of close friends, or the homophobic responses of friends and family. Since our initial assessment, we now realize that several new burdens may befall the homosexual man who is diagnosed as HIV-1 seropositive and these are likely to persist across the course of the infection (for a detailed list, see Hoffman, 1991). We have reasoned that the combination of *multiple uncontrollable burdens and declining coping resources* may overwhelm their previously adequate direct coping strategies such as active coping, positive appraisals of burdens, problem solving, and seeking social support, resulting in the adoption of more indirect strategies such as avoidance and denial on the one hand and substance use and possibly risky sexual behaviors on the other. One behavioral loop that may establish itself is that the men's awareness of the ineffectiveness of their coping modes and strategies may increase their sense of low self-efficacy, helplessness, and hopelessness, which in turn perpetuates social isolation, depression, and continued substance use and other self-destructive behaviors. Many of these psychosocial and behavioral phenomena have been associated with impairments in the immune system that could, potentially, contribute to the immunological abnormalities extant in these HIV-1 infected men.

Pathophysiological Targets: The Immune System

Although much less PNI work has been focused in the area of HIV-1 infection, evidence has begun to accumulate linking psychosocial stressors with the progression of the infection (Ironson et al., 1992). Some putative mechanisms have been offered to explain these associations, including stressor-triggered activation of latent HIV-1 to a vigorous replicating state (Glaser & Kiecolt-Glaser, 1987). Thus, some psychosocial phenomena may relate to the pathophysiology of the infection, perhaps affecting, as well, its clinical course (i.e., progression to full-blown AIDS). We have reasoned that such associations may be mediated, in part, by stress-related alterations in the immune system. Also, there is reason to believe that certain specific immunological measures may be especially important in marking or contributing to the course of HIV-1 infection.

T-Helper Lymphocyte Distribution

Even at the asymptomatic stage of the HIV infection there are decrements in CD4 cell counts and impairments in the ability of T-lymphocytes and NK cells to respond to antigenic challenge (DeMartini et al., 1988; Klimas et al., 1990). We also know from HIV epidemiological research and the clinical immunology literature that precipitous drops in CD4 cell counts—particularly when they fall below 200 cells per cubic millimeter (mm^3)—are highly predictive of the onset of physical symptoms and general clinical decline (DeMartini et al., 1988). In fact, the 1993 edition of the World Health Organization classification system for HIV spectrum disease now designates those HIV-infected individuals with CD4 cell counts less than 200 cells/mm^3 as having AIDS, regardless of their symptom status.

NK Cell Cytotoxicity

Certain high-impact psychosocial stressors such as bereavement (which happens to be quite prevalent among individuals who are HIV infected, and among members of risk groups who are not HIV infected but are at risk for becoming HIV infected) (Martin, 1988) can be associated with decreased NKCC (Irwin, Daniels, Smith, et al., 1987). This specific index of immune system status refers to the ability of certain types of lymphocytes—NK cells—to kill an experimental tumor cell line. Specifically, NKCC provides a model for how efficiently the immune system may be able to chase down a virus-infected cell or tumor for which it has not been primed or introduced to previously. Impairments in this immunological function may be especially important in the case of HIV-1 infection, where the T-helper-inducer (CD4) cells are depleted both quantitatively and qualitatively. Perhaps NK cells, in their activities, compensate to some degree for HIV-1-induced CD4 deficiencies.

Antibody Titers to Herpesviruses

Some immune measures may reflect the potential contribution of putative cofactors for HIV-1 disease progression. One set of these measures include antibody titers to herpesviruses such as Epstein–Barr virus (EBV), which are ubiquitous in this population. Although still a controversial topic, one line of reasoning suggests that these titers may indirectly reflect the degree to which the corresponding viruses have been reactivated in the host. The trailblazers for this line of thinking, Drs. Ron Glaser and Janice Kiecolt-Glaser were the first to write that certain psychosocial stressors and emotional states (as a result of their relationship to the reactivation of certain herpesviruses) might affect the course of HIV-1 infection (Glaser & Kiecolt-Glaser, 1987). Accordingly, HIV-1-infected individuals who experience elevated life stressors and who experience distress, depression, and a sense of social isolation may be at greater risk for reactivation of certain herpesviruses, which in turn may act as a cofactor for HIV progression (Rinaldo, DeBiasio, Hamoudi, Rabin, & Liebert, 1986; Rinaldo, 1990; Antoni, Esterling, Lutgendorf, Fletcher, & Schneidermen, 1995).

Neuroimmune Linkages

Although the PNI literature provided some guidelines for the psychosocial variables to target in the intervention strategy we were developing in early 1986, none of these studies had looked at the PNI of HIV-1. Nevertheless, we took that literature and formed a rationale for examining the effects of stressors and stress management on the immune system in HIV-1-seropositive individuals and how these relationships may relate to disease progression. The logic went as follows: Individuals in HIV risk groups—such as sexually active gay men—may encounter a large number of major stressors, which, based on the way they perceive them, may result in differential cognitive interpretations of and emotional responses to those stressors. These events and responses may relate to altered levels or dysregulation of certain neuroendocrine substances that have been shown to have depressive effects on lymphocytes. If this course of events is occurring, there may be decrements in certain functions of lymphocytes occurring concurrently (e.g., lymphocyte blastogenic responses to mitogens, or NKCC). If these biological events can be affected by stressors and emotional reactions, perhaps by way of a neural or hormonal process, there is the possibility that HIV-positive individuals—who have preexisting immune dysfunction—may have a faster progression of symptoms.

Immunological Changes and Health Outcomes in HIV-1 Infection

If psychological factors could affect the immune systems of HIV-infected individuals, even small changes in their immune systems might have clinical relevance. This is particularly interesting in light of one of the primary criticisms of PNI research, which has been that the immunological changes observed following stressors and psychosocial intervention are unlikely to have a clinical impact among the samples studied. This extant viewpoint seems justified given the large variability in many measures of immune status in the normal population and the high number of checks and balances and compensatory mechanisms built into the human immune system. However, if HIV-1 seropositive individuals are "teetering on the brink" of some threshold, reflecting their probable ability to deal with encountered pathogens (e.g., 200–500 CD4 cells/mm^3), small changes of unknown magnitude could quite possibly have an impact on disease onset.

With this no doubt simplified model in mind, we set forth to look at how we might be able to (1) assess and (2) "manipulate" the immune system and psychological state by observing people's responses to a salient stressor, and, we hoped, by utilizing a salient stress-reducing intervention. As a salient, naturally occurring stressor we chose to focus on the notification of an HIV-1-seropositive diagnosis. HIV-1 diagnosis, much like a cancer diagnosis, is accompanied by several well-documented psychological reactions such as anxiety and depression. These usually manifest as diagnosable adjustment disorders.

Intervention Strategy

As an intervention we chose group CBSM adapted by our laboratory for use in this particular sample. The principal aim of this work was to determine whether we could intervene behaviorally to buffer the psychological and, possibly, the immunological "impact" of informing individuals of their HIV seropositivity. Several different intervention strategies might have been effective in the context of the stressor of HIV-1 serostatus notification. Some of the approaches previously studied with medical patients tended to focus on either emotional or cathartic release of pent-up feelings, restructuring maladaptive cognitive appraisals, or learning techniques to enhance bodily relaxation. Because our goal was to offset or "buffer" the acute impact of HIV-1 serostatus notification and to facilitate initial adjustment to this diagnosis, we focused our efforts on stress management techniques. Interventions that focus on stress management as an overall goal have typically used techniques such as cognitive restructuring to increase awareness of how cognitive appraisals about stressors might affect on emotions and progressive muscle relaxation to reduce anxiety reponses to stressful events.

We wanted to utilize an intervention that was replicable and that had also been tied to changes in the immune system. Kiecolt-Glaser and colleagues (1985) observed that in both nursing home residents and medical students, relaxation training was associated with, in the case of the geriatric group, enhancement of immune functioning and, among the medical students, a "buffering" of the impact of taking a medical school examination. In the latter sample, they found that students who took the examination in the nonrelaxation control group showed substantial immune decrements, whereas those who were in the relaxation group showed much smaller immunological decreases and lower distress levels. We extrapolated that relaxation training (and perhaps other stress-reducing techniques) might modify the effects of stressful events (e.g., learning about one's seropositivity) on the immune system in HIV-1-infected individuals.

The first stressor we studied was the *anticipation* of HIV-1 antibody testing. We felt that by increasing subjects' sense of control and self-efficacy and modifying the way they felt about themselves, they might experience less anxiety, depression, and self-isolation during this stressful period. We speculated that these psychological changes might have an impact on the nervous system that could affect the peripheral levels of some immune-modulating hormones. If we could modulate the surveillance capabilities of the immune system (e.g., as reflected in increased NKCC), individuals may progress through the HIV-1 spectrum at reduced rates.

Summary

Our general model views HIV-1 infection as a chronic disease that is characterized by a progressive yet unpredictable decline in the efficacy of the immune system. Factors such as psychosocial and behavioral stressors, capable of modulating the immune system, might contribute to further immunological decrements with subsequent "complications" manifested as opportunistic infections and neoplasias and eventually death. Behavioral interventions designed to modify the impact of stressors might help such individuals to avoid extreme perturbations of hormonal regulatory systems with less subsequent impact on the immune system and possibly their health.

RESEARCH DESIGN AND METHODS

We recruited gay men from the community who were unaware of their diagnosis, had never been tested before, and were healthy. Eligible subjects had to meet several other exclusionary criteria as well (see Table 2.1). One of the primary criteria for study entry was that the men had never been tested for antibodies to HIV-1 and had no overt physical or mental signs that could

TABLE 2.1. Exclusionary Criteria for Gay Men
Participating in the CBSM Study

1. Having been tested for HIV-1 antibodies
2. Unexplained weight loss
3. Oral candidiasis
4. Lymphadenopathy
5. Fever of unexplained origin
6. Drug or ethanol abuse
7. Anabolic steroid use
8. Regular use of antihistamines
9. Age < 18 years or > 45 years
10. Participation in regular physical exercise, meditation, or relaxation regimen

serve as tipoffs that they might be seropositive. These things were verified by a physician's examination at the beginning of the study. The men could not be drug or alcohol dependent as defined by criteria under the *Diagnostic and Statistical Manual of Mental Disorders*, third edition, revised (American Psychiatric Association, 1987), and they could not be steroid users because of the effects of these substances on the immune system, For similar reasons they could not be regular users of antihistamines. All participants were required to be between the ages of 18 and 45 because the immune system is not affected to a great degree by aging within that range. Finally, the subjects could not be participating concurrently in another type of medical or behavioral intervention that might confound the effects of our experimental conditions.

To participate it was necessary that prospective subjects agree to be committed to the study for 10 weeks and also be willing to learn about their HIV serostatus some time during those 10 weeks. If a subject agreed to join the study, he was randomized to one of three experimental conditions. One condition was a CBSM group, one was aerobic exercise training—also conducted in a group format—and one was an assessment-only control group. We tested the men at baseline for several psychosocial variables (e.g., coping, distress, and social support) and behavioral "control variables" (e.g., how much they were sleeping and frequency of recreational drug use and alcohol intake). We also drew a blood sample to assess several nutritional, hormonal and immunological indices.

Five weeks later—after the subjects were engaged in one of the treatment conditions—we measured similar variables again. At this point the men were instructed that it was from this blood sample, that we would determine their HIV-1 antibody status. They were each told that within 72 hours they would attend an appointment with a licensed clinical social worker who would inform them and talk with them about their test results. The social worker utilized a standard format for conveying this information (based on Centers for Disease Control recommendations). Approximately 1 week after the appointment with the social worker the men were again assessed for psychological and immunological changes.

This design enabled us to determine the psychological and immunological effect of the "notification stressor" and the degree to which the CBSM intervention buffered these effects. The buffer hypothesis was based on the previously noted findings of Kiecolt-Glaser and colleagues using relaxation techniques to attenuate the distress and immunologic decrements during medical school examinations (Kiecolt-Glaser et al., 1986). Subsequently, we collected psychosocial data and blood samples from the men three more times over the next 4 weeks to learn how they were coping with the test results and how this differed as a function of which experimental condition they were in. We were particularly interested in how changes in coping strategies and resources over this period related to concurrent changes in their immune system. Finally, to relate intervention-related changes to longer-term health outcomes, we assessed the men again at 1- and 2-year follow-up visits and tracked changes in their health by reviewing the medical records kept by their physicians.

Psychosocial Assessments

We conducted repeated manipulation checks during the study to see how much the men were practicing, and to see whether confounds were operating (e.g., changes in health-related behaviors or commencement of other regimens). That is, we wanted to know whether, perhaps because of this intervention, they were eating differently, sleeping better, or engaging in more physical activities. Such information would be critical in interpreting any psychosocial or biological results that we obtained. In addition to obtaining self-reports on such behaviors during the 10-week intervention period, we also probed for the onset of other stressful events in their lives. To assess treatment adherence, we took attendance at the group meetings and added up the frequency with which the men practiced their progressive muscle relaxation (PMR) exercises at home each day as listed on self-monitoring cards distributed at each weekly meeting. Finally, we assayed the various blood samples the men provided for any substantial changes in diet by assessing serum albumin, a rough measure of protein/caloric malnutrition.

The key psychosocial dependent variables we measured during the immediate pre- and postnotification points were anxiety and depression using the Profile of Mood States (POMS; McNair, Lorr, & Droppleman, 1981). We also tracked changes in coping across the study with the COPE (Carver, Scheier, & Weintraub, 1989), a measure that taps 13 theoretically derived cognitive and behavioral coping strategies. Social support levels were assessed with the Social Provisions Scale (Cutrona & Russell, 1987) before and after the intervention. We assessed immunological-dependent measures which, on the one hand, were known to be associated with the pathophysiology and clinical course of HIV-1 infection and, on the other hand, were previously associated with stressors and other psychological phenomena. These included enumerations of various lymphocyte cell populations, lymphocyte proliferative responses to mitogenic challenge, and NKCC, each assayed at six time points during the 10-week period of observation.

Subject Characteristics

Subjects randomized to each of the groups did not differ in age, ethnic group membership, educational level, employment status, income, or sexual orientation. The sample was generally represented by employed, largely non-His-

panic white gay men, 95% of whom were college educated. We used the Life
Experience Survey (Sarason, Johnson, & Siegel, 1978) to see whether the
men differed in the degree to which they had experienced significant life
events in the past 6 months. There were no differences by randomization in
terms of the negatively rated stressful life events experienced over this period. There were also no differences in the amount of hours of weeknight sleep
(previous three nights) or strenuous physical activities such as rowing and
swimming.

Experimental Manipulation

Based on the self-monitoring cards that the CBSM group members took
home, we computed the frequency with which they practiced relaxation each
week throughout the study (see Figure 2.1). We instructed them to try to
practice at least two times a day. The mean at the beginning of the study was
about 6.5 times per week, persisted at this level for 4 weeks, but then dropped
somewhat the week before they were notified. This indicates fairly good adherence during the 5-week prenotification period. We also assessed the frequency of relaxation practice over this period as a predictor of postnotification outcomes.

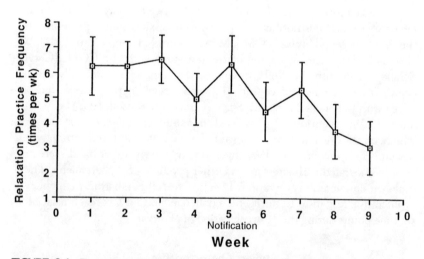

FIGURE 2.1. Frequency of self-monitored relaxation home practice (episodes per
week) in the weeks preceding and following serostatus notification for the HIV-positive gay men in the CBSM group. Week 4 contains the prenotification measurement
point and week 6 the postnotification measurement point.

Research Questions

Before summarizing the results we obtained with our CBSM program, it may be useful to restate some of the research questions we sought to address:

1. Can CBSM buffer the initial impact of a seropositive diagnosis?
2. Does CBSM affect coping strategies and resources during adjustment to HIV seropositivity?
3. Does CBSM affect the immune system during this period of adjustment?
4. Do changes in coping during adjustment to an HIV-positive diagnosis predict severity of depression, immunocompromise, and disease progression over subsequent years?
5. Does CBSM modify coping in those who have been dealing with HIV infection for some time?

1. *Can CBSM buffer the initial impact of a seropositive diagnosis?* Forty-seven healthy gay men who had never been tested for antibodies to the AIDS virus underwent an extensive physical examination and fitness evaluation, as noted previously. Approximately one-third of the men tested positive; two thirds were seronegative. Control group subjects who were found to be HIV positive showed significant increases in depression whereas HIV-positive subjects who were in the CBSM group showed little or no changes in anxiety or depression. The HIV-positive CBSM subjects showed postnotification values for depression just above college student norms, whereas the controls scored within the range for psychiatric outpatients (Antoni, Baggett, et al., 1991).

We also observed that HIV-positive controls showed slight decrements, pre- to postnotification, in CD4 cell and NK cell counts as well as the responsivity of these cells to challenge as measured with blastogenesis or cytotoxicity assays. In contrast, HIV-positive CBSM subjects displayed significant increases in CD4 and NK counts and slight increases in lymphocyte responsivity and NK CC over a similar period. Because we required our CBSM subjects to record the frequency with which they were practicing their relaxation exercises at home, we were able to relate their practice adherence to psychological and immunological changes over this period. We noted that greater treatment adherence (operationalized as frequency of PMR home practice) over the initial 5 weeks of the study predicted lower postnotification depression scores and higher CD4, and NK cell number (Antoni, Goodkin, et al., 1991). Continued relaxation practice during the acute notification period (weeks 5–7) was also correlated with these measures in a similar fashion.

2. Does CBSM affect coping strategies and resources during adjustment to HIV seropositivity? To address this question we examined the degree to which CBSM affects denial and disengaging coping strategies? As noted previously, in the coping literature, denial/disengagement coping strategies are often but not always associated with worse outcomes than involvement/engagement strategies (Folkman & Lazarus, 1980; Namir, Wolcott, Fawzy, & Alumbaugh, 1987). To the degree that the stressors are viewed as uncontrollable, the use of certain direct emotion-focused strategies (e.g., expression of pent-up angry feelings, acceptance, and seeking emotional support) may be beneficial, whereas indirect emotion-focused strategies (e.g., denial and disengagement from the stressor) may have worse health outcomes and may increase social isolation and depressed mood as well. We wanted to see whether we could decrease denial/disengagement coping strategies. Could we then increase involvement-type strategies? Would we have an effect on the men's perceptions of social support and sense of loneliness? Finally, would we be able to impact a particular immunological measure—NKCC—that provides a mechanism for defending against viruses and tumors in the general population and may compensate for the compromised cellular immune functions orchestrated by CD4 cells in the HIV-1-infected host.

To address these questions, we next studied CBSM intervention effects over the 5-week *adjustment* period following the diagnosis. Because this CBSM intervention provides subjects with alternative cognitive and behavioral coping strategies for dealing with stressors and does so in a supportive group environment, we hypothesized that intervention group members would (1) show increases in adaptive coping strategies and decreases in maladaptive strategies such as denial and disengagement, and (2) report greater levels of social support and greater use of coping strategies involving the enlistment of support networks as compared to those HIV-positive men in the control group. We used the COPE to track changes in certain maladaptive coping strategies over this period. One of these strategies was denial, or attempts to avoid acknowledgment of this stressor. Mental disengagement, another strategy, refers to attempts to distract oneself from the stressor, and behavioral disengagement refers to a "giving-up" response.

We also used the COPE to measures changes in involvement/engagement types of strategies. These included acceptance or acknowledging the stressor, active coping or behavioral attempts to deal with the stressor, planning, and positive reinterpretation and growth or reframing. In addition, we added two social support measures that cross the line between emotion- and problem-focused goals: seeking social support for emotional reasons and seeking instrumental support.

As we had anticipated, men in the control group showed significant decrements in social support and decreases in seeking instrumental and emotional social support as coping strategies over this period (Antoni, 1992). In contrast, those in the CBSM group maintained their social support levels and social-support-seeking coping strategies. The men in the CBSM group also showed significant decreases in behavioral disengagement coping (an index of helplessness) over this period. These findings suggest that this 10-week intervention may buffer the stressor of HIV-positive notification by maintaining or enhancing social support levels and providing adaptive coping strategies.

3. *Does CBSM affect the immune system during this period of adjustment?* We attempted to answer this question in two parts. First we wanted to see whether 10 full weeks of CBSM would have a significant effect on the sorts of immunological measures that it had successfully buffered during the acute impact period surrounding diagnosis and whether PMR adherence would be an important determinant of this effect. We found that HIV-positive controls showed decrements in NKCC over the 10-week period whereas CBSM subjects showed no such change (Antoni, 1992). After controlling for pretreatment immune values, relaxation practice frequency (derived from daily self-monitoring records) predicted higher posttreatment NK cell activity for the seropositive men randomized to the CBSM condition. Relaxation frequency was also correlated with decreases in depression during the 10-week CBSM period.

Second, the 10-week period allowed us to assess immunological measures that change more slowly but are more reflective of the chronic ability of the immune system to control latent herpesviruses, an important set of pathogens for HIV-1-infected persons (Rosenberg & Fauci, 1991). Previous work has suggested that reactivation of common herpesviruses such as EBV—which can occur during stressful experiences such as medical school exams (Glaser et al., 1987)—may act as a cofactor for the progression of HIV-1 infection to AIDS (for a review, see Antoni et al., 1995). Although NKCC reflects the potential of the immune system to control such pathogens, quantifying the actual antibody "titers" specific to EBV–viral capsid antigen (VCA) can suggest the degree to which the immune system is adequately controlling this virus. Here, higher titers are believed to reflect poorer control. We found that HIV-positive men had higher EBV–VCA antibody titers than those diagnosed as HIV-negative at every time point during the study with values that sat significantly above the normal range. More important, HIV-positive CBSM subjects showed significant decreases in EBV–VCA antibody titers over the course of the intervention as compared to assessment-only controls, whose antibody titers remained constant and elevated (Esterling et al., 1992).

4. *Do changes in coping during adjustment to an HIV-positive diagnosis predict severity of depression, immunocompromise and disease progression over subse-*

quent years? We evaluated the ways in which CBSM facilitated the men's ability to cope with being HIV-positive over the month following notification and how their coping changes predicted depression levels up to 1 year later. We also followed the medical progress of several of these subjects over a 2-year period and have related the ways in which they were coping during the CBSM intervention with their immunological and health status over the years. We related coping strategies used to deal with HIV-1 antibody status notification with distress levels reported 3 weeks and 1 year later (Antoni, Goodkin, et. al., 1991). We found that denial and disengagement coping strategies were associated with greater depression at both time points, whereas active coping, planning, and positive reinterpretation and growth coping strategies were related to lower depression scores.

We also related distress at diagnosis, HIV-specific denial coping (at entry to the study and at the completion of the intervention), and treatment adherence (attendance, frequency of relaxation during the 10 weeks for those in the intervention groups) to disease progression (AIDS or symptoms exclusive of persistent generalized lymphadenopathy) at 2-year follow-up for 21 HIV-positive gay men for whom physical exams and hospital records were available. At 2-year follow-up, 5 of the 21 men had developed AIDS and 9 had developed symptoms (the 5 with AIDS plus 1 with thrush and fevers, 2 with leukoplakia, and 1 with thrush). In addition, we examined two immune measures (CD4 cell counts and the proliferative response of subjects' lymphocytes to the mitogen phytohemagglutinin [PHA]) in an attempt to explain how intervention-associated changes in emotional distress related to disease progression. Interestingly, we found that distress on diagnosis of seropositivity, denial at the conclusion of the CBSM intervention, increase in denial from entry to completion of CBSM, and low treatment adherence were all significantly associated with (1) poorer immunological status (lower CD4 counts and smaller proliferative responses to PHA), and (2) greater incidence of disease progression. These findings held even controlling for men's CD4 number at entry to the study (Ironson et al., 1992, 1994).

5. *Does CBSM modify coping in those who have been dealing with HIV infection for some time?* We recently completed a pilot study examining the effects of this 10-week CBSM intervention in asymptomatic HIV-positive gay men who already knew their diagnosis at study entry. Specifically, these men had learned their diagnosis between 6 months and 2 years earlier. This pilot study was designed to test the ability of CBSM to reduce distress, depression, and denial/avoidance coping and to increase more adaptive coping strategies in men who were dealing with the chronic burden of HIV-1 infection. Results indicated significant decreases in mental disengagement, denial, and behavioral disengagement (helplessness) coping strategies. We also noted significant increases in active coping, planning, and acceptance.

These findings were similar to those obtained by Fawzy and colleagues (1990) using a similar intervention with early-stage primary melanoma patients. Because the latter study showed increasing improvements in affect and coping at 6-month follow-up, we have begun to use monthly maintenance sessions after the completion of our 10-week program. At these sessions subjects are encouraged to describe the recent stressors they have experienced and the degree to which they have been able to use CBSM strategies to deal with them. The men are also encouraged to describe alternative coping strategies they have developed and factors that seem to facilitate or obstruct their ability to cope successfully with stressors. They are asked to self-monitor their perceived stress levels and relaxation practice frequency on a weekly basis and to record this information on cards that are turned in at each monthly maintenance session. Initial results from these maintenance sessions indicate that the men are using newly learned cognitive restructuring techniques, assertiveness skills, and relaxation exercises; that they are experiencing improvements in interpersonal relationships and lower perceived stress levels; and that they enjoy the opportunity to report to the group on their frustrations and progress in using these strategies to cope with stressors. We are in the process of evaluating parallel immunological changes that occur during the course of the CBSM intervention with these groups of people.

6. *How do psychological variables affect the progression to AIDS among HIV-positive asymptomatic gay men?* Among 24 HIV-positive asymptomatic gay men we found that *lower distress* at the time of diagnosis (which was buffered by participation in the CBSM intervention) (Antoni, Baggett, et al., 1991), *less denial coping,* and greater adherence to behavioral *stress management* techniques in the weeks after initial seropositivity diagnosis *predicted a lower likelihood of progressing to symptoms or to full-blown AIDS 2 years later* (Ironson et al., 1994). This suggests that men who were able to derive more distress-reducing benefits from and make greater use of the CBSM techniques and to break through denial in the weeks surrounding notification appeared to have the slowest progression of disease during the initial 2 years after diagnosis.

7. *Can this approach be generalized to other HIV populations?* Based on the effects we observed for CBSM intervention with asymptomatic HIV-positive gay men, we have recently expanded our investigations of CBSM in two additional groups: HIV-positive gay men with symptomatic disease but prior to the onset of AIDS and HIV-positive symptomatic (pre-AIDS) African American women. During the next decade it is predicted that there will be growing numbers of individuals from these two populations who will be challenged with dealing with the unique stressors associated with the middle stages of HIV infection. Some of these stressors include a pervasive uncer-

tainty about the course of the disease, mounting medical costs (especially for the uninsured), and changes in social support networks (because of multiple bereavements and difficulties with family ties). We have recently adapted the CBSM intervention to be appropriate for each of these populations and are currently testing the effects of each as 10-week intervention protocols in two randomized clinical trials within the context of a National Institute of Mental Health (NIMH)-funded program project. Our preliminary results suggest that among symptomatic gay men, this intervention reduces dysphoric symptoms and general distress and facilitates the use of adaptive coping strategies and social support (Lutgendorf et al., 1996; Lutgendorf et al., in press) as well as modulating some aspects of immune function associated with herpesvirus reactivation (Antoni, Lutgendorf, Ironson, Fletcher, & Schneiderman, 1996). The study testing the effects of CBSM in symptomatic African American women is actively recruiting subjects—preliminary results should be ready in approximately 1 year.

A MODEL FOR STRESS MANAGEMENT

This section discusses some of the key ingredients of most of the stress management interventions we decided to employ in the studies presented previously, which we continue to use in clinical research. Stress management interventions have been proposed for groups of people dealing with a wide variety of psychological and physical disturbances ranging from anxiety and depression on the one hand to headaches and hypertension on the other. The development of interventions for this group was guided by some of the basic assumptions underlying stress management.

What Is Stress Management?

To understand the notion of stress management, it is first, of course, useful to define the thing we are trying to manage—stress. However, most behavioral scientists have a great deal of difficulty in doing so, leading to an unofficial consensus that the term "stress," despite its wide use in nonscientific circles, may have little value for research purposes. The problem here is one of precision. The term "stress" is often used to describe an external event (a stimulus), discomfort or tension (a phenomenological state), one's reaction to an event or state (a response), or the way in which all these entities interact (a process). From the standpoint of research enterprises, the ambiguity of this term makes it quite difficult for scientists to decide on just what they will call stress, even though anyone will say, "I know stress when I have it!"

Because of this definitional problem, attempts to relate stress-related variables to psychosocial and physical outcomes can be problematic. Several theorists have justifiably asked that researchers therefore shift their focus to the study of how individuals respond, adapt, or "cope" with demands and difficulties, and how these changes can be used to predict their future health status. Many have argued that in making such predictions, it is less important to know what types of a storm a person has been through than it is to know how that person got through it. This rationale is buttressed by data supporting that *individual differences* in coping actions and resources play a substantial role in amplifying, diminishing, or otherwise "moderating" a wide range of environmental burdens. Moreover, the attraction for the study of the coping process is driven by the precision with which it can be defined and measured (Justice, 1988), its empirical association with psychosocial and physical changes, its inclusion of a wide range of human experiences, and the fact that it captures the dynamic quality of the ways in which people interact or "transact" with their environments (Folkman & Lazarus, 1980).

One comprehensive model of the coping process, developed by Folkman and Lazarus (1980) and later adapted by Justice (1988), was quite instrumental in the development of the CBSM package we have been using. According to this model, the coping process can be classified into "modes and strategies" and "resources" (Justice, 1988). Modes and strategies can include "direct" and "indirect" activities, which vary in terms of the degree to which they are designed to focus precisely on the source of the burden or challenge (problem focused) or, alternatively, on the feelings evoked by the burden or challenge (emotion focused). It is not our intent to exhaust all the possibilities that result from combining all these categories; however, it is useful to list some of the modes and strategies that are common to several extant stress management packages and our CBSM package in particular.

Coping Modes and Strategies

Direct activities of the problem-focused variety include *problem-solving techniques* (e.g., learning how to go from point A to B by the shortest, least painful means), *assertive behaviors* (e.g., standing up for one's rights, expressing one's needs, and operating with effective communication skills), and *seeking out the help of external sources for information* (e.g., approaching other members of an individual's network of family or friends to get him out of a jam) (Justice, 1988). As others have pointed out, these directives operate on the external environment. Some actions, on the other hand, can directly affect an individual's internal world (i.e., private thoughts). These actions, also the focus of stress management packages such as our own, include the *correction of thinking errors* or "cognitive distortions" (Beck & Emery, 1979) and the *reforming, restructuring, relabeling or replacement of one's cognitive appraisals of burdensome stimuli*. As we highlight later, these cognitive distortions come in many forms, tend to occur "automatically" or without volition, and often precede the exacerbation of emotional discomfort. Thus, an initial target of stress management interventions that focus on cognitive aspects is to help individuals become more aware of (1) the situations in which their thinking errors have been recently evoked, (2) the particular ways in which the errors took form (e.g., magnification vs. minimization), (3) the close proximity of the cognitive appraisal to the emotional change, and (4) the ways in which these cognitive–emotional "events" shaped their outward behaviors and sense of self-efficacy. Some of the exercises used to build a greater awareness of these interlocking processes are illustrated later.

Another set of modes and strategies of coping relevant to stress management are those direct actions focused on the remediation of feelings evoked by burdens (Justice, 1988). These emotion-focused activities can be directed to tension reduction and include things such as relaxation exercises and physical (e.g., aerobic training) exercises. Alternatively, actions such as verbally ventilating anger, sadness, or fears are direct actions that an individual can take to modulate his or her emotional reactions to a burden. Emotion-focused modes and strategies including direct actions for tension reduction and emotional release are important ingredients of stress management and are incorporated in our CBSM program.

We have generally viewed the aforementioned directed activities as useful in buffering the impact of both acute challenges (e.g., learning the initial news of HIV-positive antibody status) (Antoni, Baggett, et al., 1991) and longer-term conditions (e.g., coping with the demands of a chronic disease) (Antoni, 1991). In fact, we designed our CBSM intervention package to teach individuals tangible, direct actions, some of which are problem focused (problem-solving, assertive behaviors, communication skills, and social support utilization) and some emotion focused (PMR training, aerobic exercise training). Beyond providing individuals with these new skills, we also teach them to become more aware of the environmental demands and biobehavioral stress "signals" that warrant the engagement of these modes and strategies. As well as teaching people to become more aware of situations in which direct actions can be employed, stress management interventions such as ours also teach them to become more aware of their old, less effective modes and strategies for dealing with difficulties. These activities, often classified as indirect actions, exist on both the problem-focused and emotion-focused planes. By teaching themselves to become more aware of the occurrence of these automatic reactions and habitual behaviors, people may find the entry point for replacing an old ineffective strategy with a new, more effective one.

These indirect actions can be centered around a burden or difficulty (problem focused), including such things as behavioral and cognitive avoidance. *Behavioral avoidance*, as the name implies, refers to the lengths that people will go to reroute their lives away from an uncomfortable person, place, or activity. These behaviors may range from the more extreme forms, referred to as phobias, to the much more subtle ways that people find to avoid interpersonal conflicts. *Cognitive avoidance* often takes the form of distraction from or outright denial of the problem at hand and does little to change the nature of the burden.

Other indirect action strategies tend to be focused on ameliorating the emotional sequelae of environmental burdens (indirect emotion-focused strategies). These strategies include changes in *consummatory behaviors* such as increased smoking, eating, and alcohol and recreational drug use/abuse (Justice, 1988). Indeed, these activities, at the physical level, may distract an individual from the problem at hand. Indirect strategies operating more clearly at the feeling level include giving up, feeling helpless, or, perhaps, fainting (Justice, 1988). Beyond the fact that these strategies may be ineffective for dealing with present difficulties, burdens, and challenges, some groups have gathered evidence that such strategies may increase depressed feelings and impair bodily systems (e.g., the immune system) that confer protection against certain pathogens or help to slow the progression of extant disease processes. For instance, a growing body of literature has related an attitude of giving up or hopelessness to a poorer prognosis and shorter survival time for patients with some types of cancer (e.g., Greer, Morris, & Pettingale, 1971).

One final note regarding indirect strategies is that they are often interrelated and "transperpetuating." That is, the use of indirect problem-focused strategies often gives rise to the use of indirect emotion-focused strategies, and vice versa. The following example demonstrates this loop:

> Joe is having a difficult time approaching his supervisor about some recent anxiety-arousing events in which he was discriminated against because of his ethnicity. Anticipating that he will gain no support from his supervisor, Joe avoids him, feels more anxious, and tries to distract himself from the problem, which is now recurring. As discriminatory experiences increase in frequency, Joe finds himself eating more junk food and having a few drinks at lunch to "calm down." Thus, his behaviors are now designed to avoid both the problem and his anxious feelings. These alternative consummatory activities may make Joe less likely to confront the problem because they (1) provide a temporary relief from the irksome nature of the problem, (2) provide him with a primary reinforcer or biological reward for escaping from the problem, and (3) deflate his sense of self-efficacy or "take the wind of his sail," thereby making him more likely to avoid, disengage, and distract himself in the future. Beyond these behavioral consequences, Joe may become depressed because this process also perpetuates feelings of helplessness.

Unfortunately, these events run in a closed loop or vicious reinforcing cycle—increases at one end or the other of the cycle are the rule rather than the exception because habitual coping often makes people "feel safe" and may actually be "driven" by the activities that precede and follow them. This is how people get "stuck" in maladaptive coping strategies. Simply telling people to "break their dirty habits," "stand up to their fears," and "clean up their act" often does little more than remind them of how helpless they are to change things. Interestingly, other processes may also become ignited by the vicious reinforcing cycle of indirect modes and strategies. The sense of low self-efficacy that is bred by the cycle of events may generalize to other areas of a person's competence, possibly triggering *cognitive distortions* (e.g., "I' ll always be second rate"), *nonassertive responses* (e.g., "I have no right to expect more"), and *social isolation* (e.g., "I don't need any help from anyone"). These cognitive "spin-offs" from the vicious cycle of indirect coping strategies are several of the "targets" of stress management programs such as ours. Once we help individuals to become more aware of the degree to which they use indirect strategies, and the fact that the strategies do little to control their environments but much to constrict them and that the "costs" of the strategies outweigh the "benefits," they may find themselves willing to look into more adaptive strategies. At this point, standard stress management techniques can be introduced that teach problem-solving, cognitive restructuring, and problem-focused assertiveness skills on the one hand and more emotion-focused activities such as relaxation or physical exercises on the other. The hope of programs like ours is that these active coping strategies will replace habitual, less effective indirect ones.

Coping Resources

As several authors have noted previously, it does little good to provide people with these strategies when they live in an environment that is devoid of sufficient *coping resources* (Justice, 1988). Coping resources that seem to be critical for most stress management efforts include basic *information* and *social support*. Information on stress responses (cognitive, emotional, biological, and social) make tangible the often abstract collection of sensations that people experience during periods of excessive demands and help them to become more aware of these as signals for modifying their current activities. Moreover, by providing people with information on the potentially destructive mental and physical health consequences of their old coping strategies, they may find it easier to shift to new ways of dealing with problems.

Social support, or a set of people or institutions that individuals can count on in situations ranging from minor jams to their "darkest hour," is a critical fuel for making the stress management machine work. These special people help bring an individual's attention to the way he or she looks and feels, what he or she is doing, and where he or she seems to be going, and, as such, they can alert an individual to early warning signals that he or she is missing. These people also reinforce an individual for the bravery needed to leave the safe waters of indirect coping strategies; they are there to provide the needed pat on the back for getting through difficult storms and setbacks. Finally, these significant others can provide an individual with tricks about how they learned to "plug in" to a new strategy and jettison an old one.

Of course, not all significant others or acquaintances are facilitative. Some people can batter down self-confidence with punitive, judgmental quips (often containing the words "should," "ought," "never," or "always"); others would prefer to be a drinking companion to mutually "drown sorrows" with indirect emotion-focused strategies. Although volumes of research articles have emphasized the beneficial aspects of social support, more recent literature points to some of the "toxic" elements of certain people in an individual's environment. For our purposes, to the extent that other people facilitate an individual's ability to utilize some of the more adaptive direct strategies mentioned previously, that source of social support is viewed as potentially beneficial (Zuckerman & Antoni, 1995).

Clinical researchers are becoming increasingly aware that the two coping resources mentioned so far, information and social support, may contribute as much (or more) to the success of stress management interventions as the particular modes and strategies introduced. Thus, two features of contemporary stress management interventions seem to make such interventions especially effective—an educational component that is threaded through all the topics discussed and a group format for discussions. The educational component of stress management packages such as our own includes didactic modules delivered by group leaders and written information packets that are distributed repeatedly throughout the weeks of the intervention. These materials can include assessment vehicles (e.g., wallet-size take-home self-monitoring cards) designed to help increase people's awareness of the different ways that their stress responses take form, thus making them available as cues for change. Other information media include diagrams showing the circularity of indirect coping strategies and their unhealthy consequences.

When stress management strategies are introduced in a group format, participants benefit from the joint sense that everyone is working toward a common goal. They may also benefit from observing and vicariously enjoying the successful strategies that are modeled by other group members, from the honest feedback they receive from those who witness their behaviors firsthand at close range and from the sense of warmth and security that comes from other caring humans who "know their situation." Because stress management "groups" make information and social support resources readily available, we have reasoned that this intervention format for modifying coping responses to stressors may be the most potent and long lasting. We acknowledge that coping resources in the "natural environment" (home, work, etc.) will be ever-changing and that the ambiance of the stress management group is, thus, unrealistic as a goal for structuring a postintervention environment. Thus, as part of our stress management package, we conduct in-session exercises and assign "homework" to members designed to increase their awareness and utilization of informational and social support resources in their community, job, and home.

In sum, we have developed a time-limited program that offers in a group format the possibility of emotional, social, and even physical benefits subsequent to improvements in coping strategies and coping resources. It is essential, however, to adapt the content of this stress management program to the specific needs and experiences of the population being served and observed. Following is the specific intervention program we developed for HIV-positive gay men, the effectiveness of which we reported earlier.

THE COGNITIVE-BEHAVIORAL STRESS MANAGEMENT PROGRAM AT MIAMI

Program Development

We employed several steps to arrive at the 10-module program that we ultimately used to study this cohort (Antoni et al., in press) (see Table 2.2). We looked at the literature to find the best intervention strategies for both reducing the effects of short-term acute stressors and helping people develop coping strategies to deal with future stressful events. Once we determined some of the therapeutic tools we wanted to use, we assembled relevant topic areas for discussion in the groups: areas such as the nature of the human stress response, safer sex techniques, negotiating safer sex, transmission of HIV-1, and relationships. These were stimulating topics that could be used, in the case of cognitive restructuring, for instance, to show how distorted cognitions can influence the way participants interpreted an interpersonal situation or handled a stressor in the environment. After we developed a standardized treatment scheme, we put together these things in the order we wanted to use them and pilot-tested the protocol with graduate students as

---

TABLE 2.2. CBSM Protocol Development

1. Determine relevant intervention techniques.
2. Assemble relevant discussion topic areas for study sample.
3. Develop standard treatment sequence and system for integrating across modules.
4. Prepare a training program for group leaders.
5. Supervise pilot trials of protocol.
6. Modify protocol and construct manual containing modules for each session.
7. Ongoing weekly supervision of all sessions facilitated by audiotapes.

---

our subjects. Following their impressions and our own, we modified the treatment modules and put together a manual. This manual was used subsequently to train the co-leaders who ran the groups for our study. We planned the group sessions for four to seven men led by two co-leaders. The groups were audiotaped, and we conducted face-to-face supervision on a weekly basis.

Goals and Strategies

Our overarching goal in developing a CBSM intervention is to educate people on the role that cognitive and behavioral responses to stressful events might play in maintaining their mental and physical well-being (see Table 2.3). One of the most critical elements of this program was our effort to increase the participants' awareness of the ways in which they appraised and responded to demands and burdens and the ways in which they utilized social resources to help them cope with such challenges.

First, we provided them with an easy-to-use anxiety reduction skill. We taught them PMR, using a 10-week adaptation of Jacobsonian relaxation techniques that were further developed by Bernstein and Borkovec (1973). Second, we attempted to modify the way individuals appraise stressors by using cognitive restructuring (Beck & Emery, 1979). Third, to help individuals manage interpersonal conflict and the way they express anger, we used an assertion training approach with special emphasis on the assertive expression of negative emotions. Fourth, we taught behavioral control strategies so participants could learn to bite off a little bit at a time in trying to change the behaviors pertaining to the goals just listed. Some of these strategies were taken from the work of Jeff Kelly and Jill St. Lawrence who developed a behavioral intervention for decreasing risk behaviors in gay men (Kelly, St. Lawrence, Hood, & Brasfield, 1989). Finally, we hoped to instill in participants a sense of connectedness to the group and to enhance their awareness of the social resources they have not yet utilized. These resources include those at the level of lover, family, and friends, as well as those at the institutional level.

TABLE 2.3. CBSM Program Goals and Strategies

Goals	Strategies
1. Educate on relevant topics	Didactic information provision
2. Provide an anxiety-reduction skill	Progressive muscle relaxation training
3. Modify stressor appraisal	Cognitive restructuring
4. Manage conflicts and express anger	Assertion training, anger control
5. Enhance behavioral control	Self-management and behavioral change
6. Increase utilization of social support	Group support, awareness exercises

In sum, based on the HIV-associated phenomena outlined previously, we developed a CBSM intervention designed to reduce perceived loss of control, maladaptive coping strategies, and social isolation on the one hand and to increase perceptions of self-efficacy, personal control and self-mastery, and social support on the other. We felt that such a program might enhance well-being across emotional, cognitive, and social spheres of functioning while providing a set of prophylactic coping strategies to use as "stress buffers." For the purposes of our research agenda, we reasoned that a group CBSM intervention could simultaneously address problems related to personal control, coping demands, social isolation, and depression—all relevant for individuals who are attempting to adjust to being HIV-1 seropositive. Several of these psychosocial "targets" have been shown to influence the immune system in a wide variety of healthy and clinical populations. There is evidence, for instance, that uncontrollable stressors, avoidance coping strategies, and low social support or loneliness are associated with alterations in several immunological measures including reductions in cell counts and impairments in cells' functional abilities (for a review, see Antoni et al., 1990). Thus, our research program tests the degree to which our CBSM intervention might modulate both psychosocial and immunological status of HIV-infected individuals.

Strategic Features of the Program

The CBSM program that we ultimately developed was one "arm" of the GET SMART (Graded Exercise Training and Stress Management and Relaxation Treatment) study being conducted by the departments of psychology and medicine at the University of Miami as part of a larger NIMH-funded AIDS research center. The primary aims of the CBSM intervention, as discussed earlier are as follows:

1. To provide individuals with information on HIV-1 infection and its treatment and on risk behaviors, stress responses, coping, and social support.
2. To teach anxiety reduction skills such as PMR and relaxing mental imagery.
3. To modify cognitive appraisals (e.g., cognitive distortions) using cognitive restructuring.
4. To enhance interpersonal coping skills (e.g., conflict resolution and anger expression) via assertion training.
5. To provide a supportive group environment and to help individuals utilize available social support networks.

Beyond these major aims, the program contains some less obvious features. Implicit in all the treatment modules is the importance of *increasing awareness of the automatic yet controllable nature of an individual's responses to stressors and burdens.* We tell subjects that we would like them to become "stress-perts" by the end of the program. As mentioned previously, it is difficult to adopt a new, untested coping strategy without first "stepping back" and becoming more aware of the failure of our old strategies to resolve burdens, their circular path, and their destructive spin-offs. The didactic segments and written handouts accompanying most of the weekly modules are designed to catalyze this awareness process. However, some of the most potent ways that people become more aware of these subtle processes is by doing "homework" assignments where they track their own thoughts and feelings accompanying stressful encounters and report them back to the group, and by observing other group members "do their own distorting" during the group sessions and modeling more appropriate "second takes" at formulating a coping response (Antoni et al., in press).

Another subtlety of this CBSM program is that it includes a combination of problem-focused (e.g., cognitive restructuring) and emotion-focused (e.g., relaxation training and seeking emotional support) coping options. We deemed this to be important for several reasons. First, it is well-known that people use a blend of both of these classes of coping strategies; neither is the sole answer for all situations. Thus, by weaving both types into the program we hoped to enhance its utility in real-world situations. Second, people differ (based on their core personality "style") in their preferred set of coping strategies (e.g., some are not entirely comfortable with emotion-focused strategies). Interventions that fail to offer the opportunity for a personality *style–coping strategy* match may be ineffective. We regularly encourage people to use those CBSM techniques that are most helpful to them. Third, people are likely to differ in the degree to which they perceive themselves as having personal control over current life demands. Emotion-focused strategies are believed to be most effective with uncontrollable situations and problem-focused strategies most effective with controllable situations (Folkman et al., 1991). By providing people with a blend of each type of strategy, our hope is that this CBSM program will improve individuals' ability to deal with the wide range of controllable and uncontrollable burdens that are a predictable part of having HIV-1 infection.

We ran the CBSM program in 10 modules conducted twice weekly over a 10-week period. We implemented this program using two group leaders who were trained in the specifics of the program using the treatment manual, behavioral role play, and directed readings. The program uses group leaders and group members as *coping role models*. This facilitates positive social comparisons and demonstrates an *in vivo* use of social support for informational purposes. It was our hope that people responding particularly well to this aspect of the program might leave a session with such thoughts as the following: "I saw him do it so I feel that I could also pull it off," or "I'm glad to hear that someone else has these crazy thoughts," or "It's good to know that I can rely on these people for some honest feedback and guidance." Although such responses deal mainly with the informational aspects of the group interaction process, the emotional aspects emphasized here refer more to nurturance, unconditional positive regard and reassurance of worth, and a general sense that one can rely on other group members at any time. The supportive group environment used in our program also encourages *honest expression of feelings* and provides a regular *opportunity to seek out emotional support*. Emotional support seeking is most fluid and potent in groups that possess the qualities of cohesiveness and communality (Yalom & Greaves, 1977). Group interventions directed toward groups of people attempting to manage the same chronic burden or disease have a built-in sense of community that allows for the honest expression of emotions to come more freely.

Within the group context, the program also attempts to replace feelings of powerlessness and isolation with a sense of mastery and altruism. By providing the opportunity for personal mastery experiences and observing others master their own obstacles, self-efficacy is bolstered, which may generalize to other situations. Although our instructions to people about how to change their thinking and behaviors are an important and useful blueprint, it is their own belief in their ability to overcome adversity that allows them to turn over the soil, pour the cement for the foundation, and execute the building plan. By giving them the opportunity to witness and personally experience cause–effect relationships in the group, we hope that this process is set into motion. It is also well-known that such group interventions owe much of their lasting success to the fact that they provide people with the opportunity to fulfill a very human need for becoming involved in the lives of others in an altruistic fashion. Thus, by knowing that their disclosures of old ineffective strategies and discoveries of new ones are helping their fellow group members, people in the CBSM program may feel less defensive about disclosing personal or potentially embarrassing information and may also leave the group with a renewed sense of self-worth and belongingness.

The final mission of the group is to discourage avoidance and denial of current problems and to encourage more direct actions such as cognitive restructuring, active problem solving, doing relaxation exercises, and seeking social support. This is achieved explicitly through the didactics and awareness exercises in each module and explicit feedback between group members and occurs implicitly through the more subtle aspects of cohesiveness and commonality. A salient feature of this program is that it encourages group members to monitor ongoing stressful events each week and to utilize samples of these for in-session exercises that involve all members of the group. For instance, after individuals record an incident in which they are aware of a cognitive distortion or nonassertive behavioral response, they are encouraged to reenact the situation with one other group member while the "audience"

of other members provides feedback from their observations. This reenactment increases the awareness of subtleties of different coping responses
among all those involved in the exercise. To further explicate the actual content of this program, we now walk through a more detailed description of the
sequence of weekly modules used. Each module has been adapted for use with
the target population that we have been focusing on—HIV-1-infected gay
men. However, the techniques employed are presented as tools that all people can use to improve the ways in which they deal with burdens, difficulties,
and challenges.

Content of the Weekly Modules

Relaxation Training

In one 45-minute session a week, members receive training in PMR (Bernstein & Borkovec, 1973). Briefly, this portion of the program starts by training them to relax by tensing and releasing each of 16 muscle groups in the
first session, gradually reducing muscle groups to 7 then 4 clusters, and finally
teaching them to relax their entire body through a countdown procedure.
This "progressive" aspect has the advantage of enabling people to obtain
concrete evidence of improving their ability to control tension levels across
the 10-week period. Because this approach culminates in a relatively simple,
quick, and easy-to-engage counting cue for relaxation, people may be more
likely to continue practicing it after the program has ended. We recommend
that people practice these exercises twice daily, preferably in the same location (e.g., in a quiet place at their lunch break and at home in the evening).
We also ask that people record how often they practice and indicate, along a
subjective 7-point scale, how much tension or "stress" they felt immediately
before and after doing their relaxation exercise. This information is recorded
on wallet-size cards which are turned in at the beginning of each relaxation
session. After people have completed 4 weeks of the relaxation training, they
are provided with a "beach scene" imagery component to enhance the depth
of their relaxation experience. At this point they are given an audiotape describing a peaceful beach scene and asked to use this during their twice-daily
PMR exercises. This provides more "color" to the daily exercises as well as
the opportunity for more focused relaxation due to the fact that auditory distractions become less likely.

Information Provision

In addition to the relaxation/imagery session, people also meet in an additional, longer session once weekly. In these 90-minute sessions they receive
informational didactics and learn stress management techniques such as cog-

nitive restructuring, assertion training, and social support sensitization and utilization.

Topical relevant issues such as immune system functioning, HIV-1 antibody testing, viral transmission, safer sex, and the nature of the human stress response are used for educational purposes and are catalysts for discussion and application of newly learned CBSM techniques. We have juxtaposed much of the informational aspects of the program with the specific cognitive behavioral techniques that are most relevant for the information being disseminated. For instance discussions of viral transmission and safer sex are instigated simultaneously with the introduction of assertion training, which may be important in negotiating the nature of sexual encounters.

Cognitive Restructuring

Cognitive restructuring is introduced early in the program and as in the programs developed by Beck and colleagues (e.g., Beck & Emery, 1979), group members maintain an ongoing daily program of monitoring stressful events, accompanying emotions, automatic thoughts, and physical and social "symptoms" of stress. These stress symptoms refer to evidence of their responses to burdens and are conceptualized across cognitive, emotional, behavioral, social, and physiological domains. The goal here is to increase group member's awareness of the ways in which they are dealing with burdens and difficulties and the possible cues that they may want to use as early warning signals in the future.

We also stress the interrelationship between the changes that group members experience across these five domains. Most notably, we encourage people to focus on the link between the way in which they *think* and the way they end up *feeling* (e.g., "Your emotions result largely from the way you look at things"). Before people can experience an event as, say, upsetting, they you must first process (filter, magnify, distort) it in their mind and assign it some personal meaning. So, if a person's perceptions of an event are exaggerated or distorted in some way, their emotional response may be extreme. Depression and pervasive anxiety might fall into this category of extreme responses. A handy metaphor displaying this relationship goes as follows: If music is playing on the radio and there is static, it is not faulty transistors or wiring ("you don't have a 'screw loose'"), but rather the problem is that the listener is not accurately tuned to the right frequency ("your reading of the situation is simply off target"). Because the radio is intact, correcting the situation is a matter of making a small tuning adjustment. Because an individual's cognitive faculties are intact, the individual can also make adjustments in his or her appraisals.

When conducting these types of cognitive "scans," it is important to ask the following questions: *What form do the typical cognitive distortions take? Are the key words in the individual's thoughts a clue to his distortions? What do people do once they identify such cues?* Following the work of Beck, we first introduce group members to some of the more common cognitive distortions. We provide them with a typical "book definition" of each distortion along with a tangible example of how this sort of thinking might take form in real-life situations. Next we encourage group members to contribute their own, most commonly encountered distortions and, if possible, the most recent situation in which they were aware of its occurrence and consequences.

After all members appear to have a grasp of these distortions, we have them begin a continuing weekly assignment in which they record stressful or emotionally uncomfortable events occurring in their daily experiences. For each event we ask them to note the type of emotion that they were experiencing and have them rate its severity along a 1–100 point scale. They also record the automatic thought they felt preceded the emotional experience and rate their degree of belief in that thought (0–100%). Finally, members are asked to note the physical and social symptoms that accompanied this experience so they can become more attuned to these as warning signals in future situations. To facilitate their adherence to this exercise we furnish all group members with thought-monitoring sheets similar to those developed by Beck and Emery (1979) and ask them to record at least one automatic thought each day. After members have become adept at identifying these distortions we teach them ways to constructively alter these thoughts—a technique called rational thought replacement. Excellent, easy-to-use strategies for replacing dysfunctional cognitive appraisals can be found in the work of Beck and Emery (1979) or Burns (1981).

Assertiveness Training

Assertiveness training and anger management are introduced late in the program in two separate modules and follow closely the group's discussion of such relevant interpersonal issues as sexually transmitted disease and safer sex techniques. The rationale we use for including assertion training in our CBSM package is as follows: If an individual cannot communicate his emotional reactions and behavioral intentions to others (including fellow workers, family members, friends, and romantic partners), interpersonal conflict is likely to occur and continue to persist. Because such conflict can create an acute (e.g., hostile reactions) or a chronic (e.g., resentment) burden, emotional, physical, and social symptoms of stress responses may occur. By responding assertively in such situations, these conflicts and their accompanying symptoms may be minimized substantially.

For the informational portion of the first assertion module we introduce members to three styles of communicating: nonassertive (or passive), aggressive, and, finally, assertive. We begin by defining passive behavior as activities that set up individuals to have other people make their choices. This is problematic because it fosters dependency and low self-efficacy and often results in hurt, anxiety, and resentment when others are given the power to make the individual's choices and yet are perceived as not choosing wisely. We point out that although we all know the difference between passivity and aggressiveness, it is common for people to confuse the terms "assertive" and "aggressive." Thus, an important part of training is to delineate the subtle differences between these modes. We remind people that aggressive (hostile, invasive) behavior commonly leads to others feeling put down and turned off. Because the other person's rights are denied, he or she feels hurt and offended and is likely to react aggressively toward the offender or to abandon him or her. This form of communication can be classified as closed, negotiation usually ceases, and both parties often end up feeling tense and isolated—an unpleasant and unhealthy combination. On the other hand, assertiveness involves an exercise of personal rights (e.g., to state one's opinion or feelings) simultaneously with a respect for the rights of others (e.g., hearing them out). In assertive exchanges, the communication channels are left open, messages have less of a chance of getting blocked or distorted, and the communicators remain more relaxed, even during the discussion of burdensome topics. Because stressful topics are dealt with efficiently, the opportunity exists for resolution and mastery at the earliest point in time, and there is less net strain on the relationship and on each person.

Assertion and anger management techniques are demonstrated in relation to several life situations (e.g., talking with a member's physician about a diagnosis, claiming legal rights in the workplace, and negotiating safer sex with a prospective partner). The primary goals of this experience are to help individuals learn basic communication skills, to enhance their awareness of their "interpersonal rights," and to encourage them to express their opinions and feelings to others without undue delay, avoidance, and denial. We also teach people to become more aware of the different emotional, physical, and social sequelae of each form of communication. As in the earlier modules, we stress the importance of using emotional and bodily cues of discomfort as an early warning signal that participants are in the midst of a situation that may require a shift in their appraisals and coping strategy. As such, this training comprises that part of the program that teaches skills for managing interpersonal burdens, difficulties, and challenges.

Social Support

Once subjects learn to handle interpersonal conflict more efficiently, they might find that they value frequent exchanges and crave more fulfilling social relationships. Social support enrichment is provided in several aspects of our CBSM program. The group format may increase perceptions of communality and decrease a sense of social isolation, and regular participation in role-playing exercises among group members further facilitates a cohesiveness among the men. Also, in the initial session group members are paired in a "buddy system," which remains intact throughout the 10-week program, although all members are encouraged to interact with one another and group leaders during the role-play exercises. An entire didactic session is dedicated to presenting the different "shades" of social support that some people are often unaware of as resources in their environments. For example, this module delineates various sources of social support—those who provide more or less guidance through murky times (instrumental or informational support) versus those who offer nurturance and positive regard on a regular basis (emotional support). Social support is not a single concept. It can be seen as a coping resource that is housed in many different domains, some of which facilitate one form of coping or another. For instance, financial or physical support might fuel such active coping attempts as problem solving, whereas positive regard or emotional support may help an individual to accept, vent feelings about, or cognitively reframe a difficult and inevitable situation.

Group members participate by "mapping out" the qualitative aspects of their own social support networks based on a social support utilization questionnaire (Barrera 1981). Some of these questions refer to receiving a loan from a friend, some to getting useful information when in a pinch, and even just getting cheered up by somebody when feeling down. After presenting their "maps" to the group, group members discuss strengths and weaknesses of various social support channels. We also encourage group-generated strategies for enhancing support systems. These strategies often represent a synthesis of cognitive restructuring and assertion techniques learned in the previous weeks.

Finally, we provide group members with information on the whereabouts of several formalized support organizations in the community. The focus on the value of human relationships that occur within the context of a supportive social environment sets the stage for the men's final task, the dismantling of the group. Each member is given the opportunity to share with the group what he has taken from the 10-week experience and where he plans to go next. After we make the final "rounds," we plan a party.

CONCLUSION

Our research suggests that behavioral interventions such as CBSM may reduce distress and depression (and normalize immunological status) for HIV-positive men during the stressful period immediately following notification of HIV-positive antibody status and during the adjustment period following this news. We have also identified psychosocial factors that may predict disease progression. Results suggest that these effects may be mediated by increases in social support perceptions and utilization, increased use of active coping strategies (e.g., relaxation exercises, active coping, and planning), and decreased use of denial/avoidance coping strategies.

It is critical to learn at this point whether this time-limited intervention and the implementation of a regular group maintenance program can help people adjust to the chronic burden of symptomatic HIV infection. We are also exploring the effects of CBSM with other groups of people who are dealing with long-term burdens related to immune system dysregulation and such virological factors as chronic fatigue syndrome. Behavioral modulation of psychological and immunological status may have health implications for these individuals as well as other clinical populations including those diagnosed with certain virus-associated cancers that are more prevalent in immunocompromised populations (e.g., cervical carcinoma) (Antoni & Goodkin, 1992). All these intervention strategies rest on the assumption that adjustment to these extremely demanding and chronic human conditions requires that people develop new coping strategies and resources to facilitate the preservation of both mental and physical health. Stress management, as conceptualized here, may offer the opportunity for such growth.

ACKNOWLEDGMENT

This work was supported by NIMH Grant Nos. P50MH4355, P01MH49548, and T32MH18917.

REFERENCES

Ader, R., Cohen, N., & Felten, D. (1991). *Psychoneuroimmunology* (2nd ed.). New York: Academic Press.

American Psychiatric Association. (1987). *Diagnostic and statistical manual of mental disorders* (3rd ed., rev.). Washington, DC: Author.

Antoni, M. H. (1991). Psychosocial stressors and behavioral interventions in gay men with HIV infection. *International Review of Psychiatry, 3*, 383–399.

Antoni, M. H. (1992, April). *Cognitive-behavioral stress management and coping responses to HIV+ notification: Mental and physical health implications.* Paper presented at the Society of Behavioral Medicine, Washington, DC.

Antoni, M. H., Schneiderman, N., & Ironson, G. (in press). *Stress management for HIV infection* [Society of Behavioral Medicine Clinical Research Guidebook Series]. Hillsdale, NJ: Erlbaum.

Antoni, M. H., Baggett, L., LaPerriere, A., August, S., Ironson, G., Klimas, N., Schneiderman, N., & Fletcher, M. A. (1991). Cognitive behavioral stress management intervention buffers distress responses and elevates immunologic markers following notification of HIV-1 seropositivity. *Journal of Consulting and Clinical Psychology, 59*(6), 906–915.

Antoni, M. H., Esterling, B., Lutgendorf, S., Fletcher, M. A., & Schneiderman, N. (1995). Psychosocial influences in herpesvirus reactivation in HIV-1 infection. In A. Baum & M. Stein (Eds.), *Perspectives in behavioral medicine: AIDS, aging and Alzheimer's disease*. Hillsdale, NJ: Erlbaum.

Antoni, M. H., & Goodkin, K. (1992). The interaction of viral and psychosocial factors in the promotion of cervical neoplasia. In J. ten-Have de Llabije & H. Balner (Eds.), *Coping with cancer and beyond*. Amsterdam: Swets & Zeitleiner.

Antoni, M. H., Goodkin, K., Goldstein, D., LaPerriere, A., Ironson, G., Schneiderman, N., & Fletcher, M. A. (1991). Coping responses to HIV-1 serostatus notification predict short-term affective distress and one-year follow-up immunologic status in HIV-1 seronegative and seropositive gay men [Abstract]. *Psychosomatic Medicine, 53*, 227.

Antoni, M. H., Schneiderman, N., Fletcher, M. A., Goldstein, D., Ironson, G., & LaPerriere, A. (1990). Psychoneuroimmunology and HIV-1. *Journal of Consulting and Clinical Psychology, 58*, 38–49.

Antoni, M. H., Lutgendorf, S., Ironson, G., Fletcher, M. A., & Schneiderman, N. (1996). CBSM intervention effects on social support, coping, depression and immune function in symptomatic HIV-infected men. [Abstract]. *Psychosomatic Medicine, 58*, 86.

Barrera, M. (1981). Social support in the adjustment of pregnant adolescents: Assessment issues. In B. H. Gottlieb (Ed.), *Social networks and social support* (pp. 69–96). Beverly Hills, CA: Sage.

Beck, A., & Emery, G. (1979). *Cognitive therapy of anxiety and phobic disorders*. Philadelphia: Center for Cognitive Therapy.

Bernstein, D., & Borkovec, T. (1973). *Progressive relaxation training: A manual for the helping professions*. Champaign, IL: Research Press.

Borysenko, M., & Borysenko, J. (1982). Stress, behavior, and immunity: Animal models and mediating mechanisms. *General Hospital Psychiatry, 4*, 56–67.

Burns, D. (1981). *Feeling good: The new mood therapy*. New York: New American Library.

Calabrese, J., Skwerer, R., & Barna, B. (1986). Depression, immunocompetence, and prostaglandins of the E series. *Psychiatric Research, 17*, 41–47.

Carver, C. S., Scheier, M., & Weintraub, J. K. (1989). Assessing coping strategies: A theoretically based approach. *Journal of Personality and Social Psychology, 56*, 267–283.

Cutrona, C., & Russell, D. (1987). The provisions of social relationships and adaptation to stress. In W. H. Jones & D. Perlman (Eds.), *Advances in personal relationships* (Vol. 1, pp. 37–67). Greenwich, CT: JAI Press.

DeMartini, R. M., Turner, R. R., Formenti, S. C., Boone, D. C., Bishop, P. C., Levine, A. M., & Parker, J. W. (1988). Peripheral blood mononuclear cell abnormalities and their relationships to clinical course in homosexual men with HIV infection. *Clinical Immunology and Immunopathology, 30*, 258–271.

Esterling, B. A., Antoni, M. H., Schneiderman, N., Carver, C. S., LaPerriere, A., Ironson, G., Klimas, N., & Fletcher, M. A. (1992). Psychosocial modulation of antibody to Epstein–Barr viral capsid antigen and human herpesvirus type-6 in HIV-1-infected and at-risk gay men. *Psychosomatic Medicine, 54*, 354–371.

Fawzy, F. I., Cousins, N., Fawzy, N., Kemeny, M. E., Elashoff, R., & Morton, D.

(1990). A structured psychiatric intervention for cancer patients. I. Changes over time in methods of coping and affective disturbance. *Archives of General Psychiatry, 47,* 720–725.

Folkman, S., Chesney, M., McKusick, L., Ironson, G., Johnson, D., & Coates, T. (1991). Translating coping theory into intervention. In J. Eckenrode (Ed.), *The social context of stress.* New York: Plenum Press.

Folkman, S., & Lazarus, R. S. (1980). An analysis of coping in a middle-aged community sample. *Journal of Health and Social Behavior, 21,* 219–230.

Glaser, R., & Kiecolt-Glaser, J. (1987). Stress-associated depression in cellular immunity: Implications for acquired immune deficiency syndrome (AIDS). *Brain, Behavior and Immunity, 1,* 107–112.

Glaser, R., Rice, J., Sheridan, J., Fertel, R., Stout, J., Speicher, C., Pinsky, D., Kotur, M., Post, A., Beck, M., & Kiecolt-Glaser, J. (1987). Stress-related immune suppression: Health implications. *Brain, Behavior, and Immunity, 1,* 7–20.

Greer, S., Morris, T., & Pettingale, K. W. (1971). Psychological response to breast cancer: Effect on outcome. *Lancet, 2,* 785–787.

Hoffman, M. A. (1991). Counseling the seropositive client: A psychosocial model for assessment and intervention. *Counseling Psychologist, 19,* 467–542.

Ironson, G., Antoni, M. H., Simoneau, J., LaPerriere, A., Baggett, H. L., August, S., Arevalo, F., Schneiderman, N., & Fletcher, M. A. (1992). *Distress, denial, and low compliance predict disease progression in HIV seropositive gay men.* Paper presented at the third annual Perspectives in Psychoneuroimmunology meeting, Columbus, OH.

Ironson, G., Friedman, A., Klimas, N., Antoni, M. H., Fletcher, M. A., Simoneau, J., LaPerriere, A., & Schneiderman, N. (1994). Distress, denial, and low adherence to behavioral interventions predict faster disease progression in HIV-1 infected gay men. *International Journal Behavioral Medicine, 1,* 90–105.

Irwin, M., Daniels, M., Bloom, E., Smith, T., & Weiner, H. (1987). Life events, depressive symptoms, and immune function. *American Journal of Psychiatry, 144,* 437–441.

Irwin, M., Daniels, M., Smith, T., Bloom, E., & Weiner, H. (1987). Impaired natural killer cell activity during bereavement. *Brain, Behavior, and Immunity, 1,* 98–104.

Justice, B. (1988). Stress, coping, and health outcomes. In M. L. Russell (Ed.), *Stress management for chronic disease* (pp. 14–29). New York: Pergamon Press.

Kelly, J. A., St. Lawrence, J. S., Hood, H. V., & Brasfield, J. (1989). Behavioral interventions to reduce AIDS risk activities. *Journal of Consulting and Clinical Psychology, 57*(1), 60–67.

Kiecolt-Glaser, J., Glaser, R., Strain, E., Stout, J., Tarr, K., Holliday, J., & Speicher, C. (1986). Modulation of cellular immunity in medical students. *Journal of Behavioral Medicine, 6,* 5–21.

Kiecolt-Glaser, J. K., Glaser, R., Williger, D., Stout, J., Messick, G., & Sheppard, S. (1985). Psychosocial enhancement of immunocompetence in a geriatric population. *Health Psychology, 4,* 25–41.

Lutgendorf, S., Antoni, M. H., Ironson, G., Klimas, N., Kumar, M., Starr, K., Schneiderman, N., McCabe, P., Cleven, K., & Fletcher, M. A. (in press). Cognitive behavioral stress management decreases dysphoric mood and herpes simplex virus-type 2 antibody titers in symptomatic HIV-seropositive gay men. *Journal of Consulting and Clinical Psychology*.

Lutgendorf, S., Antoni, M. H., Ironson, G., Klimas, N., Starr, K., Schneiderman, N., & Fletcher, M. A. (1996, March). *Coping and social support predict distress changes in symptomatic HIV-seropositive gay men following a cognitive behavioral stress management intervention.* Paper presented at the Society of Behavioral Medicine, Washington, DC.

Martin, J. (1988). Psychological consequences of AIDS-related bereavement among gay men. *Journal of Consulting and Clinical Psychology, 56,* 856–862.

McNair, D., Lorr, M., & Droppleman, L. (1981). *EITS manual for the Profile of Mood States.* San Diego, CA: Educational and Industrial Testing Service.

Namir, S., Wolcott, D. L., Fawzy, F. I., & Alumbaugh, M. J. (1987). Coping with AIDS: Psychological and health implications. [Special Issue: Acquired Immune Deficiency Syndrome]. *Journal of Applied Social Psychology, 17,* 309–328.

Rinaldo, C. R., DeBiasio, R., Hamoudi, W., Rabin, B., & Liebert, M. (1986). Effect of herpesvirus infections on T lymphocyte subpopulations and blastogenic responses in renal transplant recipients receiving cyclosporine. *Clinical Immunology and Immunopathology, 38,* 357–366.

Rodin, J. (1988, April). *Aging, control, and health.* Paper presented at the ninth annual scientific meeting of the Society of Behavioral Medicine, Boston.

Rosenberg, Z. F., & Fauci, A. S. (1991). Activation of latent HIV infection. *Journal of the National Institutes of Health Research, 2,* 41–45.

Sarason, I., Johnson, J., & Siegel, J. (1978). Assessing the impact of life changes: Development of the Life Experiences Survey. *Journal of Consulting and Clinical Psychology, 46,* 932–946.

Shavit, Y., & Martin, F. (1987). Opiates, stress, and immunity: Animal studies. *Annals of Behavioral Medicine, 9*(2), 11–15.

Stein, M., Miller, A. H., & Trestman, R. L. (1991). Depression, the immune system and health illness. *Archives of General Psychiatry, 48,* 171–177.

Yalom, I., & Greaves, C. (1977). Group therapy with the terminally ill. *American Journal of Psychiatry, 134,* 396–400.

Zuckerman, M., & Antoni, M. H. (1995). Social support and its relationship to psychological, physical, and immune variables in HIV infection. *Clinical Psychology and Psychotherapy, 2*(4), 210–219.

CHAPTER 3

Reducing Coronary Recurrences and Coronary-Prone Behavior: A Structured Group Treatment Approach

CARL E. THORESEN
PAUL BRACKE

In the worry and strain of modern life, arterial degeneration is not only very common but develops often at a relatively early age. For this I believe that the high pressure at which men live and the habit of working the machine to its maximum capacity are responsible rather than excesses in eating and drinking.

—*Sir William Osler* (*1987, p. 157*)

In this chapter, we discuss the Type A behavior pattern and its role in coronary heart disease (CHD), particularly in reducing recurrences in coronary patients. After an introduction to Type A behavior pattern, we comment briefly on research in Type A behavior, focusing primarily on some earlier descriptive and laboratory studies. We describe results of a controlled 4½-year intervention study and a subsequent follow-up study with more than 1,012 postmyocardial infarction patients (Recurrent Coronary Prevention Project) conducted in the late 1970s and early 1980s. After briefly citing some of the current controversies surrounding Type A behavior, in the final section we describe the clinical side of the treatment story, one seldom presented in journal articles. Throughout we also direct readers to reference materials for those interested in pursuing topics more fully.

Despite substantial advances in controlled research as well as clinical practice over the past three decades, diseases of the cardiovascular system remain the leading cause of death in the United States and other Western industrial cultures (American Heart Association, 1995). Age-specific mortality rates from cardiovascular disease, especially CHD for those less than 70 years old, have declined about 35% since the late 1960s, but the total proportion of death due to CHD has not changed significantly (Sutherland, Pershy, & Brody, 1990). Thus, fewer people younger than 70 currently die from CHD, succumbing later in life. Interestingly, in the United States, malignant neoplasms have for the first time surpassed CHD as the leading cause of death in men and women between the ages of 45 and 64. Still, CHD remains the leading overall cause of mortality in men and women, resulting in six times more death from CHD than from cancer. Further, women who suffer a myocardial infarction (MI) have twice the mortality rate compared to men (Mattsen & Herd, 1988).

THE BIOPSYCHOSOCIAL PICTURE IN CHD

Although increasingly understood, the etiology of CHD still remains unclear. In prospective (i.e., longitudinal) studies, established risk factors for CHD, including age, hypertension, diabetes, cigarette smoking, and elevated serum cholesterol, have predicted CHD but not in ways that explain the *majority* of the new cases of CHD (Jenkins, 1971; National Center for Health Statistics, 1989). The failure of standard risk factors to explain most new cases may be a result of several factors. Among these are differences in risk because of gender, geographic regions, and ethnicity as well as population density of urbanization along with level of industrialization (Rosenman, Swan, & Carmelli, 1988). That is, the relationship of standard risk factors (e.g., serum cholesterol level) and CHD may be mediated by an individual's living situation at home, at work, and in the local community.

Given the continuing failure of risk factors to explain most cases, the possible role of personality, along with behavior and social–cognitive factors, reemerged in the 1960s and remains a lively if not contentious topic (Henry & Stephens, 1977; Friedman & Ulmer, 1984). Recognition of causal relationships between human behavior, cognition, and physiology (i.e., psyche and soma) can of course be traced back to Hippocratic medicine 2,500 years ago in ancient Greece as well as in early Chinese culture.

Plato, in his *Dialogues*, cites Hippocrates as advocating cure by "treating the body as well as the soul." In the 1890s, Sir William Osler, considered by many the father of internal medicine, forcefully advanced the view that direct links existed between a person's lifestyle and atherosclerosis. He admonished medical students to treat the person with the disease, not the disease in the person. However, these clinical observations and those of others (e.g., Menninger & Menninger, 1936) went largely unheeded. It was not until the latter half of this century that researchers in CHD discovered crucial links between psyche and soma. These links launched two new fields: health psychology and behavioral medicine.

THE EARLY TYPE A STORY

In the late 1950s Meyer Friedman and Ray Rosenman proposed what they called a "specific action–emotion complex" based on extensive clinical observations in young and middle-age male coronary patients. A chronic struggle to accomplish often vague goals or acquire more and more material symbols of success seemed to dominate these patients. They appeared not to be the neurotic, anxious persons who commonly presented themselves for psychotherapy but, instead, were observed to be nonpsychologically minded extroverts whose style was often to take immediate action and not give much reflection to their problems. These persons were called Type A and were contrasted with those labeled Type B, defined as a relative lack of Type A characteristics. Rosenman et al. (1988) summarized Type A characteristics as follows:

1. Intense, sustained drive to achieve self-selected but often poorly defined goals.
2. Profound eagerness to compete and need to "win."
3. Persistent desire for recognition and advancement.
4. Continuous involvement in multiple and diverse activities under time restraints.
5. Habitual tendency to increase the rate of doing most physical and mental activities.
6. Extreme mental and physical alertness.
7. Pervasive aggressive and hostile feelings.

Rosenman et al. (1988) viewed this pattern in terms of a combination of *behavioral dispositions* (e.g., aggressiveness), *specific behaviors* (e.g., rapid and emphatic speech), and *emotional responses* (e.g., anger). Since then, other researchers (e.g., Price, 1982; Strube, 1990) have emphasized specific *cognitive processes*, including self-evaluative factors and underlying beliefs to this combination (e.g., "I must constantly prove my worth to others").

A series of studies was conducted in the late 1950s and throughout the 1960s (e.g., Friedman & Rosenman, 1959; Friedman, St. George, Byers, & Rosenman, 1960; Rosenman & Friedman, 1961). These studies established the fact that men and women classified as Type A evidenced higher levels of total serum cholesterol in the absence of any changes in diet, faster blood clotting, greater "sludging" of red blood cells after ingesting high-fat meals, and, more important, over five times more signs and symptoms of clinical heart disease than found in non-Type A persons.

Studies also demonstrated that Type A men had higher levels of norepinephrine and ACTH (adrenocorticotropic hormone) than non-Type A men. Animal studies were also conducted, demonstrating, for example, that surgical removal of part of the rat's hypothalamus prevented the animal's physiology from controlling its emotions. This emotional disruption combined with a high-fat diet caused dramatic and continuing rises in the rat's serum cholesterol compared to rats eating a high-fat diet only. Rats only on the high-fat diet showed an increase in serum cholesterol that quickly plateaued but did not continue to rise. Thus, diet plus chronic emotional disruption seemed responsible for increased levels of serum cholesterol. (For a fuller description of these studies, see Friedman & Ulmer, 1984.)

The most significant early study—the Western Collaborative Group Study (WCGS)—involved more than 3,500 healthy men between 39 and 59 followed over 8½ years (Rosenman, Brand, Sholtz, & Friedman, 1976). This prospectively designed study demonstrated that men classified as Type A by a structured interview were twice as likely to develop clinical CHD than men assessed as non-Type A. Importantly, differences found in the WCGS in CHD were not explained by differences in serum cholesterol level, blood pressure, smoking, diabetes, and other CHD risk factors. That is, Type A behavior was shown in multivariate analysis to be a significant independent risk factor for CHD. Other behaviorally mediated factors, such as higher levels of serum cholesterol and smoking, were also found to be significant independent risk factors in the WCGS. (More recently Ragland & Brand, 1988a, found that Type A behavior assessed at baseline in the WCGS failed to predict CHD over 20 years.)

Although many cross-sectional studies have often found Type A behavior to be significantly related to CHD markers (Booth-Kewley & Friedman, 1987), results from prospectively designed or longitudinal studies conducted over several years can provide more convincing evidence of a possible Type A/CHD connection. Thoresen and Powell (1992) recently concluded in reviewing the evidence that Type A behavior does significantly predict CHD in population-based studies (i.e., large, reasonably heterogeneous samples) for noncoronary white males but only when Type A behavior has been assessed by structured interview and not by brief written self-report measures of Type A behavior (see Booth-Kewley & Friedman, 1987; Matthews & Haynes, 1988; Booth-Kewley & Friedman, 1987; Miller, Turner, Tindale, Posavac, & Dugoni, 1991). However, when more homogeneous samples of males have been studied, such as postcoronary patients or those with advanced coronary artery disease, Type A behavior when assessed globally (i.e., a person rated as either Type A or Type B) has consistently not predicted

CHD when mortally is used as the outcome. There are many possible reasons for this failure to predict:

- Type A assessed as a dichotomous, "trait-like" construct is too insensitive to discriminate risk of cardiac death because there is too much variability *among* post-MI persons labeled Type A.
- Cardiac death can result from too many different physical, social, behavioral, and environmental factors for Type A to be a significant independent predictor.
- Measures of Type A may "deteriorate" in their validity and reliability over many years because people may change their degree of Type A, such as their degree of hostile thoughts and actions; all negative Type A/CHD studies reported to date have only assessed Type A on one occasion.
- Only cardiac death has been used as the coronary end point in studies failing to show a Type A relationship, not degree of disease, progression of coronary pathology (e.g., changes in coronary artery occlusion), or nonfatal recurring myocardial infarction.

The predictive power of Type A behavior gains considerably, however, when the hostility component of Type A behavior serves as the predictor rather than the global dichotomous rating of Type A. For example, Dembroski, MacDougall, Costa, & Grauditz (1989) demonstrated in a large prospective study (Multiple Risk Factor Intervention Trial) that hostility rated from the structured interview predicted CHD mortality in multivariate analyses while global Type A behavior in that study failed to predict. Others have also demonstrated that hostility predicted CHD when rated from the Type A structured interview (e.g., Hecker, Chesney, Black, & Frautschi, 1988). (See Barefoot, 1992, for an excellent discussion of the role of hostility in empirical studies.)

In all, many correlational and descriptive studies have created a portrait of CHD risk for white adult Type A males and, in a few studies, white adult Type A females (Booth-Kewley & Friedman, 1987; Burell, 1996). Type A behavior seemed associated with CHD as well as factors that increase the risk of CHD (e.g., smoking). However, evidence showing that Type A behavior was causally related to CHD was essentially lacking (see Rahe, Ward, & Hayes, 1979, for an example of an early intervention). If it could be shown that reductions in Type A behavior were directly linked to reductions in CHD factors within a controlled, experimentally designed study, support of Type A behavior as a possible causal factor in CHD would be strengthened.

THE RECURRENT CORONARY PREVENTION PROJECT

In 1972, planning started on an experimentally designed intervention study. The goals were to demonstrate that Type A behavior could be reduced and, in doing so, would reduce CHD. To accomplish this, 928 adult male and 84 adult female post-MI volunteers were recruited for a 5-year study.

Prior to treatment, all participants (n = 1,012) received a complete physical examination, including a resting 12-lead electrocardiogram (ECG), as well as the Videotaped Structured Interview (VSI) to assess Type A behavior. In addition, they completed several self-report scales, including an extensive questionnaire on Type A behavior and measures on anger, social support, work satisfaction, and self-efficacy measures about ability to relax, to slow one's rate of eating, talking and walking and other factors. Participants' average age was 53.2 years.

Participants were randomly assigned to the two treatment conditions (Type A/cardiac counseling, n = 592, or cardiac counseling, n = 270) on a two-to-one basis because a higher dropout rate was expected for the more demanding Type A treatment. Differences on 20 variables were evaluated, such as sociodemographic factors (e.g., age and marital status), CHD risk factors (e.g., degree of myocardial pathology), other CHD treatments (e.g., use of beta blockers), and CHD clinical symptoms (e.g., complex arrhythmia). None differed significantly between the two treatment groups at the beginning of the Recurrent Coronary Prevention Project (RCPP).

Cardiac recurrence was defined as a nonfatal MI or cardiac death verified by physician report, hospital records, and examination of death certificates. Nonfatal MI was defined at the time of the event as the appearance of new or abnormal Q-waves (ECG), elevation of MB isoenzyme fraction > 5% of total serum creatine kinase concentration, or both.

A total of 60 Type A treatment groups (with about 10 participants per group) met over 4½ years compared to 22 groups (about 12 per group) in the cardiac counseling condition. Mean attendance at all sessions over the 4½ years averaged almost 67% (two-thirds of all sessions). In the Type A treatment, 28 sessions of 90 minutes each were held in the first year with monthly sessions for the remaining 3½ years. A total of 62 sessions were offered.

The cardiac counseling treatment monthly sessions (a total of 33) were held over the 4½ years with a focus on discussing adherence to medication, pathophysiology of CHD, efficacy of surgical and medication treatments (e.g., bypass and beta blockers), and the role of diet and nutrition in preventing recurrences. No mention was made of chronic stress or Type A behavior, nor were specific skills taught. Attendance and dropout rates over the 4½ years did not differ significantly for the two treatments.

Major Results of RCPP

The "intention to treat" principle was used to analyze data (Peto et al., 1976). This highly conservative procedure requires all participants, once randomized to a treatment, to be counted as having received the entire treatment. Thus, even dropouts who never attended sessions or attended very few are considered as having been fully treated. In this way, any significant differences found between treatment groups provides a highly conservative estimate of relative treatment effects.

By the third year the cumulative total coronary recurrence rate (fatal and nonfatal events) was 7.2% for the Type A counseling compared to 13% in the cardiac counseling treatment ($p < .005$) (Friedman et al., 1986). The 44% difference was due primarily to fewer nonfatal events; significant differences between treatments were not found, however, for fatal recurrences.

Reductions in Type A behavior were also found to favor the Type A intervention. For example, of participants who remained active in both treatment groups, 31.7% in the Type A intervention had *markedly* reduced their Type A behavior (>1 *SD* on two separate measures) compared to only 7.2% in the cardiac counseling treatment. Furthermore, participants in both treatments who markedly reduced their Type A behavior had a total coronary recurrence rate of only 1.7% compared to 8.6% for those who showed fewer or no reductions in Type A behavior. Further, those who remained in the Type A intervention reduced their Type A behavior significantly more than those who dropped out in the first year.

At the end of treatment (4½ years), the recurrence picture was essentially the same. Figure 3.1 displays the cumulative annualized total recurrence rate for both treatments over the 4½-year course of treatment.

These reductions in coronary events paralleled reductions in Type A behavior as assessed by the VSI (see Figure 3.2). In addition, Type A rating scales for the participants were also completed by participants (self-rating) as well as by spouses and work colleagues. All yielded similar results (Friedman et al., 1986).

Bypass and Beta-Blocker Effects

One of the most surprising findings concerned participants who entered the RCPP having already undergone coronary artery bypass surgery ($n = 247$). Of those randomly assigned to the cardiac counseling treatment, 30.3% experienced coronary recurrences over the 4½ years, yet only 14% of those with bypass in the Type A treatment suffered recurrences ($p < .05$). A similar pattern was found for participants already using beta-blocker medication (propranolol). The difference in recurrence was similar: 27.4% in cardiac counseling versus 15% in Type A counseling ($p < .05$).

These findings have major implications for the rehabilitation of post-

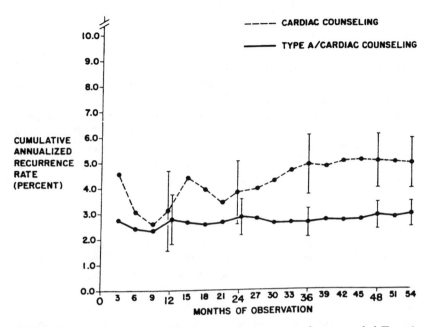

FIGURE 3.1. Cumulative annualized recurrence rate in cardiac-counseled Type A and cardiac-counseled participants calculated quarterly for 4½ years. Note that 95% confidence limits of quarterly calculated cardiac recurrence rates no longer intersect at end of 36 months. Adapted from Friedman et al. (1986). Copyright 1986 by the *American Heart Journal*. Adapted by permission.

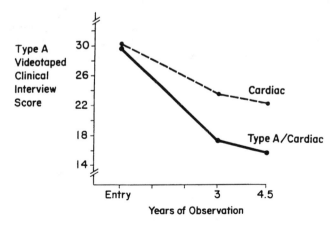

FIGURE 3.2. Reductions in observed Type A behavior at 3 years and at end of treatment (4½). Within-group and between-group changes were significant at 3 years (*p* < .001). Adapted from Friedman et al. (1986). Copyright 1986 by the *American Heart Journal*. Adapted by permission.

coronary patients. Burnell (1996) has also reported significant reductions in coronary bypass patients using a comparable but much shorter structured group treatment with 17 3-hour sessions. Clearly, a psychosocial group-oriented treatment, such as Type A modification coupled with pharmacological or surgical interventions, may offer a more powerful intervention than medications and/or surgery alone. Equally clear are the cost-effective and cost benefit implications of behavioral compared to pharmacological and surgical interventions. For example, coronary artery bypass graft (CABG) surgery may prove to be significantly more cost-effective if it is complemented with a behavioral intervention focused on altering lifestyle patterns (Thoresen & Powell, 1983; Linden, Stossel & Maurice, in press).

Changes in Other Psychosocial Factors

In a recent examination of other psychosocial changes over the 4½ years, Mendes de Leon, Powell, and Kaplan (1991) found that participants in the Type A treatment demonstrated reductions not only in Type A behavior but also in the components of Type A: hostility, time urgency, and impatience. In addition, significant improvements in self-efficacy ratings were found favoring the Type A treatment. Participants reported greater confidence, for example, in their ability to physically relax, to do one thing at a time, and to instruct themselves to act calm and relaxed in stressful situations ($p < .001$). Comparable improvements in perceived well-being, anger, depression, social support, and social contacts were also found favoring the Type A treatment.

Lower Pathological Risk and Cardiac Death

The Type A treatment failed to produce a significantly lower cardiac mortality compared to the other treatment. However, when the *degree* of coronary pathology was considered (i.e., severity of damage to myocardium by the prior infarction), those with less pathology (62% of the total RCPP sample) who received the Type A treatment had lower cardiac mortality ($p < .05$) than those in the cardiac counseling treatment (Powell & Thoresen, 1988). These results seem to parallel those of Spiegel, Bloom, Kraemer, and Gotthert (1989) for women with metastasized breast cancer. Those who survived longer after 12 monthly group sessions had less advanced cancer pathology.

Emotional Arousability

Another intriguing finding concerns a type of coronary mortality: sudden cardiac death (SCD). The issue of SCD has long been associated with intense emotional turmoil, especially for those with coronary disease. SCD appears to be an electrical accident, triggered by changes in the neocortex and affecting the heart's ability to control the rhythm of contractions (e.g., left ventricle contractions) (Lown & Wolf, 1971).

In the RCPP, an index of emotional arousability was developed from rescoring the VSI for observable behavioral factors in hopes of finding a more sensitive psychosocial indicator of cardiac risk. This arousal measure was found to predict SCD, whereas total TA scores from the VSI were not predictive. The relative risk ratio (RR) of emotional arousability was found to be 1.5 ($p < 0.2$), or 50% higher for participants showing higher emotional arousability in the initial structured interview compared to those lower on arousability (Powell, Simon, Bartzokis, Pattillo, & Thoresen, 1992). This RR was still significant in multivariate analyses when congestive heart failure, number of prior infarctions, use of antiarrhythmic drugs, smoking, and family history of CHD were controlled for in the statistical analyses. Interestingly, men with high arousability *and* higher serum cholesterol levels (> 250 mg) were almost three times more likely to suffer SCD. High-arousability participants who consumed high levels of alcohol ("several drinks a day") also had an RR of 3.81 ($p = .02$) for SCD.

These data represent post hoc findings. Most were not predicted in advance nor expected, and, as such, need to be viewed with caution. Still they offer exciting findings and deserve further study. The Type A treatment program seemed to influence a variety of psychosocial factors. Reduced coronary recurrences also appeared linked to changes in not only Type A behavior but other stress-related factors. Given these findings, the Type A treatment program could be viewed as a generalized stress/distress reduction program that lowers cardiac morbidity and mortality among certain persons and possibly reduces other disease-related factors. Currently, this possibility is being explored in a large-scale ($n = 3,000$) 10-year intervention project for healthy adults (ages 39 to 64) by the Coronary and Cancer Prevention Project at the Meyer Friedman Institute, Mt. Zion Medical Center of the University of California, San Francisco. In addition, Burell et al. (1994) have partially replicated the RCPP results in Sweden.

Follow-Up Results of RCPP

Between 4 and 5 years after the RCPP treatment program ended, a comprehensive evaluation of participants was conducted. More than 500 former participants were reexamined, including a physical examination, videotaped interview, and several self-report measures. Although these data are still being analyzed, some preliminary findings can be reported.

In terms of coronary recurrences, significant differences between the two treatments remained but at a reduced level (40% difference dropped to 29%, $p < .001$). Part of the reduced difference between treatments was due to a 12-month crossover treatment at 4½ years. All participants in the cardiac counseling treatment were invited to take part in a condensed 1-year version of the original 4½-year Type A treatment. More than 90% of those still active participated. During this 1-year treatment, few recurrences occurred, especially no deaths, for the former cardiac counseling participants, a significant reduction for these participants compared to the prior 2 years ($p < .05$).

Participants in the Type A treatment who entered the program with CABG surgery or who used beta blockers continued to show fewer coronary recurrences 4 years after treatment: 51% fewer recurrences for those with bypass and 45% fewer recurrences for those on beta blockers.

Differences between treatments in Type A level were also maintained ($p < .05$), although some relapse was observed for participants in both treatments. The mean Type A level of the cardiac counseling group members as measured by the VSI at 4-year follow-up had regressed significantly so that it no longer differed from their pretreatment level of Type A, despite their 1 year of Type A treatment. For the Type A treatment, however, participants still showed highly significant reductions compared to their pretreatment level ($p < .001$).

Psychosocial Predictors

We recently explored which psychosocial variables most accounted for reductions in coronary events. Specifically, we examined eight psychosocial measures at posttreatment (4½ years) and used these to predict coronary recurrences at 8½ years (Powell, Mendes de Leon, Thoresen, et al., 1993). These psychosocial measures included overall Type A score (VSI), hostility component score (VSI), impatience component score (VSI), self-reported depression, and several self-efficacy measures. Change scores (pretreatment minus posttreatment) were also used to predict recurrences at 8½ years.

Multivariate analyses of change scores were used to predict recurrences 4 years after treatment, adjusting for several major CHD risk factors (e.g., arrhythmia and congestive heart failure). *Only* the overall change in Type A score and the depression self-report score predicted cardiac recurrence (RR = 2.12, $p < .001$; RR = 1.57, $p < .10$, respectively). In addition, *only* the overall Type A score in multivariate analyses significantly predicted mortality from all causes (RR = 2.00; $p < .05$). (See Frasure-Smith, Lesperance, & Talajic, 1993, for influence of depression on post-MI mortality over 6 months.)

These findings may point to possible psychosocial mechanisms that could explain the reduced morbidity and mortality found in the RCPP. Participants in the RCPP who demonstrated reductions in their *overall* Type A behavior as assessed by the VSI had significantly fewer recurrences. However, reduced hostility or impatience components of Type A behavior by themselves failed to predict recurrence. Perhaps hostility, taken out of context, may not be the sole pathogenic component of the Type A behavior as believed by some investigators (see Barefoot et al., 1994; Thoresen & Powell, 1992). Alternatively, the component score of hostility used in this study may not be sensitive enough to discriminate those at greater risk. Further, changes in perceived social support, size of social network, and self-efficacy ratings (e.g., more confidence that I can relax) also failed to predict recurrences in the multivariate analyses. Again, the issue may relate to less than optimal assessment methods used in this study.

Although a clear-cut picture does not emerge from these findings, they provide a glimpse of what may facilitate reduced recurrences. Namely, to have an impact on pathophysiological factors responsible for recurrences, intervention programs may need to influence overall lifestyle rather than attempting to modify isolated components, such as hostility. This broader portrait conveys a life of reduced competitiveness, time urgency, hostile beliefs, and felt anger. Such reductions may complement an increased sense of inner peace, a greater acceptance of life's inevitable disappointments, a calmer and reflective outlook, and more emphasis on intimate social relationships and on clarifying personal and spiritual values. Perhaps overall Type A behavior proved to be predictive of reduced cardiac recurrences because it better captured changes in overall lifestyle compared to more specific measures.

Women in RCPP

What of the small number (n = 83) of female participants in the RCPP? Some data are available (Powell, Slaker, et al., 1993) suggesting the following: (1) overall Type A behavior and its components measured by VSI failed to predict cardiac recurrences; (2) being divorced and working without a college degree predicted cardiac mortality (e.g., RR = 6.9, p = .003 for being divorced); and (3) suffering arrhythmias on resting ECG at pretreatment dramatically increased risk of cardiac death (RR = 7.83, p = .003). In multivariate analyses, the level of emotional arousability, unlike males, actually reduced rather than increased risk of recurrences. Note that the small number of women involved seriously limits the generalizability of these results. Still, these results deserve careful consideration given the paucity of data on treating postinfarct women.

Thoresen and Graff-Low (1990, 1994) note that the relationship of Type A behavior and CHD for women remains ambiguous. One reason for this may be because anxiety and depression confound the relationship between Type A behavior and clinical outcomes. That is, the VSI may yield lower scores due to depressive and anxious feelings and behavior. Validated studies of Type A behavior assessed by the VSI or any interview and CHD factors do not currently exist for women. Overall, we lack a well-focused picture of Type A and other coronary-prone factors in women, especially psychosocial factors. Given the risk of CHD for women, research in Type A and other psychosocial factors clearly deserves the highest priority.

IS TYPE A STILL IMPORTANT?

In the early 1980s, the National Heart, Lung and Blood Institute declared that sufficient evidence existed that Type A behavior was a significant and independent risk factor for CHD (Review Panel, 1981). To date, no other psychosocial factor has been so identified, although evidence for social isolation, low perceived social support, and depression seems strong (see Booth-Kewley & Friedman, 1987; House, Landis, & Umberson, 1988; Friedman, Hewley & Tucker, 1994). Over the past decade, however, the validity of Type A behavior in predicting CHD has been challenged. In the 1980s, some large-scale prospective studies failed to find a significant Type A–CHD relationship with cardiac death (e.g., Ragland & Brand, 1988b; Shekelle et al., 1985), promoting the view that Type A behavior is no longer an important issue. Several reasons may have accounted for these failures, as already noted, including the inadequacy of assessing Type A behavior as a global, dichotomous concept (i.e., everyone considered as only A or B) resulting in a very heterogeneous group of persons all labeled as Type A, and the serious limits of measuring Type A behavior on only one occasion and trying to predict death over 20 to 30 years. Unlike eye color or gender, a habitual pattern of behavior such as Type A behavior may alter gradually over the decades. (For a more thorough discussion, see Thoresen & Powell, 1992.)

Some of the confusion about psychosocial factors, such as Type A and CHD factors, stems from the paucity of well-controlled intervention studies. Few treatment studies have been conducted and fewer have used rigorous experimental designs lasting over several months or years to see whether changes in Type A behavior or its components (e.g., hostility) directly relate to changes in CHD indicators. Data from well-controlled experimental studies bear more forcefully on the question of Type A behavior and its relation to CHD disease than do correlational studies, even if prospectively designed. This point was made forcefully by a distinguished medical researcher (Feinstein, 1988) who noted that the serious limitations of any correlational study, even if conducted prospectively over many years, cannot adequately control for other possible factors not examined which could explain relationships.

Type A and Interventions

The picture of a Type A–CHD connection becomes somewhat clearer when controlled intervention studies are examined. Here the evidence shows that altering Type A behavior reduces CHD morbidity (e.g., recurring MI) in patients with mild to moderate CHD pathology. After reviewing 18 Type A intervention studies using meta-analyses, Nunes, Frank, and Kornfeld (1987) noted the following:

- Roughly three out of four persons receiving treatment for Type A behavior did better than the average change for those in control nontreatment conditions (i.e., mean effect size of studies was 0.61).
- Results of controlled interventions, while very limited in sample size in most cases, strongly suggest that clinical applications of Type A interventions are warranted and should be encouraged.
- Intervention using treatments from several methods (e.g., relaxation training, self-monitoring, and cognitive restructuring) are more effective compared to those only using one or two methods (e.g., only relaxation training).
- Interventions lasting several months are clearly more effective compared to those of a few weeks (e.g., six or eight sessions).

These earlier conclusions by Nunes et al. (1987) have recently been reiterated by other reviewers (Ketterer, 1993; Linden, Stossel, & Maurice, in press). It is important to note, however, that demonstrating a reduction in morbidity and mortality by reducing Type A behavior still leaves the conceptual picture cloudy. Many questions remain unanswered, including the following:

- Who benefited the most from these multicomponent treatments, as not everyone was equally helped by those treatments?
- How does a change in Type A-related behavior or cognitions eventuate in reduced risk of cardiac events (i.e., what mechanisms account for these changes)?
- Are there other factors as yet unrecognized that covary in persons identified as Type A, that could possibly explain why psychosocial treatments reduce cardiac risk (e.g., depressive affect and cognitions may consistently covary with Type A behavior and, by being reduced, may explain improvement in cardiac status rather than reduced Type A behavior)?
- What about gender, socioeconomic status, and ethnicity issues (e.g., do African American patients reduce their risk if treated for Type A behavior; are those from lower socioeconomic status helped by psychosocial treatments comparably to higher socioeconomic status persons)?
- Would multicomponent interventions with young persons (e.g., young adolescents) identified as Type A reduce cardiac risk over the long run (i.e., would primary prevention prove useful)?

Ketterer (1993) offers an interesting perspective, in reviewing 9 controlled experimental studies, on the effectiveness of cognitive behavioral interventions for postcoronary patients when compared to persons in a control condition. Table 3.1 presents these results. The percentage of relative reduced risk for those receiving treatment is derived by comparing the treated persons with those in the nontreated condition. Using what is called a weighted summary percent relative risk reduction, Ketterer found that those treated by behavioral procedures over several studies had 39% fewer nonfatal recurring MIs and 33% fewer cardiac deaths. Although some of these studies failed to show a statistically significant reduction, often due to small sample size, taken together these studies strongly suggest that treatments focused on altering behavior and habitual lifestyle factors do reduce disease. Ketterer also notes that compared with data from medical interventions (e.g., medications and bypass surgery), the results from psychosocial/behavioral group interventions compare very favorably and are often more effective in reducing risk of recurring MI or cardiac death than are medical procedures. Further, psychosocial interventions do not produce the negative side effects common-

TABLE 3.1. Percentage of Relative Risk Reduction in Randomized Controlled Trials of Cognitive-Behavioral Therapies for Secondary Prevention in CHD

	n	Follow-up (years)	Percent relative risk nonfatal MIs	Percent reduction cardiac deaths
Friedman et al. (1986)	862	4.5	−46*	−28
Frasure-Smith & Prince (1985)	453	1.0	—	−50*
Frasure-Smith & Prince (1989)	355	7.0	−33*	−15
Ibraham et al. (1974)	105	1.5	—	−34
Rahe, Ward, & Hayes, 1979	44	3.5	−100*	−100
Patel et al. (1985)	169	4.0	−54	−100
Fielding (1979)	45	1.0	−100*	—
Horlick et al. (1984)	116	0.5	—	+60
Stern, Gorman, & Kaslow	64	1.0	+149	—
		WPRR[a] =	−39%	−33%

Note. The data are from Ketterer (1993). Reference information can be found in Ketterer (1993).

[a]WPRR refers to "weighted percent relative risk reduction" and is calculated by multiplying the percentage of relative risk reduction by the number of patients observed, summing over the column and dividing by the total number of patients. See Yusuf, Wittes, and Friedman (1988) for additional information on this procedure.

*Statistically significant difference ($p < .05$).

ly found for surgical and medication treatments. (Also see Davidson, Gidron, & Chaplin, 1996, for a similar analysis of psychosocial vs. medical interventions showing advantages of psychosocial group interventions.)

Some data suggest that cognitive-behavioral group counseling with postcoronary patients may yield cost-effective results (Linden et al., in press). Thoresen and Powell (1983) found that Type A group counseling in the RCPP over the first 3 years was dramatically more cost-effective than CABG surgery and somewhat more cost-effective than beta-blocker medication (propranolol) when cardiac events were the outcome. For example, the cost of cognitive-behavioral group counseling in the RCPP when compared to CABG surgery for postinfarction patients was roughly 50 times less costly in preventing cardiac death. In addition, the combination of group counseling for persons entering the RCPP with CABG proved to be particularly effective in reducing recurrences (Thoresen & Powell, 1983).

Neglected Cultural and Developmental Considerations

One of the most neglected issues in Type A research has been the insensitivity to social and cultural factors affecting Type A persons (Margolis, McLeroy, Runyon, & Kaplan, 1983; Thoresen & Powell, 1992). Such issues loom large for intervention studies. Type A behavior in many ways represents a culturally created and socially sanctioned style of living, an often respected way of coping with demands and challenges. Van Egeren (1991) offers an intriguing frame of reference for Type A. He argues that Type A behavior as a way of coping may have been highly adaptive in preindustrial rural/frontier 19th-century America (e.g., the fiercely self-reliant "cowboy" character) but has become very maladaptive in late 20th-century America. He asks why many Type A persons today, given their deep dissatisfactions and frequent frustrations, fail to revise their unrealistic goals, diminish their incessant struggling against time and others, and reconsider their faulty ideas of success. Why do they fail to distinguish between what is controllable and what is uncontrollable in their lives?

His answer suggests a classic approach–avoidance dilemma, what he calls a "success trap." Some of the Type A person's individualistic, hostile, and impatient thoughts and actions can produce rewarding consequences, especially in the short term. Examples include reduction of worrisome thoughts, personal fears, and anxieties; increase in social praise and recognition; and enhanced sense of power and control. But the same Type A behavior also yields many ongoing negative consequences. Thus the person becomes trapped in an inconsistent system of rewards and punishments. The chronic struggling to accomplish goals (often ill-defined) creates a great deal of dissatisfaction, if not bitter discontent. Van Egeren believes the person becomes enmeshed in a series of futile challenges and perceived threats, prompting hopeless and helpless feelings as well as deep resentment and pervasive hostility. This, in turn, drives the person to seek the reward of success experienced earlier. Thus, engaging in Type A behavior seems to reduce the threat and challenge yet, ironically, creates more perceived challenges and threats that maintain the Type A cycle.

From a treatment perspective, viewing Type A behavior as a culturally sanctioned success trap helps frame the therapeutic task. How can interventions be designed to help release participants from a culturally sanctioned trap? How can persons come to realize that excessive impatience, unbridled competitiveness, and pervasive hostility create a heavy and dangerous burden, impeding a sense of genuine satisfaction and meaningful success? We might ask what developmental factors can contribute to acquisition and maintenance of the Type A behavior as a coping lifestyle. Thoresen and Pattillo (1988) reviewed this question of how Type A behavior may develop in children and adolescents. After examining more than 50 empirical studies of Type A behavior in children and adolescents, they note, among others, the following points:

- The evidence is suggestive that Type A-like behaviors and characteristics have been observed in children as young as 4 years old.
- Lacking controlled longitudinal studies, no direct evidence exists that Type A-like characteristics in children lead to increased cardiovascular disease risk.
- Evidence exists that younger persons with Type A-like characteristics show neuroendocrine and cardiovascular responses similar to adult Type As.
- Some evidence consistently shows that Type A-like behavior in younger persons is related to higher levels of anger (expressed directly as well as "anger in") and more physical signs and symptoms of distress (e.g., headaches, gastrointestinal upset, muscle tension, reduced self-esteem, and increased negative self-evaluations).
- Children and adolescents assessed with Type A-like behaviors generally do not perform better academically than those who have fewer Type A characteristics (some exceptions include doing certain tasks faster, such as arithmetic problems).
- Developmental, psychological, and cultural theories that *may* explain the origins of Type A behavior include infant attachment theory, social cognitive theories (e.g., self-evaluative processes, including ambiguous standards to evaluate oneself, perceived control, and attributional styles), and narcissistic personality development and disorders (e.g., excessive self-referencing, grandiosity, and deeply felt insecurity).

ALTERING TYPE A: TREATMENT OVERVIEW

Viewed as a lifestyle metaphor for contemporary living in a culture greatly obsessed with time, rugged individualism, competitive success, and violence, the Type A pattern provides a useful conceptual framework for beginning to understand why such a lifestyle may create premature risk of CHD.

The group treatment program for altering Type A behavior first emerged in the 1970s, as previously mentioned, with the RCPP. Designed originally as 5-year behavioral intervention, this treatment approach has evolved over the years in at least two major ways:

1. Limitations of a more narrowly focused behavioral approach have been realized with experience, giving way to an expanded cognitive-behavioral perspective coupled with a more existential and spiritual/philosophical focus.
2. Length and format of treatment have changed to accommodate programs lasting from 9 months to 2 years rather than 4½ years. Although some participants can make meaningful changes after 9 to 12 months of group treatment, others have required ongoing participation spanning several years.

The treatment program to be described was originally created to help post-MI participants gain a better understanding of how and why Type A characteristics may affect them physically, socially, and emotionally at work, at home, and in the community. Currently, the program also serves those who are reasonably healthy yet who are trying to reduce the chronic distress and struggle characterizing their lives. To accomplish this, the program focuses on several major themes, including:

- Pathophysiology of Type A and CHD.
- Diagnostic signs and symptoms of Type A.
- Type A-related emotions, attitudes, and beliefs.
- Case examples of persons exhibiting Type A.
- Role of self-esteem and feelings of self-worth.
- Increases in sense of meaning, purpose, and connectedness.
- Reduction of excessive impatience, competitiveness, and hostility.

To deal with these themes, a changing format for group sessions has been developed. In the first few weeks, for example, the format is highly structured, focused on conveying information and increasing understanding of Type A behavior and CHD. Initially, the group leader serves primarily as a *teacher* and the group functions primarily as a group of students in a course.

As the group develops in terms of process factors, the focus shifts gradually to the experiences of participants surrounding their efforts to apply what they have discussed, observed, and read. For example, the "driving game" becomes one of their first experiential tasks, where participants become much more aware of what they experience while driving a car. These experiences include physiological changes, overt behavior, specific thoughts and feelings, and the impact of other drivers on their experience as well as the impact of passengers in their cars when they are driving.

Later, group members, as a result of a greater sense of trust and respect for others in the group, increasingly bring current problems and issues to the group, often work- or family-related concerns. Although such problems become a major focus, the group still gives attention to practicing less Type A behavior outside the group, coupled with daily relaxation practice and repeated use of the "self-monitor" (discussed later).

Besides participating, group members are asked to take action between group sessions. Participants are repeatedly reminded that the success of the program depends on what each member does *between* group sessions. It is not enough to attend sessions because the real work and benefit come from making changes in daily living. To facilitate change, both in the group sessions as well as in other settings, a variety of audiovisual and print material is used. Each participant receives a "Drill Book" (explained later) and reading material. Initially chapters are assigned in *Treating Type A Behavior and Your Heart* (Friedman & Ulmer, 1984). This reading serves as a focus for discussion.

Later, a variety of books are suggested, such as biographies of famous persons whose lives illustrate Type A behavior, such as *Lyndon Johnson and the American Dream* (Kearns, 1976). Participants also bring to the group newspaper articles and cartoons clipped from newspapers and magazines illustrating Type A characteristics. In addition, every group session commences with a brief relaxation practice (about 10 minutes), in part to model the value of taking time to slow down, to become more calm, to focus attention, and to be more alert and attentive in the group.

Group leaders take attendance at every session and typically call a participant who has missed a session to ask how things are going and to mention that the person was missed at the last meeting. The message conveyed and almost always appreciated by the participant is clear: We care about you, we missed you, and we hope you will attend the next session.

Goals of Group Treatment

The goals and therapeutic approaches of the treatment program to be described grew directly out of how the Type A person has been conceptualized. Type A persons are seen as generating chronically excessive physical, emotional, and behavioral arousal. Thus, the primary aim of treatment is to reduce the arousal that accompanies the pervasive impatience and free-floating hostility that characterizes the Type A individual. However, because Type A behavior is generated by a particular self and world philosophy, effective treatment must also help participants examine and often change their underlying attitudes and beliefs. Further, although what might be called a Type A worldview includes such qualities as suspiciousness, cynicism, and alienation, its foundation appears to be built on personal insecurity and precarious self-esteem. Reducing insecurity and enhancing self-esteem are thus seen as essential for the effective treatment of Type A persons.

Because we are seeking to help participants begin the process of changing a world view and style of coping that is often lifelong, the treatment program is aimed at the following:

- Increasing participants' awareness of the Type A behavior and its pervasive consequences.
- Developing greater self-awareness of personal manifestations of Type A (e.g., by using the self-monitor).
- Teaching participants strategies for physical and psychological relaxation.
- Providing behavioral exercises by which participants can develop healthier behaviors.
- Helping participants recognize and modify Type A attitudes, thoughts, and beliefs.
- Reducing participants' insecurity and fostering healthier ways of maintaining self-esteem.

Although these goals are necessary to achieve significant and lasting change, we have continually observed that the rate and process of change remain exquisitely idiosyncratic. For instance, some participants are able to initiate significant changes surprisingly soon after developing the ability to observe and monitor their Type A behavior. Others, however, need repeated and intensive work to examine and modify underlying attitudes and beliefs. Unfortunately, some participants seem hopelessly trapped and enslaved by their Type A behavior, regardless of their best efforts to facilitate change. A profound fear of relinquishing control and letting go enough to change seems to surround them. Still, the vast majority who make a genuine commitment and show patient effort succeed in making life-enhancing, and in many instances life-saving, changes.

Treatment Format and Approach

The Type A person is best treated in a small-group format using an approach that combines elements of cognitive-behavioral and existential–humanistic orientations (e.g., Bandura, 1986; Powell & Thoresen, 1987; Bugental & Bracke, 1992). The small group (approximately 10 to 12 participants), meeting in sessions of 1½ to 2 hours, offers the following advantages over individual treatment:

- The small group provides an excellent opportunity to experience the benefits of ongoing social support.
- Participants' learning is enhanced vicariously by listening to the problems and successes of others.
- Almost all participants need to improve their weak "active listening" skills to be successful.
- Feedback from several persons (peers) is often perceived as more valid than feedback from only one person, especially a professional.

The optimal atmosphere in the group of mutual trust, respect, and support must, however, be persistently cultivated by the group leader, given the abundance of a well-established hostile and cynical outlook of many participants.

Essential Qualities of Effective Group Leaders

More than any other elements, the talent and humanity of the group leader determine the success of treatment. Although effective group leaders may come from a variety of theoretical orientations, they must share some common essential qualities.

1. To convey expertise and authority to often hypercritical Type A participants, a group leader needs a substantial basic understanding of the pathophysiology of CHD, especially as related to the Type A person.
2. To help direct, motivate, and support participants' efforts to reduce their Type A behavior, the leader needs expertise in the principles of behavioral change.
3. A thorough understanding of Type A, by the leader, particularly when that understanding develops from being actively involved in modifying his or her own Type A behavior.

Personal understanding by leaders of their own Type A dynamics enables them to empathize with participants' problems in trying to change. It also facilitates recognition of the attitudes and beliefs underlying participants' Type A behavior. Effectiveness can be severely undermined if leaders lack insight into their own behavior, are not willing to disclose these insights to their group, and are not actively committed and involved in modifying their own Type A behavior.

The personal qualities of a group leader, such as level of sensitivity and flexibility, become even more important because the role of the leader changes over time. In the course of group treatment over several months, the leader assumes the roles of *teacher, consultant, guide,* and *companion.* All roles remain essential but some predominate at different phases of treatment. Initially, for example, the leader functions primarily as a caring teacher. After a few months, the role gradually shifts to that of a consultant and guide. Each role requires different expertise and personal qualities. Given these requirements, group leaders selected for the RCPP were experienced clinicians who were able to present themselves as mature, respected, and successful professionals. They avoided technical jargon, communicated in a simple and sincere manner, and exhibited the same gentle sense of humor about their own foibles and incongruities as they did toward those of participants. Indeed, the necessity for an easy and comfortable sense of humor proved invaluable if not essential to promoting change.

Because alteration of Type A behavior requires improvement of participants' self-esteem, a group leader needs to experience and actively express a genuine caring attitude toward group members. This can be a formidable challenge when confronted with the often hypercritical hostility of some participants, especially in the first few months. Thus, group leaders' caring must often have the qualities of disciplined compassion—the ability to set limits and engage in firm confrontations while still retaining empathy and understanding. Helping others to change their Type A behavior consistently challenges the leader to intervene with as much presence, caring, and respect as is humanly possible. In effect, the leader needs to process his or her experiences in the group with a "Type B mind-set" (Price, 1988).

Developing Greater Awareness

To develop increased subjective awareness and understanding, the Type A self-monitor is employed. More than most, those with a Type A style seem to have lost much of their innate ability to be subjectively aware of themselves. The most serious consequence of this loss is that participants too often direct their lives in mindless attempts to please, impress, or protect themselves from others. Many participants have chronically suppressed feelings, such as exhaustion, insecurity, and loneliness, to aggressively strive for more professional status and economic gain. They often appear "numb" to these feelings. To change, participants need to develop the ability to access and remain aware of their unique internal experience. We try to accomplish this through an ongoing combination of meditation and relaxation, self-monitoring exercises, and the supportive feedback of group members and the group leader.

"Bombs and Fuses"

Initially, participants often deny that the Type A exists as a distinct syndrome and doubt its contribution to CHD risk. Or, they believe it only exists in others (Powell & Thoresen, 1987). As a means of confronting participants' denial and increasing adherence to the treatment regimen, the "bomb and fuses" metaphor was developed (Friedman & Ulmer, 1984). The "bomb" was identified as participants' original infarction, their occluded coronary arteries, and their "cardiac denial." The bomb was also portrayed as being subject to detonation by any of the several "fuses" (i.e., physical or behavioral risk factors). These included Type A behavior, especially anger and impatience, physical exertion at an excessive altitude (i.e., above 3,000 feet), excessive prolonged physical activity, one heavy-fat meal, becoming mentally/emotionally exhausted, excessive caffeine, and excessive alcohol. Group leaders consistently inquired about each participant's avoidance of these fuses, especially if a member "lit a fuse," asking him or her to describe the situation to the group and how situation might be avoided in the future.

Just as the Type A obscures awareness of a person's subjective state, it also blinds many participants to their Type A behavior at home, at work, and in the community. Without an accurate and reliable awareness of their own Type A behavior, participants are seriously hampered in making informed choices about how they wish to respond to the situations they encounter. The cultural glamour and hype sometimes afforded the Type A person can be eliminated by reducing the Type A behavior pattern to its essential features and effects. To do this, the therapeutic acronym AIAI (anger, irritation, aggravation, impatience) was created in part to facilitate a greater awareness of Type A behavior by participants.

Self-Monitor (Inner Voice)

Derived from behavioral research on self-monitoring (Thoresen & Mahoney, 1974) the Type A self-monitor procedure was developed to help participants detach from the personal distress in a situation by refocusing their attention on the occurrence of distress itself. For example, when a person is impatiently waiting in a slow bank line, the person's Self may start criticizing the incompetence of the teller or the bank's deplorable understaffing. The person's self-monitor would ideally intervene at this point with the awareness that the Self is acting impatient and hypercritical and that patience, not criticism, is a more desirable response. The self-monitor might, for example, note, "Waiting in line gives me the opportunity to reflect on some interesting thing I could do this weekend or could remind me to observe specific Type A signs and symptoms of others waiting in line." Essentially, the participant develops a sort of meta-cognition, an observing and more impartial third-person perspective, one that has an intimate awareness of the participant's emotional responses, fears, and rationalizations as well as behaviors (Powell & Thoresen, 1987).

Development of a self-monitor begins with group discussions that comprehensively describe the specific behavioral signs and symptoms of the Type A person. Videotapes and audiotapes to illustrate speech and psychomotor behaviors provide concrete examples. In addition, participants complete a variety of self-monitoring exercises. Perhaps the most effective means of developing the self-monitor comes from the immediate feedback that participants receive from others as they discuss provocative topics, such as reactions to a rude driver or to a critical colleague at work. A primary responsibility of the group leader in this process is to cultivate an atmosphere of trust, respect, and mutual support so that participants can give and accept feedback on their behavior and explore possible underlying beliefs.

Relatedly, the group leader must also establish that both impatience and anger are natural emotional phenomena that only become destructive of health and well-being when they are intense, prolonged, and chronic. Unless they can accept this view of anger and impatience, many participants suppress and deny their Type A behavior to impress the group leader and to compete with other participants. The consequence of such denial and premature suppression creates a crucial loss of opportunities to examine and modify the basic emotional reactions that stimulate Type A behavior. The self-monitor we seek to develop is one that is respectful, curious, and interested in understanding the self, rather than the harsh, rigid, and perfectionistic critic that usually lies at the core of the Type A psyche. A useful self-monitor is one that observes behavior, attitude, and emotion and chooses to respond in a patient, calm, and reassuring manner.

Relaxation Training

Developing the ability to reduce the physical and emotional arousal that Type A behavior creates is highly beneficial both directly and indirectly. The health value of using relaxation and meditative strategies to reduce physiological hyperarousal has been consistently demonstrated for a number of stress-related diseases (Henry & Stephens, 1977). Many participants who exhibit Type A have great difficulty in modulating their "engines at full speed ahead" and easing off their hard-driving behavior. They need systematic training in relaxation strategies (Price, 1988). The chronic sympathetic nervous system hyperarousal associated with Type A can be significantly reduced by practicing relaxation in a systematic fashion. Progressive muscle relaxation, for example, has been shown to reduce factors associated with sympathic arousal, including accelerated heart rate and elevated blood pressure (Cottier, Shapiro, Julius, & Johnston, 1985). Several other procedures (e.g., autogenic training, breath meditation, and guided imagery) are also effective.

However, it is unrealistic to expect that all participants possess the motivation and discipline necessary to practice formal relaxation procedures on a daily basis. Typically, at first, only one or a few in any group make the effort. Thus, relaxation training can be used as a "primer" with less ambitious goals. Group sessions can begin with some form of relaxation exercise that helps focus attention, create physical comfort, and provide an experience of calm and peacefulness that usually contrasts dramatically with the physical and emotional tension that infuse the experience of most participants. Because many have become deeply habituated to the tense feelings of chronic arousal, doing relaxation often sensitizes participants to the experiential differences between arousal and relaxation.

Typically, the group leader initially demonstrates a particular relaxation procedure to instruct and model the most effective use of a procedure. Because relaxation of any type is usually an unfamiliar feeling, participants often experience some discomfort during initial relaxation exercises ("I feel more tense than I did before!"). The group leader can use this discomfort to discuss possible resistance to slowing down. After a relaxation strategy has been demonstrated and practiced at a group session, members are instructed to practice the procedure between group sessions daily and discuss their experience at the next meeting.

Group leaders present a variety of relaxation strategies, including deep abdominal breathing, progressive muscle relaxation, health meditation, autogenics, and guided imagery, to allow participants to select a procedure or combination of procedures that work for them. The goal is to help each participant develop a proficient personal style of relaxing to use in reducing arousal that arises from daily situations that often invite impatient, depressed, or angry thoughts and behaviors.

Daily Drills ("One-a-Day Behavior")

Replacing the time-urgent and hostile behaviors associated with the Type A person requires that participants experience and practice healthier alternative behaviors. A set of daily drills developed in RCPP provide participants with structured exercises that involved acting and thinking in healthier ways.

Figure 3.3 illustrates a page from the participants' Drill Book. The daily drills include exercises aimed at modifying actions and attitudes in the areas of impatience (e.g., leave watch off and eat more slowly), hostility (e.g., purposely say, "Maybe I'm wrong"), self-esteem (e.g., contemplate positive achievements for 10 minutes), and improving relationships (e.g., ask family members about their day's activities and verbalize affection to spouse). In addition to the daily exercises, each week's drills are accompanied by a weekly philosophical/spiritual concept that participants are asked to reflect on and discuss at group sessions.

January (First year)	
Monday:	Alter one of your usual habits or ways of doing things.
Tuesday:	Ask member of family about his or her day's activities.
Wednesday:	Leave watch off.
Thursday:	Walk more slowly.
Friday:	Verbalize affection to spouse/children.
Saturday:	Eat more slowly.
Sunday:	Practice smiling as you remember two or three happy events of the past.

1. "For every minute you are angry, you lose 60 seconds of happiness." —Ralph W. Emerson
2. "Contempt for others is a weed that can flourish in only one very special kind of soil, that composed of self-contempt."—Anonymous
3. "One can stroke persons with words."—F. Scott Fitzgerald
4. "When a fixed idea makes its appearance, a great ass also makes its appearance."—Friedrich Nietzsche

FIGURE 3.3. Example from RCPP Drill Book used in structuring daily behavioral exercises.

The group leader plays an essential role in helping participants develop and maintain the motivation and discipline needed to complete the drills consistently. Initially, participants' motivation can be increased by presenting the rationale behind the drills in general and the particular value of completing specific exercises. In addition, the group leader points out that while completing all drills is most beneficial, the difficulties and resistances that participants often encounter are important to observe and understand, even if a specific drill has not been completed. Through this guidance, members become increasingly aware of their own personal version of the Type A behavior pattern as well as *how* they resist changing. Time is reserved in group sessions for discussing of experiences during drills to emphasize the positive effects that members report, provide support, and share suggestions on how difficult drills might be successfully accomplished. Throughout these discussions, the group leader can reiterate the importance and rationale for completing drills and provide ongoing encouragement and reinforcement. In time, participants create their own drills, tailored to their particular problems and concerns.

Reducing Time Urgency

In addition to the daily drills, group discussions and specific exercises are needed to reduce participants' chronic impatience. Initially, the nature of time urgency, its causes, and its destructive effects are discussed to promote self-awareness and motivation to change. Time urgency, the frenetic drive to accomplish an unrealistic number of tasks in progressively less time, is believed to be the result of covert insecurity and an unstable or inadequate level of self-esteem (Friedman & Ulmer, 1984). This insecurity arises in part from an individual's fear that he or she will be unable to cope with a task and will consequently lose status with peers, superiors, or family.

The general manifestations of this insecurity include the following:

- A chronic inability to reject others' requests to do unnecessary tasks.
- An inability or refusal to delegate tasks and to reduce overall workload.
- An apparent greed to acquire an unrealistic number of responsibilities, material possessions, or symbols of achievement in trying to prove self-worth.
- A preoccupation with personal shortcomings and "weaknesses" coupled with a devaluing of strengths and positive feedback from others.

By contrast, it is crucial that the time pressure of excessive tasks and deadlines actually imposed by superiors be validated by the group leader as "real." The effect of Western culture's increasing movement toward becoming a cult that worships speed and hurriedness must also be included when discussing factors that promote time urgency and impatience.

To help reduce time urgency, participants must first develop an awareness of their own specific manifestations of impatience and become sensitized to the oppressive subjective experience that characterizes "hurry sickness." This is best accomplished through self-observation exercises, group discussion of specific impatient behaviors, and the examination of participants' experience of greater calmness created through relaxation. That is, participants are asked to report on the subjective experience of relaxation as compared to the tension of chronic time urgency. Identifying the specific time-urgent behaviors of participants that occur in the group itself is an extremely potent means of developing self-awareness.

Similarly, discussions are used to expose the consequences of chronic impatience that participants are unaware of or deny. For instance, many participants deny the likelihood that impatience actually promotes errors rather than greater productivity. This is especially true when participants employ polyphasing (i.e., doing more than one task at a time). Crucially, participants are confronted with the reality that their impatience often encourages them to view others as "obstacles" in their way, thus promoting hostile behavior. This hostility, in turn, erodes or destroys relationships with others, depriving them of social support, a critical source of self-esteem. This vicious cycle lies at the root of the Type A behavior pattern and perpetuates it. Although discussions such as these are useful, the crucial factor lies in increasing participants' awareness of their *personal* time urgent behaviors and their unique causes. Without this awareness, significant change will not occur.

Specific exercises are employed to help participants become aware of their personal beliefs that generate time urgency and, more important, to develop more realistic attitudes and healthier strategies for coping with demands. Cognitive restructuring is based on the principle that an emotional reaction is produced by demands in the environment and by one's perception of those demands (Bandura, 1986). Because participants' perceptions play a major role in their emotional arousal and coping behavior, exposing, examining, and modifying these Type A-related perceptions is essential for successful treatment. For example, participants are asked to list the causes of a major professional or personal success. Through such analyses, members realize that they have succeeded *despite* their impatience and that time urgency actually impedes, never enhances, a career.

Through other exercises, participants realize that their reluctance to delegate is often due to an excessive need to retain control in a misguided effort to raise self-esteem. Participants examine such Type A-related beliefs as:

1. "My worth depends on the quantity not the quality of my achievements."
2. "I must constantly prove my worth again and again, because my past accomplishments don't count."
3. "I must do more than others to be worthy."

Through such awareness and reflection, participants begin to develop and apply healthier and more personally congruent beliefs that help them to reduce chronic overscheduling and underdelegating.

Similarly, the necessity to engage in *genuine* prioritizing of activities is established by exercises that illustrate the fallacious nature of "Type A prioritizing": *All* tasks are crucial and *must* be accomplished *today!* Role-play exercises are used to develop participants' ability to assertively reject the unrealistic demands of others and, more importantly, of themselves. Covey, Merrill, and Merrill (1994) offer a helpful model of demands as important or unimportant and urgent or not urgent. Too much is misconstrued as urgent and important at the expense of important but not urgent activities. (See also Ulmer & Schwartzburd, 1996.)

Reducing Anger and Hostility

Research examining the components of the Type A behavior pattern suggests that hostility may be its most toxic element (e.g., Matthews & Haynes, 1986; Williams, Barefoot, and Shekelle, 1984). Although it is clear from a clinical perspective that time urgency and hurry sickness are pervasive antecedents of hostility and must be modified, the treatment program does consider the reduction of hostility as the program's predominant goal. Because we are seeking to help participants modify a hostile Type A world view and style of coping, treatment must focus on the following:

1. Increasing the individual's understanding of Type A hostility.
2. Developing a pervasive awareness of personal manifestations of hostility.
3. Identifying specific situations that evoke hostility.
4. Understanding and modifying the personal beliefs that generate hostility.
5. Developing, practicing, and applying healthier methods of dealing with provocative situations.

Initially, the nature and specific behavioral manifestations of Type A hostility needs to be comprehensively described and discussed. The group leader needs to establish, as already noted, that anger is a naturally occurring and often healthy emotional response to challenge and frustration. It is important to avoid the tendency of many to suppress and deny their hostile reactions so that they may appear to be "reasonable and in control." Thus, it is important for participants to learn that the problem with Type A anger is not simply that anger occurs but that it occurs more frequently, often more intensely, and lasts for longer durations. Group leaders must emphasize the abuse of anger and how some have become "addicted" to the immediate energies (physiological arousal) resulting from the emotion of anger.

Groups begin by discussing the essential features of Type A anger and hostility:

- A hypercritical world view, cynicism, distrust, suspiciousness, blame, and attribution of malevolence by others.
- To avoid participants' defensiveness about their hostile attitudes, initial discussions focus on the primary behavioral signs and symptoms in others and gradually move to the identification of participants' own hostile behaviors.
- To monitor their Type A hostility, participants must become aware of more subtle manifestations of hostility, such as sarcasm, biting humor, facial grimacing, hypercritical generalizations about groups (e.g.,

other races, women, and professions), persistent chiding and teasing, and explosive or jarring laughter.

A particularly fertile microcosm that may be used to identify participants' anger and hostile beliefs concerns driving ("the driving game"). Group members describe provocative driving experiences with the goal of identifying specific signs and symptoms of anger, exposing underlying hostile attitudes, and developing alternative ways of perceiving and responding to the automotive idiosyncrasies of others. They are asked to practice more cooperative, friendly, and calm approaches to driving, such as driving in the slow lane and yielding to oncoming traffic. The continued development and pervasive use of the self-monitor cannot be overemphasized as an essential process in reducing anger and hostility.

The Hook Metaphor

One of the most useful therapeutic metaphors is that of "bait and hooks" (Powell & Thoresen, 1987; Powell, 1996). Participants learn that as they move through the unpredictable waters of daily life, they encounter, like fish, obstacles and provocative situations ("bait") that invite hostile responses. The crucial concept that participants come to realize is that the "hook" is their own *perception* of an event or situation and how they interpret its meaning is what evokes their hostility. To increase awareness of provocative situations, participants examine a series of situations that often evoke Type A hostility with the goal of assessing which "baits" are most personally provocative. The increased awareness and reflection that such exercises produce help many participants to start avoiding certain situations when possible or to employ healthier responses. Examples of a "bait and hook" exercise are presented in Table 3.2. It is essential that participants become aware of the personal beliefs that hook their hostility through such exercises as well as self-monitoring and group discussion.

The Narcissistic Connection

Much Type A hostility appears to arise from an excessive sense of entitlement, a hypersensitivity to perceived disapproval, and an exaggerated need for control (Thoresen & Pattillo, 1988). Lasch (1978) describes the "neonarcissism" that characterizes much of the Type A perspective: fiercely competitive for approval, superficially cooperative while restraining a deep anger, demanding immediate gratification yet perpetually unsatisfied. Within this context, Type A hostility seems understandable. If an individual is exhausting him- or herself to complete more and more productive tasks and trying to

TABLE 3.2. Examples of "Bait-and-Hook" Metaphor

Bait situations	Others making trivial mistakes.
Examples	Spouse forgets to pick up shirts from laundry. Colleague makes insignificant error in the office.
Type A "hook" attitude	"How dare you make a mistake that inconveniences me! Your mistake clearly indicates your general incompetence and my general superiority."
Bait situations	Ideology (political, religious, etc.).
Examples	Friends express different political views. Patient reads article describing the religious or cultural beliefs of a different group.
Type A "hook" attitude	"How can these people be so incredibly stupid to believe that stuff? How dare these people question my beliefs by believing differently from me?"
Bait situations	Being pressed for time or under a deadline.
Examples	Project deadline at work; struggling to arrive for an appointment on time.
Type A "hook" attitude	"I have the right to push everything and everyone out of my way. It's grossly unfair that I don't have all the time I need."

do so in less and less time but still feeling unloved and unappreciated if not ignored, hostility and cynicism seem justified (Bugental & Bracke, 1992).

Although these beliefs are idiosyncratic, examples of typical implicit assumption in the narcissistic Type A include the following:

1. "I need hostility in order to succeed."
2. "My hostility is unalterable."
3. "My anger is caused by the ignorance and incompetence of others."
4. "Giving and receiving love and affection is a sign of weakness."
5. "It's a dog-eat-dog world and people are not to be trusted."

As with time urgency, interventions used in the group support participants in reconsidering their hostile beliefs and subsequently in developing healthier attitudes and beliefs based on understanding, compassion, and forgiveness.

Becoming More Assertive

In addition to examining and modifying personal beliefs, participants learn how to respond assertively rather than aggressively. Participants are confronted with the reality that although hostile responses may achieve short-term compliance from others, the long-term consequences of hostility are often severe. Hostility promotes counterattacks, rejection, and feelings of guilt. Assertiveness requires that participants learn to reduce the emotional intensity of their responses, take time to consider a situation, and respect both their needs and those of the other. Further, participants learn to monitor the psychomotor phenomena that accompany their assertive responses: to use appropriate volume and emphasis in their speech, be conscious of facial expressions, and structure requests in a manner intended to resolve a conflict (Bower & Bower, 1976). Assertive responses are best developed and practiced in group sessions using actual conflict situations that participants bring up in their daily experiences. Participants are encouraged to respond assertively to situations marked by clear moral and ethical transgressions. Our goal is to enable participants to mindfully choose from an expanded range of response options.

ENHANCING SELF-ESTEEM AND DEVELOPING A HEALTHY PHILOSOPHY FOR LIVING

Because many Type A persons appear to be motivated by a covert insecurity or low self-esteem, enhancing self-esteem remains essential for effective treatment. Self-esteem appears to comprise two major components: (1) the perception of some degree of control (Glass, 1977) and self-efficacy (Bandura, 1982) in one's life and (2) a positive perception of one's worth as a person (Branden, 1969). Treatment enhances participants' perceptions of control and self-efficacy by increasing their ability to do the following:

1. Identify and reduce unwanted Type A behaviors.
2. Reduce physical tension and create calmness by applying relaxation strategies.
3. Improve relationships, including social support, and resolve conflicts using assertiveness training.
4. Identify, examine, and mindfully alter Type A beliefs.

Participants' feelings of self-worth are enhanced through a variety of exercises and processes. Because the self-worth of many participants is excessively dependent on career achievement, participants are encouraged to identify and develop other sources of self-esteem (e.g., family relationships and broadening esthetic interest in hobbies, music literature, and art). Group leaders promote greater self-acceptance through a realistic evaluation of achievements and performance expectations. Although many participants have already accomplished a great deal, their self-esteem has received little nourishment. This is probably due to perfectionistic expectations and excessively harsh self-criticism (Bracke & Thoresen, 1996). The relationship between self-esteem, achievements, and expectations was described by William James (1890) as follows:

$$\text{Self-esteem} = \text{Achievements/expectations}$$

Thus, an individual can raise esteem by either increasing achievements or reducing expectations. This becomes the focus of group discussions and exercises designed to help participants focus on their daily achievements and reflect on developing realistic expectations.

The supportive and caring environment of the group accompanied by the comparatively unconditional acceptance of the group leader provides a powerful boost for participants' self-esteem. Within this context, participants begin to reflect on the broader issues and values in their lives and to develop a healthier and more authentic personal if not spiritual philosophy. Although behavioral drills and cognitive restructuring exercises as commonly used are extremely effective in reducing the destructive effects of the Type A behavior pattern, such approaches may be limited in helping participants create more meaningful and satisfying lives (Bugental & Bracke, 1992). As treatment progresses, participants begin to explore basic philosophical and spiritual questions. For example, "Do I believe in a higher power or force in the world?" "What are my responsibilities to others, to the earth?" "Am I living a spiritually healthy life?" The final goal is to help participants develop a healthy personal philosophy for living that will maintain and extend after treatment the progress made during the group program.

The closing affirmation read aloud to end all group sessions as participants stand, holding hands, illustrates this dimension of treatment:

> We are here because we realize that we all need more help than we can give ourselves. We need each other. So may all our efforts be of benefit to each one. And may friendship and love bring enrichment to all our lives, and to all those whose lives are in our care. We this acknowledge gratefully. Amen.

Although it is extremely important for participants who have chronically struggled with life to reach the point where they ask, "Is this worth dying for?" it is truly crucial that they also ask, "What is worth living for?"

A CONCLUDING WORD

The promising yet tentative results of the group treatment described in this chapter and the work of others in applying psychosocial group interventions with coronary patients and other chronic diseases deserve careful consideration. We need to provide more programs that in effect show patients how to act in more health-enhancing ways, and that reduce the expensive and at times questionable costs of invasive surgery and costly lifetime medications. We also need to recognize that we have a great deal to learn about how to best structure group treatments for people of color, male and female. One size does not fit all when it comes to group treatment for CHD (Thoresen & Powell, 1992; Thoresen & Graff-Low, 1994; Graff-Low, Thoresen, King, Pattillo, & Jenkins, 1995). As we have urged in this chapter, we also need to recognize much more the powerful part played by philosophical, spiritual, and religious issues in the lives of patients and people in general (Thoresen, in press).

ACKNOWLEDGMENTS

We are very appreciative of the encouragement and leadership of Meyer Friedman, M.D., the Principal Investigator of the Recurrent Coronary Prevention Project, as well as the help of our many colleagues at the Meyer Friedman Institute, Mt. Zion Medical Center, University of California, San Francisco. The views expressed here remain ours and are not the responsibility of those who have supported our work. The help of Dorothy Farana and Ada Glucksman in preparing this manuscript is also greatly appreciated.

Support in part for the research discussed here was provided by NHLBI (NIH) Grant No. 2ROIH34396 to Carl E. Thoresen as well as by a grant from the John D. and Catherine T. MacArthur Foundation.

REFERENCES

Allan, R., & Scheidt, S. (1996). *Heart and mind: The practice of cardiac psychology.* Washington, DC: American Psychological Association.

American Heart Association. (1995). *Heart facts.* Dallas, TX: Author.

Bandura, A. (1982). Self-efficacy mechanism in human agency. *American Psychologist, 37,* 122–147.

Bandura, A. (1986). *Social foundations of thought and action: A social cognitive theory.* Englewood Cliffs, NJ: Prentice Hall.

Barefood, J. D. (1992). Developments in the measurement of hostility. In H. Friedman (Ed.), *Hostility, coping and health* (pp. 13–31). Washington, DC: American Psychological Association.

Barefood, J. C., Patterson, J. C., Harey, T. L., Cayton, T. G., Hickman, J. R., & Williams, R. B. (1994). Hostility in asymptomatic men with angiographically confirmed coronary artery disease. *American Journal of Cardiology, 74,* 439–442.

Booth-Kewley, S., & Friedman, H. S. (1987). Psychosocial predictors of heart disease: A quantitative review. *Psychological Bulletin, 101,* 343–362.

Bower, G., & Bower, S. (1976). *Asserting yourself: A practical guide for positive change.* Boston: Addison-Wesley.

Bracke, P. E., & Thoresen, C. E. (1996). Reducing Type A behavior patterns: A structured-group approach. In R. Allan & S. Scheidt (Eds.), *Heart and mind: The practice of cardiac psychology* (pp. 255–290). Washington, DC: American Psychological Association.

Branden, N. (1969). *The psychology of self-esteem*. New York: Bantam.

Bugental, J. F. T., & Bracke, P. E. (1992). The future of existential–humanistic psychotherapy. *Psychotherapy, 29*, 28–33.

Burell, G. (1996). Group psychotherapy in Project New Life: Treatment of coronary-prone behaviors for patients who have had coronary artery bypass graft surgery. In R. Allen & S. Scheidt (Eds.), *Heart and mind: The practice of cardiac psychology* (pp. 291–310). Washington, DC: American Psychological Association.

Burell, G., Ohman, A., Sundia, O., Strom, G., Ramrend, B., Cullhed, I., & Thoresen, C. E. (1994). Type A behavior pattern in post-myocardial infarction patients: A route to cardia rehabilitation. *International Journal of Behavioral Medicine, 1*, 32–54.

Cottier, C., Shapiro, K., Julius, S., & Johnston. (1984). Treatment of mild hypertension with progressive muscle relaxation: Predictive value of indexes of sympathetic tone. *Archives of Internal Medicine, 144*, 1954–1958.

Covey, S. R., Merrill, A. R., & Merrill, R. R. (1994). *First things first*. New York: Simon and Schuster.

Davidson, K. D., Gidron, Y., & Chaplin, W. F. (1996). *Statistical significance versus clinical significance and the evaluation of medical and psychological interventions for post-MI patients*. Unpublished manuscript, Dalhousie University, Halifax, Nova Scotia, Canada.

Dembroski, T. M., MacDougall, J. M., Costa, P. T., & Grauditz, G. (1989). Components of hostility as predictors of sudden death and myocardial infarction in the Multiple Risk Factor Interventon Trial. *Psychosomatic Medicine, 51*, 514–572.

Feinstein, A. P. (1988). Scientific standards in epidemiologic studies of the menaces of daily life. *Science, 242*, 1257–1263.

Frasure-Smith, N., Lesperance, F., & Talajic, M. (1993). Depression following myocardial infarction: Impact on 6-month survival. *Journal of American Medical Association, 270*, 1819–1825.

Friedman, M., Hawley, P. H., & Yucker, J. H. (1994). Personality, health, and longevity. *Current Directions in Psychological Science, 3*, 37–41.

Friedman, M., & Rosenman, R. H. (1959). Association of specific overt behavior pattern with blood and cardiovascular findings. *Journal of American Medical Association, 169*, 1286–1296.

Friedman, M., St. George, S., Byers, S. O., & Rosenman, R. H. (1960). Excretion of catecholamines, 17-ketosteroids, 17-hydroxycorticoeds, and 5-hydroxyindole in men exhibiting a particular behavior pattern (A) associated with high incidence of clinical coronary artery disease. *Journal of Clinical Investigation, 39*, 758–764.

Friedman, M., Thoresen, C. E., Gill, J., Ulmer, D., Powell, L. H., Price, V. A., Brown, B., Thompson, L., Rabin, D. D., Breall, W. S., Bourg, W., Levy, R., & Dixon, T. (1986). Alternation of Type A behavior and its effect on cardiac recurrences in post-myocardial infarction patients: Summary results of the Recurrent Coronary Prevention Project. *American Heart Journal, 112*, 653–665.

Friedman, M., & Ulmer, D. K. (1984). *Treating Type A behavior and your heart*. New York: Alfred A. Knopf.

Glass, D. C. (1977). *Behavior patterns, stress, and coronary disease*. New York: Wiley.

Graff-Low, K., Thoresen, C. E., King, A., Pattillo, J. R., & Jenkins, C. (1995). Anxiety, depression and heart disease in women. *International Journal of Behavioral Medicine, 1*, 305–319.

Hecker, M. H. L., Chesney, M. A., Black, G. W., & Frautschi, G. (1988). Coronary-prone behaviors in the Western Collaborative Group Study. *Psychosomatic Medicine, 50*, 153–164.

Henry, J., & Stephens, P. (1977). *Stress, health and the social environment*. New York: Springer-Verlag.

House, J. S., Landis, K. R., & Umberson, D. (1988). Social relationships and health. *Science, 241*, 540–545.

James, W. (1890). *The principles of psychology* (Vols. I & II). New York: Dover.

Jenkins, C. D. (1971). Psychologic and social precursors of coronary disease. *New England Journal of Medicine, 294*, 974–994.

Ketterer, M. (1993). Secondary prevention of ischemic heart disease: The case for aggressive behavioral monitoring and intervention. *Psychosomatics, 34*, 478–484.

Lasch, C. (1978). *The culture of narcissism: American life in an age of diminishing expectations*. New York: Norton.

Linden, W., Stossel, C., & Maurice, J. (in press). Psychosocial interventions for patients with coronary artery disease: A meta-analysis. *Annals of Internal Medicine*.

Lown, B., & Wolf, M. (1971). Approaches to sudden death from coronary heart disease. *Circulation, 44*, 130–142.

Margolis, L. H., McLeroy, K. K., Runyon, C. W., & Kaplan, B. H. (1983). Type A behavior: An ecological approach. *Journal of Behavioral Medicine, 6*, 245–258.

Matthews, K. A., & Haynes, S. G. (1986). Type A behavior pattern and coronary disease risk: Update and critical evaluation. *American Journal of Epidemiology, 123*, 923–960.

Mattsen, M. E., & Herd, J. A. (1988). Cardiovascular disease. In E. Bleichman & K. Brownell (Eds.), *Handbook of behavioral medicine for women* (pp. 160–174). New York: Pergamon Press.

Mendes de Leon, C. F., Powell, L. H., & Kaplan, B. C. (1991). Changes in coronary-prone behaviors in the Recurrent Coronary Prevention Project. *Psychosomatic Medicine, 53*, 407–419.

Menninger, K. A., & Menninger, W. C. (1936). Psychoanalytic observations in cardiac disorders. *American Heart Journal, 11*, 10–11.

Miller, T. Q., Turner, C. W., Tindale, R. S., Posavac, E. J., & Dugoni, B. L. (1991). Reasons for the trend toward null findings in research on Type A behavior. *Psychological Bulletin, 110*, 469–485.

National Center for Health Statistics. (1989). *Health, United States, 1988*. (USD-HHS [THS] 89-1232). Washington, DC: U.S. Department of Health and Human Services.

Nunes, E. V., Frank, K. A., & Kornfield, D. S. (1987). Psychologic treatment for Type A behavior pattern and for coronary heart disease: A meta-analysis of the literature. *Psychosomatic Medicine, 48*, 159–173.

Osler, W. (1897). *Lectures on angina pectoris and allied states*. New York: Appleton & Co.

Powell, L. H. (1996). The hook: A metaphor for gaining control of emotional reactivity. In R. Allan & S. Scheidt (Eds.), *Heart and mind: The practice of cardiac psychology* (pp. 313–328). Washington, DC: American Psychological Association.

Powell, L. H., Mendes de Leon, C., Thoresen, C. E., Simon, S. S., Pattillo, J. R., & Kaplan, B. H. (1993). *Mechanisms of treatment effectiveness in the Recurrent Coronary Prevention Project.* Manuscript submitted for publication.

Powell, L. H., Simon, S. S., Bartzokis, T. C., Pattillo, J. R., & Thoresen, C. E. (1992). *Emotional arousability predicts sudden cardiac death in post-myocardial infarction men.* Unpublished manuscript, Rush–St. Luke's–Presbyterian Medical School, Chicago.

Powell, L. H., Slaker, L. A., Jones, B. A., Vaccarino, L. V., Thoresen, C. E., & Pattillo, J. R. (1993). Psychosocial predictors of mortality in 83 women with premature acute myocardial infarction. *Psychosomatic Medicine, 55,* 426–433.

Powell, L. H., & Thoresen, C. E. (1987). Small group treatment of Type A behavior. In J. A. Blumenthal & D. C. McKee (Eds.), *Applications in behavioral medicine and health psychology: A clinician's source book* (pp. 174–208). Sarasota, FL: Professional Resource Exchange.

Powell, L. H., & Thoresen, C. E. (1988). Effects of Type A behavioral counseling on severity of prior acute myocardial infarction on survival. *American Journal of Cardiology, 62,* 1159–1163.

Price, V. A. (1982). *Type A behavior pattern: A model for research and practice.* New York: Academic Press.

Price, V. A. (1988). Research and clinical issues in treating Type A behavior. In B. H. Houston & R. Snyder (Eds.), *Type A behavior pattern: Current research and future trends* (pp. 275–311). New York: Academic Press.

Ragland, D. R., & Brand, R. (1988a). Coronary heart disease mortality in the Western Collaborative Group Study. *American Journal of Epidemiology, 127,* 462–475.

Ragland, D. R., & Brand, R. (1988b). Type A behavior and mortality from coronary heart disease. *New England Journal of Medicine, 318,* 65–69.

Rahe, R. H., Ward, H. W., & Hayes, V. (1979). Brief group therapy in myocardial infarction rehabilitation: Three to four-year follow-up of a controlled trial. *Psychosomatic Medicine, 41,* 229–242.

Review Panel on Coronary-Prone Behavior and Coronary Heart Disease. (1981). Coronary-prone behavior and coronary heart disease: A critical review. *Circulation, 63,* 1199–1215.

Rosenman, R. H., Brand, R. J., Sholtz, R. I., & Friedman, M. (1976). Multivariate prediction of coronary heart disease during 8.5 year follow-up in the Western Collaborative Group Study. *American Journal of Cardiology, 37,* 903–910.

Rosenman, R. H., & Friedman, M. (1961). Association of specific behavior pattern in women with blood and cardiovascular findings. *Circulation, 24,* 1173–1184.

Rosenman, R. H., Swan, G. E., & Carmelli, D. (1988). Definition, assessment, and evolution of the Type A behavior pattern. In B. K. Houston & C. R. Snyder (Eds.), *Type A behavior patterns: Research, theory, and intervention* (pp. 8–31). New York: Wiley.

Shekelle, R. B., Hulley, S. B., Neston, J. D., Billings, J. H., Borboni, N. O., Gerace, T. A., Jacobs, D. R., Lasser, N. L., Mittlemark, M. B., & Stamler, J. (1985). The

MRFIT behavior pattern study: Type A behavior and incidence of coronary heart disease. *American Journal of Epidemiology, 122,* 559–570.

Spiegel, D., Bloom, J. R., Kraemer, H. C., & Gottheil, E. (1989). Effect of psychosocial treatment on survival of patients with metastatic breast cancer. *Lancet, 2,* 888–891.

Strube, M. J. (Ed.). (1990). *Type A behavior.* Corte Madera, CA: Select Press.

Sutherland, J. E., Pershy, V. W., & Brody, J. A. (1990). Proportionate mortality trends: 1950 through 1986. *Journal of American Medical Association, 264,* 3178–3184.

Thoresen, C. E. (in press). Spirituality and health: Some intriguing connections. In S. Roth-Romer, S. Kurpius Robinson, & C. Carmin (Eds.), *The emerging role of counseling psychology in health care.* New York: Norton.

Thoresen, C. E., & Graff-Low, K. (1990). Women and the Type A behavior pattern: Review and commentary. In M. Strube (Ed.), *Type A behavior* (pp. 117–133). Corte Madera, CA: Select Press.

Thoresen, C. E., & Graff-Low, K. (1994). Psychosocial interventions in female cardiovascular disease patients. In S. M. Czajkowski, D. R. Hill, & Y. B. Clarkson (Eds.), *Women, behavior, and cardiovascular disease* (NIH Publication No. 94-3309, pp. 329–342). Rockville, MD: National Institutes of Health.

Thoresen, C. E., & Mahoney, M. J. (1974). *Behavioral self-control.* New York: Holt, Rinehart & Winston.

Thoresen, C. E., & Pattillo, J. R. (1988). Exploring the Type A behavior pattern in children and adolescents. In B. K. Houston & C. R. Snyder (Eds.), *Type A behavior pattern: Research, theory and intervention* (pp. 98–145). New York: Wiley.

Thoresen, C. E., & Powell, L. H. (1983, August). *Cost-effectiveness in reducing morbidity and mortality in post-infarction patients: Some preliminary findings.* Paper presented at the annual meeting of the American Psychological Association, Anaheim, CA.

Thoresen, C. E., & Powell, L. H. (1992). Type A behavior pattern: New perspectives on theory, assessment and intervention. *Journal of Consulting and Clinical Psychology, 60,* 595–604.

Ulmer, D. K., & Schwartzburd, L. (1996). Treatment of time pathologies. In R. Allan & S. Scheidt (Eds.), *Heart and mind* (pp. 329–362). Washington, DC: American Psychological Association.

Van Egeren, L. F. (1991). A "success trap" theory of Type A behavior: Historical background. In M. Strube (Ed.), *Type A behavior* (pp. 45–58). Corte Madera, CA: Select Press.

Williams, R. B., Barefoot, J. C., & Shekelle, R. B. (1984). The health consequences of hostility. In M. A. Chesney & R. H. Rosenman (Eds.), *Anger, hostility and behavioral medicine* (pp. 173–186). New York: Hemisphere/McGraw-Hill.

Yusuf, S., Wittes, J., & Friedman, L. (1988). Overview of results of randomized clinical trials in heart disease, I. *Journal of American Medical Association, 269,* 2088–2093.

PART III

COPING WITH
LIFE-THREATENING ILLNESS

CHAPTER 4

Brief, Coping-Oriented Therapy for Patients with Malignant Melanoma

FAWZY I. FAWZY
NANCY W. FAWZY
CHRISTINE S. HYUN
JENNIFER G. WHEELER

The bad news is that there are currently more than 8 million Americans who have a history of cancer. The good news is that these 8 million are still alive and more than 4 million have survived for 5 years or longer (American Cancer Society, 1992). In the not too recent past, the focus for psychological and emotional support was on terminal care and bereavement. Today there is an encouraging trend toward helping people live with the psychosocial aspects of cancer. Much research has been done that helps us to understand the psychological distress that patients with cancer and their families experience (Weisman, 1979a, 1979b; Cohen, Cullen, & Martin, 1982). Five phases of the cancer experience each with its own particular concerns as well as a number of diagnosis specific psychosocial issues have been delineated. Reports have also appeared in the literature regarding differing interventions aimed at helping individuals to deal with the diagnosis and treatment of cancer (see Fawzy, Fawzy, Arndt, & Pasnau, 1995). The most exciting aspect of these reports is that some of these interventions may contribute significantly to both psychological and physical health outcome possibly via the immune system (Spiegel, Bloom, Kraemer, & Gottheil, 1989; Ornish et al., 1992; Greet, 1991; Fawzy et al. 1993). A short-term structured psychiatric intervention program consisting of health education, stress management, coping skills training, and psychological support is offered as a comprehensive, cohesive, and effective model of care for newly diagnosed patients with cancer.

PSYCHOSOCIAL PHASES

The issues that cancer patients struggle with can be divided into five phases: prediagnostic phase, diagnostic phase, initial treatment phase, recurrence phase, and terminal phase (Fawzy & Fawzy, 1982; Fawzy & Natterson, 1994). Within each phase lies normal/adaptive behavioral responses and abnormal/maladaptive behavioral responses.

Prediagnostic Phase

In the prediagnostic phase, an adaptive response includes fear of cancer based on real symptoms. A maladaptive response would be inappropriate preoccupation or hypervigilance over one's body.

Diagnostic Phase

The diagnosis of cancer often produces a profound psychological reaction. Shock and disbelief are the most common initial responses in the diagnostic phase. Immediate denial or, more appropriately, minimization of the fact may be a protective mechanism against overwhelming anxiety, allowing the patient to gradually comprehend the painful news. Anger (sometimes directed toward the physical or family members), sadness, depression, and personal grief may follow. Usually there is a gradual acceptance of reality. Anxiety, helplessness/hopelessness, guilt, insomnia, irritability, and inability to concentrate are normal throughout this time. Feelings of persecution ("Why me?") are also common. The degree and quality of this perturbation are dependent on many factors such as personality, coping style, experiences with previous stresses in one's life, social support, attitude, and knowledge about the treatment and prognosis of their particular cancer. Maladaptive responses to the cancer diagnosis include excessive denial, despair, depression, and seeking out alternative therapy. These maladaptive responses are especially significant if they cause a person to delay or even to refuse standard medical treatment.

Treatment Phase

Depending on the type of treatment involved, cancer treatment brings different reactions. Surgical procedures often generate feelings of fear and grief. Maladaptive responses include avoidance, seeking out alternative therapy, postoperative reactive depression, or severe, prolonged postoperative grief reaction. Chemotherapy may cause anticipatory anxiety, changes in body image, and feelings of altruism especially if done as part of a clinical trial. Abnormal responses to chemotherapy include delirium/organic brain syndrome and isolation-induced psychotic disturbances. Radiation therapy may bring up fears about abandonment, the machine, and side effects. If the fear of radiotherapy is severe, maladaptive responses may include such psychotic-like responses as frank delusions and hallucinations.

Recurrence Phase

The psychological reaction to recurrence of cancer is similar to the feelings encountered during the diagnostic phase (i.e., feelings of shock, disbelief, denial, anxiety, anger, and/or depression). However, as a result of the failure of curative therapy, the situation may be more difficult for the patient. Trust in health care personnel is likely to diminish significantly and seeking out alternative therapies is even more likely at this point.

Terminal Phase

Once patients have reached this phase, they are usually aware of the progressive and irreversible nature of the cancer. Fear is the most common feeling at this stage. This includes fear of abandonment by the health care team; fear of loss of composure; bodily function, and dignity; fear of pain; and fear of leaving unfinished business.

PSYCHOSOCIAL ISSUES

In terms of identifying the psychosocial issues of cancer, the most frequently studied group has been women with breast cancer. Breast cancer patients have been found to manifest greater anxiety and depression than general surgery patients (Maguire, 1976) or women with benign breast tumors (Maguire et al., 1978; Morris, Greer, & White, 1977). Worden and Weisman (1977) reported that among 40 newly diagnosed breast cancer patients, 20% were notably depressed based on psychological tests and clinical interviews. In addition to increased anxiety and depression, other life changes have been described in this patient population. For instance, Maguire et al. (1978) found that mastectomy patients experienced more sexual problems than did a control group of benign breast tumor patients at 4 and 12 months postoperatively. Meyerowitz (1980), after comprehensively reviewing the literature on psychological correlates of breast cancer, summarizes the typical responses of this patient group as "a) some degree of depression, anxiety and/or anger; b) disruption in everyday life patterns, including marital and/or sexual relationships; and, c) considerable fear regarding the danger and mutilation of cancer and mastectomy" (p. 114).

Other cancer patient groups have not been studied nearly as extensively from a psychosocial viewpoint, nor has the impact of other types of cancer treatment been investigated thoroughly. Some work has been done recently on the effects of chemotherapy (e.g., Meyerowitz, Sparks, & Speers, 1979; Nerenz, Leventhal, & Love, 1983) and radiation therapy (e.g., Cassileth, Volckmar, & Goodman, 1980; Forester, Kornfield, & Fleiss, 1978; Holland, Rowland, Lebovitz, & Rusalem, 1979). Larger studies, involving a broader spectrum of patients, include those by Gordon et al. (1980) and Worden and Weisman (1977).

Gordon et al. (1980) followed 308 breast, lung, and melanoma patients through the first 6 months of their disease. The most often noted problems at the time of initial hospitalization were in the area of worry about the disease itself. Negative affect became the predominant concern in the period follow- ing discharge. Later, at 3 and 6 months postdischarge, a broader array of prob- lems was noted such as physical discomfort, concern about medical treat- ment, dissatisfaction with health care service, lack of mobility, financial concerns, family and social problems, worry about the disease, negative af- fect, and body image difficulties. Worden and Weisman (1977) found that site of cancer was a significant factor in adjustment. Different site groups (lung, breast, colon, melanoma, Hodgkin's) had peak distress periods at dif- ferent times during the first 3 months of their illness.

Identifying and prioritizing the psychosocial needs of cancer patients are important steps in helping cancer patients improve the quality of their lives. A recent study (Liang, Dunn, Gorman, & Stuart-Harris, 1990) asked 188 cancer patients (129 female, 59 male) with various solid tumors to rank areas of need. The patients ranked the areas of worry in the following ascending order: family issues, dealing with emotional stress, getting information, mon- ey problems, work issues, social life, sex life, and dealing with hospital staff. Patients with head and neck or breast cancer reported the most distress and females reported more distress than males.

Another recent study (Dunkel-Schetter, Feinstein, Taylor, & Falke, 1992) found that among 603 cancer patients, fear or uncertainty about the future was the number one concern (41%), followed by limited physical abil- ity (24%) and pain (12%). This study also assessed how patients coped with cancer and identified five coping patterns: seeking/using social support, fo- cusing on the positive, distancing, cognitive escape/avoidance, and behav- ioral escape/avoidance. Interestingly, specific concerns about cancer (e.g., fear, limited physical ability, and pain) were not associated with how patients coped. However, perceptions about the stressfulness of the situation were sig- nificantly associated with more coping through use of social support, cogni- tive escape/avoidance, and behavioral escape/avoidance.

TYPES OF INTERVENTIONS

Advances have been made in the field of psychosocial therapy for oncology patients and others who are medically ill (Fawzy & Fawzy, 1982; Fawzy, Pasnau, Wolcott, & Ellsworth, 1983; Fawzy et al., 1993, 1995; Cohen et al., 1982). Different intervention models have been utilized as part of the psychosocial response to the needs of cancer patients and those with other catastrophic disease (Bloom, Ross, & Burnell, 1978). The goals of these interventions, according to Holland (1989), are to decrease feelings of alienation by talking to others in a similar situation, reduce anxiety about the treatments, assist in clarifying misperception and misinformation, and lessen feelings of isolation, helplessness, and being neglected by others. Interventions are designed to help the person to feel less helpless and hopeless and perhaps to take more responsibility for getting well or for complying with medical regimens. The public is well aware of many psychosocial therapeutic interventions for cancer patients, and with the popularity of some approaches (such as hypnosis and guided imagery), patients may often specifically request such services.

The four most common forms of psychosocial intervention for medically ill patients are education, behavioral training, and supportive individual and group therapy. Examples of each of these intervention categories are reviewed here.

Education

In general, educational interventions are often insufficient for changing attitudes and improving coping (Zimbardo & Ebbeson, 1970). One study (Gordon et al., 1980) examined the effects of a program of education combined with counseling on 157 patients with different types of cancer. Evaluations conducted 3 and 6 months after hospital discharge revealed that there was a decrease in depression, hostility, and anxiety, as well as a greater return to activities of daily living and activities outside the home than with 151 patients in two control groups. Education alone failed to show the same benefits.

Pruitt et al. (1993) randomized radiation therapy patients with mixed diagnoses to either a three-session intervention or a standard control group. The education consisted of information about radiation therapy and cancer, coping strategies, and communication skills. Knowledge levels were unchanged in both groups, and depression was the only measure of affective state found to improve.

Brandberg et al. (1994) investigated knowledge and satisfaction with knowledge of malignant melanoma patients participating in an information program. After the program, patients in the information group demonstrated a higher level of knowledge and were significantly more satisfied with their information as compared to controls. No differences were found on psychological and psychosomatic variables.

However, several education programs have shown more positive results. Ali and Khalil (1989) assessed the effects of a psychoeducational intervention program on reducing anxiety among a group of patients with bladder cancer. The experimental group showed significantly less anxiety at both 3 days postoperation and just before hospital discharge compared to the control group.

Finally, Richardson, Shelton, Krailo, and Levine (1990) randomly assigned newly diagnosed hematology patients to either a control group or one of three educational intervention groups. Using regression analysis, it was concluded that low severity of disease, assignment to an educational program (any one), plus high allopurinol compliance were predictive of increased survival in patients with newly diagnosed hematological malignancy.

Behavioral Training

Behavioral training utilizes a variety of techniques including hypnosis, guided imagery or visualization, relaxation training, and biofeedback. Relaxation training and hypnosis have been described as effective in reducing nausea, emotional distress, and physiological arousal following chemotherapy (Burish & Lyles, 1981; Burish, Snyder, & Jenkins, 1991).

Bridge, Benson, Pietroni, and Priest (1988) conducted a randomized study to determine whether relaxation and imagery training could decrease the level of distress in early-stage (I and II) breast cancer patients. The intervention program lasted 6 weeks and was divided into three groups: (1) a control group in which patients were encouraged to talk about themselves, (2) a relaxation group in which patients were taught muscle relaxation techniques, and (3) a relaxation and imagery group in which patients were taught both muscle relaxation and guided imagery. In addition, both the second and third groups were given cassette tapes repeating the intervention instructions and told to practice once a day. At the end of the 6 weeks, there was significantly lower total mood disturbance in the intervention groups (with the relaxation and imagery group reporting less disturbance than the relaxation-only group) than in the control group.

Gruber et al. (1993) randomly assigned breast cancer patients to either an immediate treatment group, which received relaxation, guided imagery, and biofeedback training, or a delayed treatment control group. Pre- and posttreatment measures included blood samples, psychological testing, and a computerized psychophysiological stress evaluation. Results showed that the only psychological difference was in anxiety levels, which were reduced shortly after each group began the intervention. Immune system parameters were significantly improved and directly correlated with the behavioral interventions.

Finally, Baider, Uziely, and De-Nour (1994), studied the effects of progressive muscle relaxation and guided imagery training on cancer patients. This study found notable improvement on the Brief Symptom Inventory and the Impact of Events Scale for all patients who completed the behavioral intervention. This improvement was maintained up to the 6-month follow-up period. This finding supports the findings of other investigators who showed that psychological improvement was maintained long after the interventions were completed.

Supportive Therapy: Groups

The stresses of having a disease such as cancer and the mode of its treatment create the need for emotional support. Support groups are frequently employed in psychosocial interventions. There is some evidence to suggest that social support groups are associated with better psychosocial adjustment to illness (Fawzy, Wellisch, & Yager, 1977; Fawzy et al., 1990a, 1993; Gordon et al., 1980; Spiegel, Bloom, & Yalom, 1981; Bloom, 1982; Spiegel & Bloom, 1983; Cain, Kohorn, Quinlan, Latimer, & Schwartz, 1986; Cunningham & Tocco, 1989).

A prospective randomized study by Greer et al. (1992) found that adjuvant psychological therapy improved psychological distress among 174 cancer patients. The authors looked at anxiety, depression, and adjustment in patients with primary diagnosis or first recurrence of cancer. Compared to the control patients, the experimental patients scored significantly higher in fighting spirit and significantly lower in anxiety, anxious preoccupation, helplessness, and fatalism. Some of the effects were still observable at 4-month follow-up.

Another randomized study examined the effects of an early intervention program (immediately following diagnosis) versus later intervention (4-month delay) in newly diagnosed cancer patients and followed these patients for a 12-month period (Edgar, Rosenberger, & Nowlls, 1992). The intervention consisted of five 1-hour sessions with a nurse in which problem-solving techniques, goal setting, cognitive reappraisal, relaxation training, and effective use of resources were taught. The intervention program, which was developed from a review of the literature and the authors' own clinical experiences, sought to decrease distress in cancer patients by increasing knowledge, enhancing personal control, strengthening coping skills, and reducing emotional arousal. No significant differences were found between the early intervention or the later intervention until 8 months follow-up, where the later intervention group ($n = 102$) scored significantly lower in depression, anxiety, and worry, and felt in more control than the early intervention group (n = 103). At 12-month follow-up, the later intervention group continued to worry less than the early intervention group.

Spiegel et al. (1981) reported improved mood, increased coping, and less fear in female breast cancer patients who participated in group therapy once a week for a year when compared to randomly selected controls. The weekly discussion sections focused on practical coping problems associated with terminal illness, feelings and attitudes toward death, and interpersonal relationships with family, friends, and physicians. Patients were assessed at 4-month intervals for a 1-year period. In a 10-year follow-up, the authors found that patients in the experimental group had increased survival time (36.6 months) compared to the patients in the control group (18.9 months).

Cella, Sarafian, Snider, Yellin, and Winicour (1993) detailed an 8-week support group for cancer patients in a local community. There was no random selection or a control group in this study. As expected, self-reported quality of life improved significantly by the final session, compared to reports completed at the start of the intervention. Community and peer support was noted by participants as the most helpful aspect of the program and the group evaluations showed high satisfaction levels in all areas.

Berglund, Boland, Gustaffson, and Sjoden (1994) established a prospective randomized study with cancer patients who took part in a 7-week rehabilitation program. The intervention focused on "starting again" and consisted of physical training, coping skills, and information. Subjects in the experimental condition improved significantly in physical training, physical strength, fighting spirit, body image, sufficient information, and decreased sleeping problems when compared to control patients. All three goals of the intervention were met, and results indicated that the "starting again" program has many beneficial effects for cancer patients.

Finally, Cunningham, Edmonds, Jenkins, and Lockwood (1995) compared two different formats of a brief, group psychoeducational program for cancer patients. Patients were randomly assigned to either a standard (six weekly 2-hour sessions) intervention or a "weekend-intensive" intervention group. At 19 weeks following the intervention, the two formats were found to have comparable effects on mood and quality of life. Quality-of-life improvement appeared to be somewhat greater for the standard 6-week intervention group.

Supportive Therapy: Individual Counseling

There is some evidence for the value of one-on-one supportive counseling for patients with cancer. Linn, Linn, and Harris (1982) randomly assigned 120 men with end-stage cancer (various primary sites) to an intervention condition (ongoing, client-centered supportive therapy) or to a control condition (evaluation only). Patients were assessed before assignment to treatment arm and at 1, 3, 6, and 12 months. Measures included quality-of-life variables (depression, alienation, life satisfaction, and self-esteem), functional status, and survival time. Functional status and survival did not differ between groups, but patients receiving counseling showed significantly better quality-of-life scores at 3 months. Among those who survived, these differences held up through the 1-year follow-up. These findings are important because quality-of-life issues are key concerns for terminal patients.

Moorey and colleagues (1994) completed a 1-year follow-up of patients with cancer who had received individual adjuvant psychological therapy (i.e., a brief cognitive-behavioral treatment). The experimental patients exhibited less anxiety and depression than controls at 1 year following treatment.

Fawzy (1996) investigated the efficacy of a psychoeducational nursing intervention to enhance coping and affective state in newly diagnosed malignant melanoma patients. The intervention consisted of 3 hours of individualized teaching and emotional support by an oncology nurse and included health education, stress management, and coping skills training. At 3-month follow-up, patients in the intervention group demonstrated less psychological distress and decreases in Brief Symptom Index somatization and were using less ineffective passive resignation coping strategies than the control group.

As interesting as these studies are, much more research is needed to clearly identify which modalities or combination of modalities, directed toward what outcomes, with which patients, and administered by whom, are effective. It is clear that each of these intervention modalities has something to offer in helping individuals to deal with their diagnosis and treatment. It appears that such interventions can have a positive effect on coping, affective state, and overall quality of life. It is also being hypothesized that there may be positive correlations between coping, affective state, and certain immune system parameters which could in turn effect disease states. Although this field of study is still in its infancy, some interesting information has emerged.

COPING AND THE IMMUNE SYSTEM

Ader (1981) suggests the possibility that coping styles or personality attributes may mediate changes in immune function, thereby influencing morbidity and mortality. For example, Pettingale, Greer, and Tee (1977) reported higher levels of serum IgA (associated with metastatic spread) in breast cancer patients showing extreme suppression of anger compared with "normals." A recent study by Levy, Herberman, Malvish, Schlien, and Lippman (1985) suggests that breast cancer patients who exhibit passivity and depression ("poor copers") have decreased levels of spontaneous (natural killer, or NK) cytotoxicity and a higher rate of tumor metastasis. In an experimental study, writing about (i.e., expressing) emotionally traumatic events that had not previously been disclosed to others was associated with increased proliferative capacity in response to the mitogen phytohemagglutinin (PHA) (Pennebaker, Kiecolt-Glaser, & Glaser, 1988). A study of individuals with genital herpes showed that low use of problem-oriented coping and high use of more passive avoidant strategies to deal with adverse life situations over a 6-month period were associated with low CD8 levels and a high rate of herpes recurrence (Kemeny, Cohen, Zegans, & Conant, 1989).

STRESS, AFFECTIVE STATE, AND THE IMMUNE SYSTEM

Research studies have documented a relationship between exposure to various forms of stressful life experience and changes in the immune system in both animals and humans. Human studies have measured the impact of both induced and naturally occurring stressors on the immune system. Changes in measures of immune function have been detected following exposure to *major* stressful events such as spousal bereavement or marital disruption. Bartrop, Luckhurst, Lazarus, Kiloh, and Penny (1977) reported significantly decreased *in vitro* cell proliferation in response to stimulation by the mitogens PHA and concanavalin A (CON A) in bereaved spouses at 6 weeks. In a prospective study of 15 spouses of women with advanced breast cancer, Schleifer, Keller, Camerino, Thompson, and Stein (1983) showed that there was a significant depression in response to PHA, CON A, and Pokeweed (PWM) mitogens during the first 2 months following the death of a spouse compared with prebereavement levels. Irwin, Daniels, Bloom, Smith, and Weiner (1987) reported that bereaved women showed reduced NK activity and hypercortisolemia as compared to controls. Kiecolt-Glaser et al. (1987a, 1988) conducted two studies looking at marital disruption and immunity. In the first study, marital disruption among women was associated with significantly poorer proliferation response to PHA and CON A, significantly lower percentages of NK cells and helper cells, and significantly higher antibody titers to Epstein–Barr virus (EBV). In the second study, separated/divorced men were more distressed and lonely. They also reported significantly more recent illnesses than did married men. These individuals showed significantly poorer values on antibody titers to two herpesviruses. Individuals experiencing more *minor* stresses such as medical student examinations have been found to have significantly lower levels of NK activity, fewer NK cells, and lowered production of gamma interferon (Kiecolt-Glaser et al., 1984a). Dorian and colleagues (1982) showed a transiently elevated number of T and B lymphocytes and impaired plaque-forming cells and mitogen responsiveness in a highly stressed group of trainees prior to their exams. These values normalized shortly after the exams were over. One notable study (Kiecolt-Glaser et al., 1987b) on the family caregivers of Alzheimer's disease victims showed that the *chronically* stressed caregivers had significantly lower percentages of total and CD4 (helper-inducer) T-lymphocytes than controls as well as lower CD4/CD8 (suppressor/cytotoxic) T-cell ratios. They also had higher anti-body titers to EBV, while the percentages of NK cells and CD8 T-lympho-cytes were not significantly different. Subjects exposed to experimentally in-duced combat-like stress (77-hour vigil) showed a heightened ability of their lymphocytes to produce interferon in response to sendai virus but reduced phagocytosis (Palmblad et al., 1976). In another example of induced stress (elective inguinal herniorrhaphy), Linn and Jensen (1983) reported that re-sponses to PHA and CON A were significantly lower than controls at 5 days following operation and responses to CON A were still significantly de-creased 30 days postoperatively.

A number of studies investigating affective states (e.g., depressed mood) and affective disorders (e.g., major depression) in relation to immune status have been done (Albrecht, Helderman, Schlesser, & Rush, 1985; Kronfol et al., 1983, Kronfol, Turner, Nasrallah, & Winokur, 1984; Kronfol, 1987; Krueger, Levy, Cathcart, Fox, & Black, 1984; Linn, Linn, & Jensen, 1984; Stein, Keller, & Schleifer, 1987). For example, Schleifer and associates (1984) found that hospitalized patients with a diagnosis of major depressive disorder had lymphocytes with a diminished capacity to proliferate in re-sponse to mitogens such as PHA when compared to matched controls. How-ever, this group of investigators was unable to replicate these findings in a larger, more heterogeneous sample (Schleifer, Keller, Bond, Cohen, & Stein, 1989). Overall, studies have failed to provide consistent evidence of im-munological changes associated with major depression. A few studies have reported associations between normal affective states such as depressed mood and loneliness and aspects of the immune system such as decreased percent-age of CD8 cells (Kemeny et al., 1989) and decreased NK cell activity (Glaser, Kiecolt-Glaser, George, Speicher, & Holliday, 1985; Kiecolt-Glaser et al., 1984b).

PSYCHOSOCIAL INTERVENTION EFFECTS
ON THE IMMUNE SYSTEM

Immune function has been reported to have been enhanced by psychosocial interventions in the form of hypnotic/relaxation training for medical stu-dents exposed to examination stress (Kiecolt-Glaser et al., 1986) and relax-ation training in the elderly (Kiecolt-Glaser et al., 1985). Gruber, Hall, Hersh, and Dubois (1988), in a pilot study of relaxation and imagery for can-cer patients, found increases in mitogen response, NK cell activity, Inter-leukin II, erythrocyte-Rosette Assay, and serum levels of IgG and IgM. Several other studies involving hypnotic suggestion, guided imagery, and/or conditioning suggest possible psychological modulation of delayed hypersensitivity reactions in humans. Delayed hypersensitivity (sometimes referred to as a Type IV reaction) is primarily a T-cell-mediated response. Cutaneous testing in previously sensitized individuals is a well-established method for monitoring the Type IV reaction (Thestrup-Pedersen, 1975). Black, Humphrey, and Niven (1963) showed that the Mantoux (purified protein derivative of tuberculin) reaction may be inhibited by suggestions given during hypnosis. Smith and McDaniel (1983) gave tuberculin-positive volunteers monthly injections of tuberculin from a colored vial in one arm and saline from a different colored vial in the other arm. For 5 months the contents of the colored vials were held constant. In the sixth month the colors of the vials were switched and the tuberculin reaction was significantly reduced but saline did not produced a false positive. Zachariae, Bjerring, and Arendt-Nielsen (1989), in a well-controlled study, were the first to show that the Type IV reaction could be enhanced as well as diminished via guided imagery during hypnosis. All these studies suggest a connection between the central nervous system and the immune system.

Examination of immune cell differentiation and function is of particular interest in cancer patients undergoing psychological intervention therapy. The body's defense against cancer is thought to have a major immunological component, yet the stress and depression most cancer patients experience during their illness may well suppress immunity (Fauman, 1982; Klein & Klein, 1985). Alleviation of these negative psychological factors may act to enhance crucial immunological mechanisms or at least to attenuate the adverse effects of stress and depression.

STRUCTURED PSYCHIATRIC INTERVENTION MODEL

Previous research indicates that some individual types of therapies had some effects but the variance accounted for by each of these therapies alone was small. Therefore, based on a review of the lierature and our clinical experience, we selected specific portions of those interventions that were found to be effective and appropriate and combined them. This combined intervention was first used in a group of 50 gay men with acquired immune deficiency syndrome (AIDS) (Fawzy, Namir, & Wolcott, 1989). All participants were within 3 months of diagnosis, with 72% being diagnosed with Kaposi's sarcoma and 28% with opportunistic infections. Data were gathered and analyzed on these 50 gay men with AIDS before and after a 10-week structured group intervention aimed at reducing psychological distress and improving coping skills.

The subjects were divided into groups consisting of 7 to 10 participants who met for 2 hours each session for 10 weeks. In each group session, according to a preset format, subjects were taught stress management techniques, relaxation training, problem-solving skills, and effective coping methods. A series of pictures illustrating common dilemmas were shown to the patients to initiate discussion that would lead to effective solutions to the problems. This approach included learning to problem solve, practicing the process in the group, applying the approach to problems, and discussing the resolution of the problems. In addition, members received and gave emotional support to each other.

The group interventions had an impact on the mood states of the AIDS patients. Group participants had lower mean scores on every scale of the Profile of Mood States (anxiety, depression, anger, lack of vigor, fatigue, and confusion) following the 10-week intervention than they did prior to the interventions. In addition, the group interventions were likely to help patients use more active coping methods and less avoidant coping ones.

The intervention model was then used for a group of newly diagnosed malignant melanoma patients who had undergone standard surgical treatment of their tumors (consisting of wide excision of the primary site and regional lymphadenectomy when indicated (Fawzy et al., 1990a, 1990b). The short- and long-term effects of the intervention on psychological states and immunological functions were measured. Patients were assigned to either a control group receiving routine medical care or an experimental group receiving the same kind of routine medical care plus the psychoeducational group intervention below.

PSYCHOEDUCATIONAL INTERVENTION

The experimental patients participated in a 6-week structured group intervention that was tailored to encompass health education, stress management modalities, and coping skills. Groups of 7 to 10 patients met for 1½ hours weekly for 6 weeks. The group meetings, which were primarily led by a psychiatrist, were structured yet supportive.

Health Education

The health education component of the intervention is composed of easily understood health care information specific to the diagnosis of skin cancer. Melanoma patients are taught about their disease, including information on risk factors that appear to be influencing the dramatic increase in skin cancer. These factors include ultraviolet radiation, skin pigmentation, genetic factors, hormonal factors, and immunological factors. These risk factors are further delineated in the intervention manual. In addition to educational information, patients learn about preventive measures to avoid future sun exposure by reducing ultraviolet radiation exposure, by wearing protective clothing, and by using sunscreens. Finally, warning signs and the terms and definitions of malignant melanoma are presented. A pretest at the beginning of the health education section helps the patients to assess their level of knowledge and to use as a guide to their reading. An identical posttest is provided at the end to allow the patients to determine their own level of progress. Answers to these tests are provided in the back of the manual. In addition, booklets are provided from the American Cancer Society and the National Cancer Institute on nutrition and the immune system.

Stress Management

The stress management component is divided into two main sections. First, the patients are taught about stress awareness. Awareness has two subcategories: identifying the sources of stress and identifying the personal reactions to stress, including the physiological, psychological, and behavioral reactions. The second component of stress awareness is the actual management of stress. This has four subcomponents. The first two involve eliminating or modifying the source of stress through problem solving. The third subcomponent is changing the attitude or perception toward the stressor by trying to look at the situation in a "new light." The last subcomponent involves changing the physical reaction to the stressor through relaxation response. Patients are taught simple relaxation exercises (e.g., progressive muscle relaxation followed by guided imagery of a pleasant scene) that take approximately 15 to 20 minutes to perform. Patients are encouraged to use these techniques on a daily basis (to help them relax, to learn what a state of relaxation feels like, and to learn how to achieve it) and to help them fall asleep at night or to return to sleep if they should wake up during the night. In addition, patients are taught how to use an abbreviated form of this exercise when they find themselves in an acutely stressful situation. Stress monitor questionnaires covering signs and symptoms of stress as well as sources of stress are included in the intervention manual, as are worksheets for the patients to increase awareness about their stress.

Coping Skills

An important aim of the coping skills component is to increase the patient's awareness of what Weisman (1979a) termed the "key ingredients of good coping": (1) optimism (the expectation of positive change), (2) practicality (learning that options and alternatives are seldom completely exhausted), (3) flexibility (changing strategies to reflect the changing nature of perceived problems), and (4) resourcefulness (developing the ability to call on additional information and support to strengthen coping).

In the coping skills component of the intervention, patients are first taught the five steps of problem solving:

1. *Relaxation.* Patients are encouraged to use the relaxation techniques and collect their thoughts before launching into problem solving. This helps to bring the emotional arousal down to a level that is better for optimal performance.
2. *Identification of the problem.* Identifying the real problem may not always be clear. Patients are taught to separate out the presenting problem from the underlying problem. For example, a patient may state that he hates his job. The real problem may be related to numerous things associated with the job, including the boss, the coworkers, the type of job, or even the commute necessary to get to the job. Patients learn to identify the issues that affect them and to distinguish content (the matter requiring action) from process (feelings about the problem).
3. *Brainstorming.* This step involves having patients list all possible solutions, however practical or ridiculous. This process may help to reduce tension by generating possible steps for action. After the list is complete, patients are instructed to consider the positive and negative implications of each possible solution.
4. *Selection and implementation of an appropriate strategy.* With the list developed from the brainstorming step, patients select and implement the solution that appears to be the most feasible and the most likely to succeed.
5. *Evaluation.* Patients are then encouraged to determine whether it is effective or not. If it is not effective, patients are taught to return to step 1 and proceed through the process once more.

Patients are then introduced to the concept of coping methods and strategies. Three general theoretical methods of coping have been identified; the first two are helpful; the third is usually detrimental:

1. *Active–behavioral methods.* One tries to improve some aspect of the illness by active means such as exercise, use of relaxation techniques, and frequent collaborative consultations with the physician.
2. *Active–cognitive methods.* One tries to understand the illness and accepts its effect on life by focusing on positive rather than negative changes that have occurred since the onset of illness. In general, patients who use active–behavioral and active–cognitive coping methods report more positive affective states, higher levels of self-esteem, and fewer physical symptoms.
3. *Avoidance methods.* One avoids being with others, hides feelings

about the illness, and refuses to think about the illness. Those patients who use more avoidance coping usually have higher levels of psychological distress such as anxiety, indirectly expressed anger, depression, and lower quality of life.

Cognitive and behavioral responses (which have the best association with improved psychological health) may be even more specifically defined as the following strategies (Namir, Wolcott, Fawzy, & Alumbaugh, 1987):

1. *Active–positive strategies*, which involve increasing patients' involvement in their own care, planning action, and enjoying life "one day at a time."
2. *Active–expressive strategies*, which include talking with others to gain information or to offer support to others with cancer.
3. *Active–reliance strategies*, which involve seeking a friend or relative for instrumental or emotional help or a physician for intervention.
4. *Cognitive–positive strategies*, which include seeking understanding of the illness, finding some meaning attached to having the illness, and thinking about positive changes.
5. *Distraction strategies*, which consist of going out more socially or doing something nice for one's self.

The cognitive and behavioral strategies that generally do not result in making people feel better come under the avoidance category and include:

1. *Cognitive–passive strategies*, which involve ruminating or daydreaming about better times and doing nothing in the hope that would make a difference.
2. *Avoidance–solitary strategies*, which include avoiding others, taking drugs, and eating, smoking, or sleeping more than usual.
3. *Passive–resignation strategies*, which involve preparing for "the worst," keeping feelings secret from others, and letting the physician take all responsibility for decisions and care.

Patients are given a more complete list of strategies that people use to cope with stress. Some are identified as being more effective than others for people who are coping with serious illnesses. The patients are told that, in general, a specific strategy is not good or bad but that its effectiveness is determined by the situation. They are also told that the strategies identified as less or not effective can occasionally be used and be effective (e.g., yelling to ventilate emotions) but if used to the exclusion of all else can cause more problems than they solve.

The final part of the coping skills component involves integrating the stress management and problem-solving techniques with the information on coping methods and strategies and applying these to specific situations. The method used was modeled after Project Omega (Sobel & Worden, 1982; Weisman, Worden, & Sobel, 1980), which teaches positive coping strategies as a way of diminishing stress and enhancing coping. It included learning an approach to problem solving, practicing the approach theoretically, and applying the approach to personal problems via a series of pictures. The researchers at Project Omega developed and evaluated problem-solving interventions for cancer patients. They found highly distressed patients used fewer coping strategies, employed less effective ones, had more problems and concerns, and achieved poor resolutions when attempting to solve critical illness-related concerns (Weisman et al., 1980; Sobel & Worden, 1982). The authors compared two interventions, one involving clarification, emotional expression, and individual problem identification with a cognitive skills training intervention. Both interventions were effective in reducing emotional distress during a 6-month follow-up period when compared to controls.

A new series of pictures illustrating 10 common problems/situations encountered by cancer patients was developed (Fawzy et al., 1990a). Pertinent psychosocial issues include loneliness/isolation, fear/apprehension, physician–patient relationships, changes in body image, sexuality/personal contact, communication, social alienation, and depression. Each situation is represented by two different pictures. The first picture generally shows the patient coping ineffectively and the second picture depicts more effective coping behavior. The first picture is introduced and the patients are asked to identify the negative coping methods or strategies. Further discussion is encouraged that, it is hoped, will clarify why such coping is ineffective and will generate more positive options. The second picture is then introduced with the patient coping more effectively. Correct coping techniques identified by the group discussion are validated and reinforced. Any effective techniques not thought of by the group members are presented and explained by the group leader. The patients are then encouraged to apply these theoretical pictured situations to their own real-life situations. Patients are given a manual containing the coping scenarios and written descriptions of the situations and the coping techniques involved. They keep these manuals, allowing them to review the scenarios again as needed and to share them with significant others who may not have attended the meetings.

Figure 4.1 is an example of what one coping scenario (the physician–patient relationship) looks like in the manual. The first picture describes the patient's fear and anxiety about his diagnosis and about his relationship with his physician. Despite many questions and concerns, the patient avoids dealing with his condition and keeps his feelings locked inside. He relinquishes all decision-making power to his physician, thereby increasing the level of

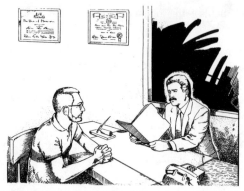

Steve has many fears and concerns about his condition. However, he has a very hard time talking with his doctor. His doctor seems distant and remote. Steve thinks he understands what the doctor tells him but when he gets home he does not remember what was said or realizes that he really did not understand. At home, Steve thinks of questions to ask his doctor but once he gets there he cannot remember what it was he was going to say. He also thinks the doctor will think he is stupid for asking about things that the doctor has already explained. As a result, Steve keeps his thoughts and feelings to himself and trusts his doctor to know what is best and to make all the decisions about his care. However, Steve is feeling more and more anxious about his condition.

What kind of coping is Steve using?

Steve is avoiding dealing with the problem directly. He is keeping his feelings to himself and giving up all decision-making powers to his doctor instead of establishing a collaborative relationship between them. He is being very solitary and passive.

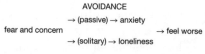

AVOIDANCE

→ (passive) → anxiety

fear and concern → feel worse

→ (solitary) → loneliness

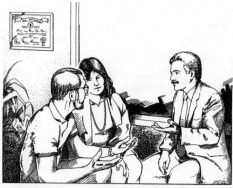

Steve finally talks to his wife, Susan, about how anxious he is and the trouble he has talking to his doctor. Susan suggests that they make a list of his questions and that they go see the doctor together. With Susan providing support, Steve is able to tell the doctor about his feelings and to ask his questions. Once the doctor realizes how Steve is feeling he takes extra time to reassure him and answer all the questions. The doctor also encourages Steve to ask more questions and even the same questions again if feels he needs more explanation. The doctor says that they would both feel better if they made decisions about Steve's treatment together. Steve feels much less anxious after this visit. He has a sense of being more in control of his life, and he feels that a positive supportive alliance has been established between himself and his doctor.

What kind of coping is Steve using now?

Steve is now using three forms of active–behavioral coping. He is becoming actively and positively involved by forming a plan of action (making a list, getting wife's support, confronting the doctor). In talking to both his wife and the doctor he is actively expressing his feelings and actively relying on their help in dealing with the problems.

ACTIVE–BEHAVIORAL

→ (active–positive) → sense of control

fear and concern → feel better

→ (active–expressive) → ventilation of feelings

→ (active–reliance) → sense of support and hope

FIGURE 4.1. Coping scenario example of a doctor–patient relationship.

anxiety and loneliness. The second picture describes a positive, collaborative relationship between the patient and his physician. Instead of keeping his thoughts and feelings inside, the patient expresses his concerns and fears to his physician. The patient writes down his questions so that he will remember to ask his doctor and brings his significant other for support. The patient is actively involved with his medical care thereby increasing his sense of control and reducing his anxiety level.

Psychological Support

Psychological support is inherent throughout the intervention and is initiated with an introductory talk describing the normal assumptive world, the forward-life trajectory of most people, and the way in which a life-threatening illness interrupts this forward-life trajectory (see Figures 4.2 and 4.3). The underlying philosophy is that with the proper medical and psychiatric treatment, a new assumptive world can be developed and the forward-life trajectory resumed (see Figure 4.4). The introductory talk ends with an analogy of how a person's support resources are similar to a building's support columns. Just as a building needs four support columns to stand, so too does a person have four sources of support. There are self, family and friends, coworkers and/or schoolmates, and religion (Figure 4.5).

Self refers to the positive facets of a person that he or she brings to an experience. These include personality, successful past experiences, coping abilities, and positive attitudes toward life. Family and friends are significant sources of both instrumental and emotional social support. Recent literature has shown the importance of this type of support to an individual facing an illness. Coworkers and/or schoolmates can also be a valuable source of sup-

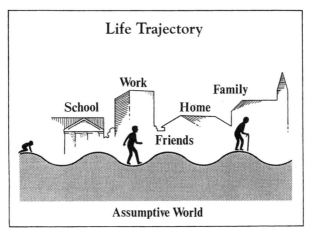

FIGURE 4.2. The normal assumptive world and forward life trajectory.

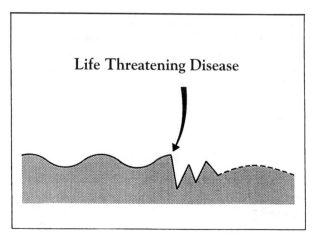

FIGURE 4.3. Interruption of the normal assumptive world and forward life trajectory.

port. They are more likely to be supportive if they are kept informed of what is happening to the person and are given some idea of how they can be helpful (time off for medical care, temporary assistance while a person is recovering from a surgery, organizing a card or letter campaign to cheer up a person in the hospital, etc.). Religion can be helpful in providing psychological and emotional support. Formal religious organizations are often sources of instrumental support (e.g., delivering meals to homes, transportation services, visi-

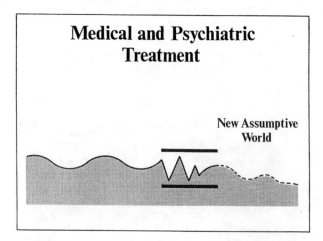

FIGURE 4.4. Development of a new assumptive world and resumption of the forward life trajectory.

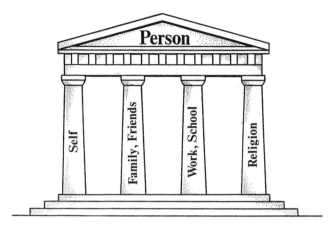

FIGURE 4.5. Support resources.

tation, and phone call networks to maintain social networks). The basic tenets of some formal religions are also helpful to some individuals in accepting and dealing with the emotional aspects of the diagnosis and treatment of cancer (e.g., "It's God's will and He will take care of me"). Many people do not have a formal religion but rather a belief in some higher power to whom they can turn for help.

Members then discuss the many topics generated by the 10 coping scenarios (see Table 4.1), ranging from illness-related concerns, family problems, and communication with physicians.

The advantages of this program are that the patients are taught to collaborate with the health team and to cope actively with increased responsibility for their own health care program. Another advantage, if the intervention is successful, is that the patients take away with them valuable skills that will enable them to deal more effectively with future problems.

RESULTS

Affective State

All the patients in the melanoma study reported moderate to high levels of psychological distress at baseline comparable to other cancer patients. However, at the end of the 6-week structured group intervention, the experimental subjects (n = 38) exhibited significantly lower levels of distress than did the control subjects (n = 28) (see Figure 4.6). Six months following the intervention, the group differences were even more pronounced. The experimental group reported significantly lower levels of confusion, depression, fa-

TABLE 4.1. Coping Scenarios

Prediagnosis
- Worries and concerns about the possible implications of the condition

Diagnosis
- Accepting the diagnosis
- Informing family and friends

Doctor–patient relationship
- Developing a collaborative partnership
- Opening up clear lines of communication

Treatment issues
- Feelings of fear and isolation
- Dealing with the overwhelming technological environment

Body image
- Surgical scars
- Loss of body parts
- Hair and weight loss

Depression
- Coping with varying degrees of depression

Communication issues
- Communicating feelings and perceptions with significant others

Dealing with coworkers
- Communicating with one's extended social network

Returning to "normal"
- Reentering everyday life
- Participating in previously enjoyed activities

Planning for the future
- Resuming "forward-life trajectory"

tigue, and total mood disturbance, and higher levels of vigor on the Profile of Mood States (POMS) (see Figure 4.7). Participation in the group intervention appeared to reduce the psychological turmoil associated with cancer diagnosis. At the 1-year follow-up, the experimental group continued to show significantly lower confusion and higher vigor.

Coping Methods

Immediately following the 6-week structured intervention, the experimental subjects showed significantly greater use of active–behavioral coping methods than did the control subjects. In addition, the experimental subjects used significantly more active–positive, active–expressive, active–reliance, cognitive–positive, and distraction coping strategies (see Figure 4.8). Six months following the intervention, the experimental patients continued to use sig-

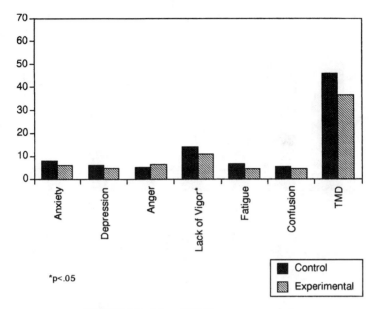

FIGURE 4.6. Mean POMS scores at week 6.

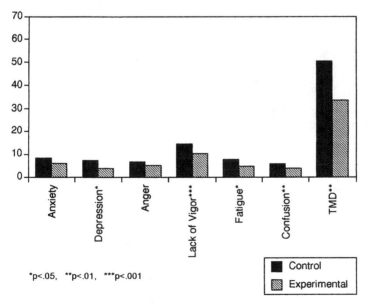

FIGURE 4.7. Mean POMS scores at month 6.

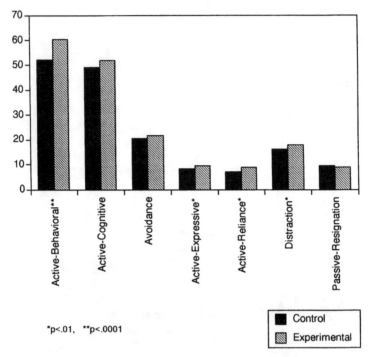

FIGURE 4.8. Mean coping method and strategy scores at week 6.

nificantly more active–behavioral coping methods as well as more active–cognitive coping methods than did the controls (see Figure 4.9). At the 1-year follow-up, active–behavioral and avoidance coping methods (specifically distraction) were significantly higher in the experimental patients compared to controls.

Immune Function

Along with a reduction in levels of psychological distress and greater use of active coping methods, the intervention patients showed a number of immune changes. Dual-color flow cytometry was used to define subsets of NK cells (CD56 and CD16) and large granular lymphocytes (LGLs) (CD57). At the end of the 6-week intervention, there was a significant increase in the percentage of LGLs (defined as CD57 with Leu7) (see Figure 4.10). Six months following the intervention, there continued to be an increase in the percentage of LGLs (defined as CD57 with Leu7) as well as increases in NK cells (defined as CD16 with Leu11 and CD56 with Leu19) and interferon alpha-augmented NK cell cytotoxicity (see Figure 4.11). The results indicate

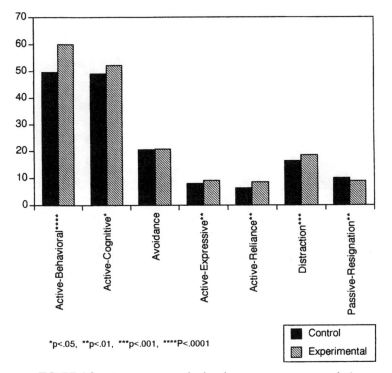

*p<.05, **p<.01, ***p<.001, ****P<.0001

FIGURE 4.9. Mean coping method and strategy scores at month 6.

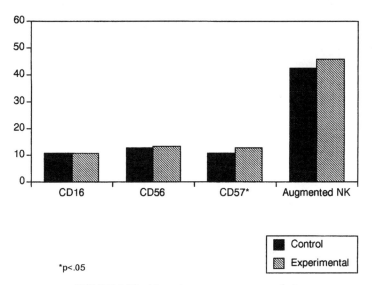

*p<.05

FIGURE 4.10. Mean immune scores at week 6.

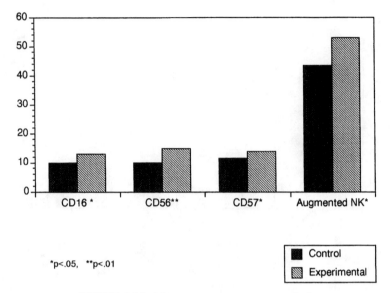

FIGURE 4.11. Mean immune scores at month 6.

that this short-term structured psychiatric group intervention for malignant melanoma patients with a good prognosis was associated with longer-term changes in affective state, coping, and the NK lymphoid cell system (Fawzy et al., 1990a, 1990b).

Affective State and Quality of Life

In both experimental and control subjects combined, quality of life was strongly negatively correlated with anxiety ($p = .0001$), depression ($p = .0001$), anger ($p = .007$), confusion ($p = .0001$), and total mood disturbance ($p = .0001$) at 6-month follow-up. As negative affective state decreased (through lower levels of anxiety, depression, anger, confusion, and total mood disturbance), the quality of life of these patients increased.

CONCLUSION

The psychological and medical problems encountered by cancer patients are numerous and unique. Patients are usually distressed, anxious, and unable to effectively utilize their normal coping styles. Based on a review of the literature and the authors' own clinical and research experience, it appears that a short-term, structured intervention consisting of health education, stress management/behavioral training, enhancement of coping skills including problem solving, and group psychosocial support offers significant benefits. The advantages of such a program include easy implementation and replication, promotion of important illness-related problem-solving skills, and increased participation in decision making and active coping. In addition, a psychoeducational intervention offered early in the course of cancer diagnosis and treatment and offered as an integral component of their overall care may be less stigmatizing and more readily accepted by both patients and staff. Such psychiatric interventions should be used as an adjunct to competent, comprehensive medical care and not as an independent treatment modality for cancer.

REFERENCES

Ader, R. (1981). *Psychoneuroimmunology*. New York: Academic Press.

Albrecht, J., Helderman, H. J., Schlesser, M. A., & Rush, A. J. (1985). A controlled study of cellular immune function in affective disorders before and during somatic therapy. *Psychiatry Research, 15*, 185–193.

Ali, N., & Khalil, H. (1989). Effects of psychoeducational intervention on anxiety among Egyptian bladder cancer patients. *Cancer Nursing, 12*(4), 236–242.

American Cancer Society. (1992). *Cancer Facts and Figures—1992*. Atlanta, GA: Author.

Baider, L., Uziely, B., & De-Nour, A. K. (1994). Progressive muscle relaxation and guided imagery in cancer patients. *General Hospital Psychiatry, 16*, 340–347.

Bartrop, R. W., Luckhurst, E., Lazarus, L., Kiloh, L. G., & Penny, R. (1977). Depressed lymphocyte function after bereavement. *Lancet, 1*, 834–836.

Berglund, G., Bolund, C., Gustafsson, U., & Sjoden, P. (1994). A randomized study of a rehabilitation program for cancer patients: The "starting again" group. *Psycho-Oncology, 3*, 109–120.

Black, S., Humphrey, J. H., & Niven, J. S. (1963). Inhibition of mantoux reaction by direct suggestion under hypnosis. *British Medical Journal, 6*, 1649–1652.

Bloom, J. R. (1982). Social support systems and cancer: a conceptual view. In J. Cohen, J. Cullen, & R. L. Martin (Eds.), *Psychosocial aspects of cancer* (pp. 129–149). New York: Raven Press.

Bloom, J. R., Ross, R. D., & Burnell, G. M. (1978). Effect of social support on patient adjustment following breast surgery. *Patient Counsel on Health Education, 1*, 50–59.

Brandberg, Y., Bergenmar, M., Bolund, C., Michelson, H., Mansson-Brahme, E., Ringborg, U., & Sjoden, P. (1994). Information to patients with malignant melanoma: A randomized group study. *Patient Education and Counseling, 23*, 97–105.

Bridge, I. R., Benson, P., Pietroni, P. C., & Priest, R. G. (1988). Relaxation and imagery in the treatment of breast cancer. *British Medical Journal, 297*, 1169–1172.

Burish, T. G., & Lyles, J. N. (1981). Effectiveness of relaxation training in reducing adverse reactions to cancer chemotherapy. *Journal of Behavioral Medicine, 4*, 65–78.

Burish, T. G., Snyder, S. L., & Jenkins, R. A. (1991). Preparing patients for cancer chemotherapy: Effect of coping preparation and relaxation interventions. *Journal of Consulting and Clinical Psychology, 59*(4), 518–525.

Cain, E., Kohorn, E., Quinlan, D., Latimer, K., & Schwartz, P. (1986). Psychosocial benefits of a cancer support group. *Cancer, 57*(1), 183–189.

Cassileth, B., Volckmar, D., & Goodman, R. L. (1980). The effect of experience on radiation therapy patients desire for information. *International Journal of Radiation Oncology, Biology, and Physics, 6*, 493–496.

Cella, D. F., Sarafian, B., Snider, P. R., Yellen, S. B., & Winicour, P. (1993). Evaluation of a community-based cancer support group. *Psycho-Oncology, 2*, 123–132.

Cohen, J., Cullen, J., & Martin, L. (1982). *Psychosocial aspects of cancer.* New York: Raven Press.

Cunningham, A. J., Edmonds, C. V. I., Jenkins, G., & Lockwood, G. A. (1995). A randomized comparison of two forms of a brief, group, psychoeducational program for cancer patients: Weekly sessions versus a "weekend intensive." *International Journal of Psychiatry in Medicine, 25*, 173–189.

Cunningham, A. J., & Tocco, E. K. (1989). A randomized trail of group psychoeducational therapy for cancer patients. *Patient Education and Counseling, 14*, 101–114.

Dorian, B. J., Garfinkel, P. E., Brown, G., Shore, A., Gladman, D., & Keystone, E. (1982). Aberrations in lymphocyte subpopulations and functions during psychological stress. *Clinical and Experimental Immunology, 50*, 132–138.

Dunkel-Schetter, C., Feinstein, L. G., Taylor, S. E., & Falke, R. L. (1992). Patterns of coping with cancer. *Health Psychology, 11*(2), 79–87.

Edgar, L., Rosberger, Z., & Nowlis, D. (1992). Coping with cancer during the first year after diagnosis: Assessment and intervention. *Cancer, 69*, 817–828.

Fauman, M. A. (1982). The central nervous system and the immune system. *Biological Psychiatry, 17*(2), 1459–1482.

Fawzy, F. I., Cousins, N., Fawzy, N. W., Kemeny, M. E., Elashoff, R., & Morton, D. (1990a). A structured psychiatric intervention for cancer patients: I. Changes over time in methods of coping and affective disturbance. *Archives of General Psychiatry, 47*, 720–725.

Fawzy, F. I., & Fawzy, N. W. (1982). Psychosocial aspects of cancer. In D. Nixon (Ed.), *Diagnosis and management of cancer* (pp. 111–123). Menlo Park, CA: Addison-Wesley.

Fawzy, F. I., Fawzy, N. W., Arndt, L. A., & Pasnau, R. O. (1995). Critical review of psychosocial interventions in cancer care. *Archives of General Psychiatry, 52*, 100–113.

Fawzy, F. I., Fawzy, N. W., Hyun, C. S., Guthrie, D., Fahey, J. L., & Morton, D. L. (1993). Malignang melanoma: Effects of an early structured psychiatric intervention, coping, and affective state on recurrence and survival 6 years later. *Archives of General Psychiatry, 50*, 681–689.

Fawzy, F. I., Kemeny, M. E., Fawzy, N. W., Elashoff, R., Morton, D., Cousins, N., & Fahey, J. L. (1990b). A structured psychiatric intervention for cancer patients: II. Changes over time in immunologic measures. *Archives of General Psychiatry, 47*, 729–735.

Fawzy, F. I., Pasnau, R. O., Wolcott, D. L., & Ellsworth, R. G. (1983). Psychosocial management of cancer. *Psychiatric Medicine, 1*(2), 165–180.

Fawzy, F. I., Namir, S., & Wolcott, D. L. (1989). Structured group intervention model for AIDS patients. *Psychiatric Medicine, 7*(2), 35–46.

Fawzy, F. I., & Natterson, B. (1994). Psychological care of the cancer patient. In R. B. Cameron (Ed.), *Clinical oncology: A Lange clinical manual* (pp. 40–44). San Mateo, CA: Simon & Schuster.

Fawzy, F. I., Wellisch, D., & Yager, J. (1977). Psychiatric liaison to the bone-marrow transplant project. In C. E. Hollingsworth & R. O. Pasnau (Eds.), *The family in mourning* (pp. 181–189). New York: Grune & Stratton.

Fawzy, N. W. (1996). A psychoeducational nursing intervention to enhance coping and affective state in newly diagnosed malignant melanoma patients. *Cancer Nursing, 18,* 427–438.

Forester, B. M., Kornfield, D. S., & Fleiss, J. (1978). Psychiatric aspects of radiotherapy. *American Journal of Psychiatry, 135,* 960–963.

Glaser, G., Kiecolt-Glaser, J. K., George, J. M., Speicher, C. E., & Holliday, J. E. (1985). Stress, loneliness, and changes in herpes virus latency. *Journal of Behavioral Medicine, 8,* 249–260.

Gordon, W. A., Freidenbergs, I., Diller, L., Hibbard, M., Wolf, C., Levine, L., Lipkins, R., Ezrachi, O., & Lucido, D. (1980). Efficacy of psychosocial intervention with cancer patients. *Journal of Consulting and Clinical Psychology, 48,* 743–759.

Greer, S., Moorey, S., Baruch, J. D. R., Watson, M., Robertson, B. M., Mason, A., Rowden, L., Law, M. G., Bliss, J. M. (1992). Adjuvant psychological therapy for patients with cancer: A prospective randomized trial. *British Medical Journal, 304,* 675–680.

Gruber, B. L., Hall, N. R., Hersh, S. P., & Dubois, P. (1988). Immune system and psychological changes in metastatic cancer patients using relaxation and guided imagery: A pilot study. *Scandinavian Journal of Behavior Therapy, 17,* 25–35.

Gruber, B. L., Hersh, S. P., Hall, N. R. S., Waletzky, L. R., Kunz, J. F., Carpenter, J. K., Kverno, K. S., & Weiss, S. M. (1993). Immunological responses of breast cancer patients to behavioral interventions. *Biofeedback and Self-Regulation, 18*(1), 1–21.

Holland, J. C. (1989). Historical overview. In J. C. Holland & J. H. Rowland (Eds.), *Handbook of psychooncology: Psychological care of the patient with cancer* (pp. 3–12). New York: Oxford University Press.

Holland, J. C., Rowland, J., Lebovits, A., & Rusalem, R. (1979). Reactions to cancer treatment: Assessment of emotional response to adjuvant radiotherapy as a guide to planned intervention. *Psychiatric Clinics of North America, 2,* 347–358.

Irwin, M., Daniels, M., Bloom, E., Smith, T., & Weiner, H. (1987). Life events, depressive symptoms, and immune function. *American Journal of Psychiatry, 144,* 437–441.

Kemeny, M. E., Cohen, F., Zegans, L. S., & Conant, M. A. (1989). Psychological and immunological predictors of genital herpes recurrence. *Psychosomatic Medicine, 51,* 195–208.

Kiecolt-Glaser, J. K., Fisher, L. D., Ogrocki, P., Stout, J., Speicher, C., & Glaser, R. (1987a). Marital quality, marital disruption, and immune function. *Psychosomatic Medicine, 49,* 13–34.

Kiecolt-Glaser, J. K., Garner, W., Speicher, C., Penn, G. M., Holliday, J., & Glaser, R. (1984a). Psychosocial modifiers on immunocompetence in medical students. *Psychosomatic Medicine, 46*, 7–14.

Kiecolt-Glaser, J. K., Glaser, R., Dyer, C., Shuttleworth, E., Ogrocki, P., & Speicher, C. E. (1987b). Chronic stress and immunity in family caregivers of Alzheimer's disease victims. *Psychosomatic Medicine, 49*, 523–535.

Kiecolt-Glaser, J. K., Glaser, R., Strain, E., Stout, J., Tarr, K., Holliday, J., & Speicher, C. E. (1986). Modulation of cellular immunity in medical students. *Journal of Behavioral Medicine, 9*, 5–21.

Kiecolt-Glaser, J. K., Glaser, R., Williger, D., Stout, J., Messick, G., Sheppard, S., Ricker, D., Romisher, S., Briner, W., Bonnell, G., & Donnerberg, R. (1985). Psychosocial enhancement of immunocompetence in a geriatric population. *Health Psychology, 4*, 25–41.

Kiecolt-Glaser, J. K., Kennedy, S., Malkoff, S., Fisher, L., Speicher, C. E., & Glaser, R. (1988). Marital discord and immunity in males. *Psychosomatic Medicine, 50*, 213–229.

Kiecolt-Glaser, J. K., Ricker, D., George, J., Messick, G., Speicher, C., Garner, W., & Glaser, R. (1984b). Urinary cortisol levels, cellular immunocompetence, and loneliness in psychiatric patients. *Psychosomatic Medicine, 46*, 15–23.

Klein, G., & Klein, E. (1985). Evolution of tumors and the impact of molecular oncology. *Nature, 315*, 190–195.

Kronfol, Z. (1987). Depression and the immune system. In O. D. Cameron (Ed.), *Presentations of depression: Depressive symptoms in medical and other psychiatric disorders* (pp. 341–353). New York: Wiley.

Kronfol, Z., Silva, Jr., J., Greden, J., Dembinski, S., Gardner, R., & Carroll, B. (1983). Impaired lymphocyte function in depressive illness. *Life Science, 33*(3), 241–247.

Kronfol, Z., Turner, R., Nasrallah, H., & Winokur, G. (1984). Leukocyte regulation in depression and schizophrenia. *Psychiatry Research, 13*, 13–18.

Krueger, R. B., Levy, E. M., Cathcart, E. S., Fox, B. H., & Black, P. H. (1984). Lymphocyte subsets in patients with major depression: Preliminary findings. *Advances: Journal of the Institute for the Advancement of Health, 1*, 5–9.

Levy, S. M., Herberman, R. B., Maluish, A. M., Schlien, B., & Lippman, M. (1985). Prognostic risk assessment in primary breast cancer by behavioral immunological parameters. *Health Psychology, 4*(2), 99–113.

Liang, L. P., Dunn, S. M., Gorman, A., & Stuart-Harris, R. (1990). Identifying priorities of psychosocial need in cancer patients. *British Journal of Cancer, 62*, 1000–1003.

Linn, B. S., & Jensen, J. (1983). Age and immune response to a surgical stress. *Archives of Surgery, 118*, 405–409.

Linn, M. W., Linn, B. S., & Harris, R. (1982). Effects of counseling for late stage cancer patients. *Cancer, 49*, 1948–1055.

Linn, M. W., Linn, B. S., & Jensen, J. (1984). Stressful events, dysphoric mood, and immune responsiveness. *Psychological Report, 54*, 219–222.

Maguire, P. (1976). The psychological and social sequelae of mastectomy. In J. G. Howells (Eds.), *Modern perspectives in the psychiatric aspects of surgery* (pp. 390–421). New York: Brunner/Mazel.

Maguire, P., Lee, E. G., Bevington, D. J., Kuchemann, C., Crabtree, R. J., & Cornell, C. E. (1978). Psychiatric problems in the first year after mastectomy. *British Medical Journal, 1*, 963–965.

Meyerowitz, B. E. (1980). Psychosocial correlates of breast cancer and its treatment. *Psychological Bulletin, 87*, 108–131.

Meyerowitz, B. E., Sparks, F. C., & Spears, I. K. (1979). Adjuvant chemotherapy for breast carcinoma: Psychosocial implications. *Cancer, 43*, 1613–1618.

Moorey, S., Greer, S., Watson, M., Baruch, J. D. R., Robertson, B. M., Mason, A., Rowden, L., Tunmore, R., Law, M., & Bliss, J. M. (1994). Adjuvant psychological therapy for patients with cancer: Outcome at one year. *Psycho-Oncology, 3*, 39–46.

Morris, T., Greer, H. S., & White, P. (1977). Psychological and social adjustment to mastectomy: a two-year follow-up study. *Cancer, 43*, 1613–1618.

Namir, S., Wolcott, D. L., Fawzy, F. I., & Alumbaugh, M. J. (1987). Coping with AIDS: Psychological and health implications. *Journal of Applied and Social Psychology, 17*, 308–328.

Nerenz, D. R., Leventhal, H., & Love, R. R. (1983). Factors contributing to emotional distress during cancer chemotherapy. *Cancer, 50*(5), 1020–1027.

Ornish, D., Brown, S. E., Scherwitz, L. W., Billings, J. H., Armstrong, W. T., Ports, T. A., McLanahan, S. M., Kirkeeide, R. L., Brand, R. J., & Gould, K. L. (1992). Can lifestyle changes reverse coronary heart disease? *Lancet, 336*(8708), 129–133.

Palmblad, J., Cantell, K., Strander, H., Froberg, J., Karlson, C., Levi, L., Granstrom, M., & Unger, P. (1976). Stressor exposure and immunological response in man: Interferon producing capacity and phagocytosis. *Journal of Psychosomatic Research, 20*, 193–199.

Pennebaker, J. W., Kiecolt-Glaser, J. K., & Glaser, R. (1988). Disclosure of traumas and immune function: Health implications for psychotherapy. *Journal of Consulting and Clinical Psychology, 56*(2), 239–245.

Pettingale, K. W., Greer, H. S., & Tee, D. E. H. (1977). Serum IgA and emotional expression in breast cancer patients. *Journal of Psychosomatic Research, 21*, 345–349.

Pruitt, B. T., Waligora-Serafin, B., McMahon, T., Byrd, G., Besselman, L., Kelly, G. M., Drake, D. A., & Cuellar, D. (1993). An educational intervention for newly-diagnosed cancer patients undergoing radiotherapy. *Psycho-Oncology, 2*, 55–62.

Richardson, J. L., Shelton, D. R., Krailo, M., & Levine, A. M. (1990). The effect of compliance with treatment on survival among patients with hematologic malignancies. *Journal of Clinical Oncology, 8*(2), 356–364.

Schleifer, S. J., Keller, S. E., Bond, R. N., Cohen, J., & Stein, M. (1989). Major depressive disorder and immunity: Role of age, sex, severity, and hospitalization. *Archives of General Psychiatry, 46*, 81–87.

Schleifer, S. J., Keller, S. E., Camerino, M., Thompson, J. C., & Stein, M. (1983). Suppression of lymphocyte stimulation following bereavement. *Journal of the American Medical Association, 250*(3), 374–377.

Schleifer, S. J., Keller, S. E., Meyerson, A. T., Raskin, M. J., Davis, K. L., & Stein, M. (1987). Lymphocyte function in major depressive disorder. *Archives of General Psychiatry, 144*, 437–441.

Smith, G. R., & McDaniel, S. M. (1983). Psychologically mediated effect on the delayed hypersensitivity reaction to tuberculin in humans. *Psychosomatic Medicine*, *45*, 65–70.

Sobel, H. J., & Worden, J. W. (1982). *Helping cancer patients cope: A problem-solving intervention for health care professionals* [audio cassette]. New York: Guilford Press.

Spiegel, D., & Bloom, J. R. (1983). Pain in metastatic breast cancer. *Cancer, 52*, 341–345.

Spiegel, D., Bloom, J. R., Kraemer, H. C., & Gottheil, E. (1989). Effect of psychosocial treatment on survival of patients with metastatic breast cancer. *Lancet*, *2*(8668), 888–891.

Spiegel, D., Bloom, J. R., & Yalom, I. D. (1981). Group support for metastatic cancer patients: A randomized prospective outcome study. *Archives of General Psychiatry, 38*, 527–553.

Stein, M., Keller, S. E., & Schleifer, S. J. (1985). Stress and immunomodulation: The role of depression and neuroendocrine function. *Journal of Immunology, 135*, 827s–833s.

Thestrup-Pedersen, K. (1975). Suppression of tuberculin skin reactivity by prior tuberculin skin testing. *Immunology, 28*, 342–348.

Weisman, A. D. (1979a). *Coping with cancer*. New York: McGraw-Hill.

Weisman, A. D. (1979b). A model for psychosocial phasing in cancer. *General Hospital Psychiatry, 1*(3), 187–195.

Weisman, A. D., Worden, J. W., & Sobel, H. J. (1980). *Psychosocial screening and intervention with cancer patients* (Project Omega, Grant No. CA-19797). Boston: Harvard Medical School, Massachusetts General Hospital.

Worden, J. W., & Weisman, A. D. (1977). The fallacy in postmastectomy depression. *American Journal of Medical Science*, *273*(2), 169–175.

Zachariae, R., Bjerring, P., & Arendt-Nielsen, L. (1989). Modulation of type I immediate and type IV delayed immunoreactivity using direct suggestion and guided imagery during hypnosis. *Allergy, 44*(8), 537–542.

Zimbardo, P., & Ebbeson, E. B. (1970). *Influencing attitudes and changing behavior*. Reading, MA: Addison-Wesley.

CHAPTER 5

Existential Group Psychotherapy for Advanced Breast Cancer and Other Life-Threatening Illnesses

JAMES L. SPIRA

Most descriptions of group therapy for the medically ill emphasize discussing specific topics related to adjusting to having the disease or teach specific coping skills for patients who are trying to cope with early stages of life-threatening illnesses or who have specific issues with milder forms of chronic illnesses (Spira, Chapter 1, this volume). Such approaches are appropriate within a brief or short-term format where coping with specific functional aspects of their disease can be addressed one at a time through psychoeducational or cognitive-behavioral methods of intervention (Antoni, Chapter 2, this volume; Fawzy, Fawzy, Arndt, & Pasnau, 1995; Fawzy, Fawzy, Hyun, & Wheeler, Chapter 4, this volume; Thoresen & Bracke, Chapter 3, this volume). However, patients with more advanced disease not only face the task of coping with functional aspects of their illness but also are confronted with more fundamental and generalized aspects of living, and dying, with their illness. For these patients, directly addressing such existential considerations appears to be both relevant and supportive of their psychological, psychophysical, and health status (Spira & Spiegel, 1993).

In contrast to most forms of psychotherapy, existential psychotherapy does not exclusively aim to correct psychopathology. Rather, existential psychotherapy attempts to:

1. *Understand* an individual's situation in light of (a) the human condition in general and (b) his or her personal and historical context.

2. *Enhance personal development* toward the individual's optimal potential for living fully in each moment, with the greatest degree of authenticity and meaning possible.

These goals require people to have an increased awareness of their cognitive beliefs and behavioral habits, along with a willingness to accept suffering and joy.

Why existential group psychotherapy for the medically ill? No previous publication has been dedicated to the applications of existential group psychotherapy for medically ill patients. This lack of attention to the modality is not surprising, because existential psychotherapy has rarely been considered within a group format. Yet, more important, existential psychotherapy is usually considered to be a long-term, in-depth modality for highly motivated and intellectually minded persons concerned with examining meaning in their lives and the direction their life is taking—hardly the type of thing managed care providers are willing to support. In a time of increased need to demonstrate "medical necessity" before treatments are approved, brief structured therapies are being supported in the medical and psychotherapeutic community, not esoteric therapies geared toward ameliorating nonpathological concerns. However, as this chapter should make evident, existential group psychotherapy for persons with advanced illness has the following characteristics. It is:

- *Effective* in improving both quality of life and quite possibly physical health as well.
- *Efficient* because it is provided in a group format compared to individual therapy. In addition, although patients may be on government medical aid (Medicare/Medicaid), making individual therapy less attractive to the practitioner, groups of 10 to 12 such persons mixed in with others can provide a more satisfactory source of revenue to therapists, and patients can find this copayment more affordable.
- *Experiential* rather than esoteric. Because of the pressing issues of life and death, there is no need for abstract consideration of living in the face of dying. For these patients, existential issues are a reality they need little encouragement to address. Certainly, discussion of issues can be stimulated by carefully chosen structured exercises. But, in truth, such stimulus is rarely required. All that is needed is to have patients meet together to discuss their major concerns, along with a well-trained therapist who, rather than fleeing from such issues, is able to draw out patients' authentic expression about their concerns as well as their hopes for living fully in the face of dying.
- *Relevant and appealing to a wide range of persons* with advanced illness (and their family members). These patients are highly motivated and are likely to commit to ongoing therapy. It is relevant for all personality types—

people who would never have otherwise sought psychotherapy or interpersonal development attend these groups as a result of an existential crisis. Narcissists seek therapy when their world is shattered; persons with Type A personality attend when their fears about their own demise overshadow their fears about exposing their inner self; shy, compliant persons may present for therapy because they are told to; persons whose lives have been spent living up to others' expectations come to receive advice on how to proceed with their life; persons who are otherwise content with their lives attend the group in this time of extreme discontent.

It should be clear that this form of therapy is *not* merely for a few intellectually reflective persons concerned with a "midlife crisis." Instead this approach is appropriate for the vast majority of persons with life-threatening illness.

This chapter discusses the theoretical foundations of existential group psychotherapy, the process of facilitating this approach for persons with advanced-stage illness (e.g., advanced cancer, incurable cardiac illness, and acquire immune deficiency syndrome), and the benefits to patients that might be expected based on research that has examined this style of intervention. Specifically, existential group psychotherapy for patients with advanced illness is intended to assist them to better cope with their diagnosis, adjust to living with the illness, and live more fully in the time they have left.

RESEARCH INTO THE EFFICACY OF EXISTENTIAL GROUP PSYCHOTHERAPY

Briefly, existentialism is the study of living life to its fullest. Almost all people have experienced times in their lives when they were able to derive maximum meaning, purpose, and value from each moment of their day. The experience of love or of helping another person to live more fully are two examples commonly associated with this experience. At such times, people report that they feel open and honest in relationship to themselves, others, and the world, able to feel comfortable and focused in the moment. This experience leads people to feel as if they are living as fully as possible, able to go to sleep knowing that their life is complete. This type of experience contrasts sharply with reports of poor quality of life, as indicated by any of the following: feeling isolated or hopeless, being easily distracted by worries about the future, suppressing one's feelings and thoughts, making an effort to be in complete control over uncontrollable events, or being unable to accept what is happening. These experiences have been identified as contributing to disease incidence, progression, and survival.

Only a few studies have actually been conducted utilizing existential principles and methods. However, there is sufficient indication from the literature of the need for this approach to warrant its widespread use. Such support comes from studies that identify psychosocial factors which correspond to existential principles as contributing to health outcomes and psychosocial interventions utilizing existential methods associated with increased psychological and physical health of patients.

Not surprisingly, persons diagnosed with a life-threatening illness undergo substantial changes in mood, psychophysical functioning, and existential aspects of their lives. The way that patients cope with their illness influences their emotional state and their ability to adjust to living with the illness (Dunkel-Schetter, Feinstein, & Taylor, 1992; Goldstein & Antoni, 1989). Moreover, it is also possible that psychosocial factors may be of influence in the course of the disease itself (Greer, 1991). Specifically noteworthy is research emphasizing the importance of social support versus isolation in survival (Berkman & Syme, 1979; House, Landis, & Umberman, 1988; Cohen, in press; Reifman, 1995), open expression of affect versus inhibition of expression (Temoshok, 1985; Greer, Morris, & Pettingale, 1979; Esterling, Antoni, Fletcher, Margulies, & Scheiderman, 1994; Lutgendorf, Antoni, Kumar, & Scheiderman, 1994) or uncontrolled hostility (Shekelle, Gale, Ostfeld, & Paul, 1983), honest expression of cognitive concerns versus denial/avoidance (Dunkel-Schetter et al., 1992; Greer & Watson, 1987; Esterling, Antoni, Kumar, & Scheiderman, 1993), and active coping versus passive compliance (Fawzy et al., 1990; Watson, Greer, Pruyn, & Van Den Borne, 1990; Antoni, Chapter 2, this volume). In brief, avoidance of feelings, denial of concerns, feeling helpless or passive compliance with others' demands, and social isolation are bound to result in poor quality of life, if not increased risk of disease incidence, progression, or survival. On the other hand, open honest expression of affective and cognitive concerns to another person in an effort to actively improve one's condition clearly corresponds to higher quality of life and also appears to be related to one's physical health (Fox, in press; Orth-Gomer & Unden, 1990).

Fortunately, all these psychosocial factors can be improved through the existential group psychotherapy format. Many descriptions of group therapy for medically ill patients that exist in the literature have some features of existential psychotherapy (Winick & Robbins, 1977; Wood, Milligan, Christ, & Liff, 1978; Frenkel & Torem, 1981; Cella, Sarafian, Snider, Yellen, & Winicour, 1993). However, although descriptions of group therapy formats are helpful, relatively few of these descriptions have been prospective randomized designs attempting to demonstrate specific benefits with specific interventional styles. Although in-depth reviews of group intervention studies can be found elsewhere (Trijsburg, van Knippenberg, & Rijpma, 1992; Spira & Spiegel, 1993; Fawzy et al., 1995; Forester, Kornfelf, Fleiss, & Thompson, 1993), it is valuable at least to note that empirical studies of group intervention illustrated the benefit of group therapy for cancer, human immunodeficiency virus (HIV), and cardiac patients.

Beginning in the late 1970s, research has consistently demonstrated the benefits of group therapy for improving cancer patients' quality of life (such as mood, coping, psychophysical distress, and physical functioning) and increasing patients' familiarity about the disease and treatment. With one exception, all reported studies of group therapy have been short term (less than 12 meetings), for the most part following a cognitive-behavioral format combining educational information, coping skills, and emotional/social support (Weisman, Worden, & Sobel, 1980; Vachon, Lyall, Rogers, Cochrane, & Freeman, 1982; Heinrich & Schag, 1985; Berglund, Bolund, Gustafsson, & Sjoden, 1994; Fawzy, Fawzy, & Hyun, 1994). The exception was a research group based on the existentially oriented work of Irvin Yalom (1985; Yalom & Greaves, 1977) which met weekly for an entire year and emphasized a more inductive interactive, emotionally supportive therapeutic style (Spiegel, Bloom, & Yalom, 1981; Spiegel & Spira, 1991; Spira & Spiegel, 1993). Another existentially oriented intervention was conducted by Mulder and associates (1994, 1995) with HIV patients. In a 16-session intervention, they found improved quality of life and immune system buffering for treatment patients compared to control groups. This study is important as it shows that, at least for medically ill patients, briefer existentially oriented therapy can be effective in improving quality of life.

Four studies indicate that group therapy that addresses existential issues to various extents may also be effective for improving physical health.

Supportive evidence for the benefits of group therapy containing some existential focus on reduction of disease recurrence and improved survival comes from a study of malignant melanoma patients conducted by Fawzy et al. (1990, 1993) and a study of patients with HIV by Antoni and associates (Antoni, Schneiderman, Fletcher, Goldstein, Ironson, & LaPerriere, 1990; Antoni, Chapter 1, this volume). In these studies, brief structured interventions urged patients to confront maladaptive coping strategies and encouraged open discussion of their concerns. Investigators found not only improved mood and coping but less immune disruption as well in treatment patients for up to 1 year following treatment. These studies also found improved survival for treatment patients at later follow-ups.

Friedman and associates took a large cohort of Type A postmyocardial infarction patients, and randomized half to long-term therapy, meeting weekly for the first year and then monthly thereafter (Friedman et al., 1986). They attempted to uncover habitual personality patterns that have been socially and developmentally shaped (e.g., Type A patterns of hostility and competitiveness, etc.; Friedman & Rosenman, 1974) and addressed issues of living more fully and authentically in relationship with other features of intervention central to existential psychotherapy. Investigators found decreases in Type A behaviors and a concomitant reduction in recurrent cardiac events (Thoresen & Bracke, Chapter 3, this volume).

The yearlong group therapy based on Yalom's existential approach to group psychotherapy found in a retrospective follow-up analysis that patients with recurrent breast cancer who had been randomly assigned to receive group therapy lived an average of 18 months longer from study entry than did control patients (Spiegel, Bloom, Kraemer, & Gottheil, 1989). However, Fox (in press) has pointed out that the treatment group lived only as long as the national and local average whereas the control group died at a faster than expected rate, suggesting that statistical sampling error accounted for the survival effect. Further research of this method is being conducted to verify the effectiveness of this method for patients with cancer (Spiegel & Spira, 1991; Spira & Reed, 1996) and HIV (Reed & Stanton, 1996). Whether or not the intervention had an effect on patient's quantity of life, the effects on quality of life are notable. Intervention patients were found to have had less mood disturbance and psychophysical distress. A replication of the earlier study found that in an environment of group support and therapeutic facilitation, patients were able to both raise and address existential issues in an open and honest fashion (Spiegel & Spira, 1991; Spira, 1991). The protocol for this existential group psychotherapy approach is described in detail later.

It must also be noted that initial blunting of feelings and avoidance of what the diagnosis entails may be *initially* helpful to buffer extreme distress (Miller, Brody, & Summerton, 1988; Reed, Kemeny, Taylor, Wang, & Visscher, 1994; Taylor, 1984). However, these studies suggesting the beneficial effects of covering up distress were interested in assessment only, not intervention. It is reasonable to assume that persons who need to avoid such distress may not have had ample external social support or internal resources to deal with the event (Spira, 1996b). Persons without such support may indeed benefit from temporary initial blunting but may be at greater risk for subsequent posttraumatic stress disorder, especially following a diagnosis of disease progression (Spira, 1993; Passick & Redd, in press). On the other hand, the intervention studies described earlier, which offered group therapeutic support to such persons, indicate that those who receive interventive support do better than those who do not. Yet the type of intervention is important. Should the supportive intervention encourage expression of distress or further covering up of one's fears?

A group based on the work of Bernie Siegel failed to find survival benefits for treatment subjects (Gellert, Maxwell, & Siegel, 1993). A major distinction between this study and the others that show positive survival outcomes lies in the style of therapy. The Siegel groups emphasized considering a more positive future without dwelling on the negative, whereas the group based on Yalom's approach and coping skills encouraged expression of distress as well as considering active coping strategies (Siegel, Spira, & Ulmer, 1992).

This difference parallels the literature, which suggests that confronting distress in an open and honest manner rather than avoiding feelings and thoughts may contribute to improved health outcomes (Watson & Greer, in press; Pennebaker, Kiecolt-Glaser & Glaser, 1988). The remainder of this chapter is devoted to the existential approach: to elicit openness and discourage avoidance in medically ill patients.

THEORY OF EXISTENTIALISM

Existentialism is the study of the experience of living. This includes attempting to understand oneself, one's relationship to others and the world, and meaning, purpose, and commitment in one's life. Moreover, existential writers have described how one's relationship to life has been conditioned and automatically/habitually conducted, diminishing one's experience, and how it is possible to more fully live a conscious, authentic and more valued existence. Different existential writers have emphasized various aspects of human experience. A brief review of existential philosophy and various related schools of thought will help readers appreciate the applications of these philosophical ideals to psychotherapy for medically ill patients.

Several modern philosophical disciplines study human experience. These include hermeneutics, phenomenology, mutualism/Marxism, and existentialism—all disciplines stimulated by Hegel in 19th-century Europe. The American equivalent would be the study of pragmatism, founded by Charles Peirce and elaborated on by William James (psychology), John Dewel (education), and George Herbert Mead (sociology). The oldest traditions that attempt to understand human experience and relationship to life are found in religious mysticism—that aspect of every religion in which adherents attempt to experience God firsthand rather than merely believe in church doctrine as law. (The various influences on existentialism, existential psychotherapy, and existential group psychotherapy for medically ill patients are represented in Figure 5.1.)

Of course, the whole of world history has bearing on existential thought. Its place in the history of philosophy is that it stems from an experiential tradition as opposed to an objectivist/rationalist school of thought. Approaches aligned with a *monist* tradition, which emphasizes direct experience as opposed to reflective rationalism, all have bearing on the development of existential thought. Landmark philosophers in this tradition include pre-Socratics Thales, Anaximander, and Parmenides (Wheelwright, 1996); Hellenistic philosopher Plotinus; and late Renaissance philosophers such as British empiricists Berkeley, Locke, and Hume (Copleston, 1946). However, the major influences that most directly shaped current existential psychotherapy commenced with the turn of the 19th century.

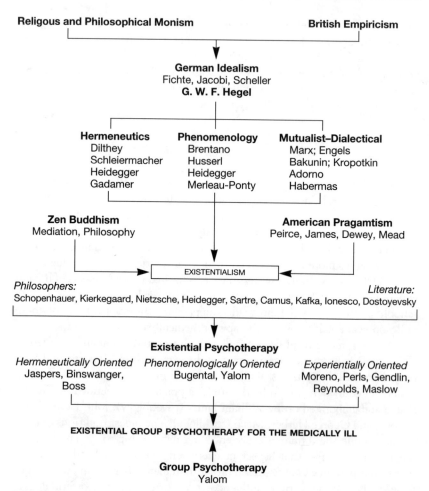

FIGURE 5.1. The influences on existentialism, existential psychotherapy, and existential group psychotherapy for the medically ill.

Early Influences on Existentialism

Several important philosophical and social science traditions influenced the formation of existentialism and existential psychotherapy. These include idealism, hermeneutics, phenomenology, pragmatism, and Buddhism. Although volumes have been written on each of these rich traditions, those aspects that have direct bearing on existential psychotherapy are highlighted here.

G. W. F. Hegel (1807/1967) laid the foundation for most of the social sciences that arose in the 19th century and are currently studied today. Following in the footsteps of the German idealist tradition (Fichte, 1794/1982;

Jacobi, 1799/1987; Schelling, 1803, cited in Behler, 1987), and in stark con-trast to the popular science of the times, which held that existence was com-prised of separate entities, Hegel argued that all existence is fundamentally unified as Spirit (*Geist*). Ego (self-awareness) is nothing more than Spirit turning in on itself and taking itself as an "object" separate from itself. As soon as self-awareness occurs, awareness of the world as separate from oneself occurs. However, this sense of separation between self and other is merely a mental construction and has no basis in reality. All we can truly know is what lies within our experience—any effort to form concepts about the world outside direct experience is merely a mental projection. From Hegel comes the importance of appreciating personal experience and the unity that binds all persons, despite our conscious minds believing us to be separate from each other and our world.

The field of hermeneutics (Schleiermacher, 1912, cited in Copleston 1946; Dilthey, cited in Rickman, 1979; Heidegger, 1927/1962) extends ideal-ist philosophy into the science of interpreting an individual's experience through studying the way the individual expresses him- or herself. Under-standing a person's meaning can only occur, these philosophers claim, from a consideration of both the individual *expressor* and the social–historical con-text within which the expression occurred. Although initially hermeneutics concerned itself with interpretation of written expression (Palmer, 1969), later work applied hermeneutic methodology to *any* manifested activity, whether verbal (Ricoeur, 1979) or nonverbal (Levin, 1985). Modern hermeneutic writers (Gadamer, 1976; Habermas, 1976) take this approach even further, arguing that the hermeneutic context of the *perceiver* must also be considered. They claimed that all one can possibly know is the *interaction* between the perceiver and the expressor. From the hermeneutic tradition comes the importance of allowing personal expression of meaning to arise within a personal and social context rather than an analysis, which imposes an "objective" interpretation on a person's life.

Phenomenology (Brentano, 1990, cited in Husserl, 1900; Husserl, 1900; Merleau-Ponty, 1962), in fact, is the study of how we tend to impose our in-terpretations on the world we perceive, and what our world is like once we suspend interpretation. As opposed to the popular use of the term, "phenom-enology" is not mere subjectivity but rather a rigorous methodology attempt-ing to understand the way we construct a meaningful world. Modern cogni-tive science informs us that the mental construct to which we consciously attend (working memory) is in fact a combination of stimulation of our sens-es which triggers previously conditioned associations (bottom-up, data-dri-ven processes) and what we expect to occur given the ongoing context (top-down, concept-driven processes) (Spiegel, Frischoltz, & Spira, 1993). Yet we assume that the mental construct we attend to corresponds directly to what exists in the world, separate from our "interpretation of it"—what Husserl

(1931) referred to as our "natural attitude." The top-down expectation and the bottom-up associations are nothing more than unconscious assumptions that form our meaningful world. One way to recognize our unconscious assumptions is to "bracket" them—that is, to examine an object from every different perspective imaginable. What remains after all interpretations are bracketed is the "object as it is." Interpretations are also revealed when there is a "breakdown" of normal functioning (Heidegger, 1927/1962). When some aspect of our world suddenly ceases to function in the intended fashion, our assumptions about that object are suddenly revealed, and we may gain a brief glimpse into that object as it is, distinct from our intentions for it. From the phenomenological tradition comes the notion that there is an authentic basis of experience beneath our usual assumptions conditioned by habit and society. Further, through effort or happenstance, it is possible gain insight into the nature of life free from our usual conditioned way of experiencing the world.

Pragmatism (Peirce, 1931–1935) is the philosophical tradition that states that consciousness, understanding, and meaning occur through interaction. It has roots in American transcendentalism as well as in European mutualist–dialectical social philosophy. Because of its "pragmatic" nature this tradition has gone well beyond mere philosophical speculation to become the foundation for modern psychology (James, 1890), education (Dewey, 1910), and sociology (Mead, 1938). Pragmatists look upon the process of thinking, learning, and interacting as more substantial than the belief that there is a fixed individual who thinks, learns, and interacts. Our experience of life develops through associations made by interacting with the environment (James, 1890). These associations become unconscious assumptions that we assume represent the workings of the world (not simply our experience of it—hence Husserl's "natural attitude"). Such habits are useful to some extent in that we can allow certain functions to occur without effort (walking, eating, talking, etc.). However, too often unconscious habit operations begin to interfere with our optimal performance and growth (habitual movements limit sports or bring on injury, habitual eating may lead to obesity, habitual relating may bring on divorce, etc.). Rather than operating from a sense of a fixed, unwavering self, being open to change allows individuals to interact more fully with their environment, and this is the basis of continued growth (Dewey, 1910). Therefore, in all manifestations of this discipline, the self as defined by dialectical interactive activity is examined (Mead, 1938). From the pragmatic tradition comes the importance of interaction and action to develop one's experience (and thus one's self) to the fullest extent possible.

Zen Buddhism (Bodhidharma, 560 A.D./1987; Suzuki, 1934; Spira, 1994b) shares characteristics with each of the traditions mentioned earlier. Steeped in 2,500 years of Eastern religious tradition, its principles and practices have been difficult to translate to non-Eastern cultures. Yet, since it was first studied by Western philosophers in the 19th century, and especially since World War II, the influence of Zen on existentialism and psychotherapy has become increasingly apparent. A few tenets are worth mentioning here. First, suffering stems from considering one's constructed image of self or other to be real (the thing in itself). Freedom from suffering entails suspending one's interpretive activity to return to one's natural foundation of interpretless unity with existence (Spirit, or *Geist*, in Hegel's terms). Only from experiencing this foundation can an individual emerge in full authentic relationship with and commitment to life. Zen differs from most Western traditions in that it involves experiential action rather than relying purely on intellectual reflection. Unlike Western traditions, which attempt to understand *one* object or expression by either understanding the context within which this expression occurs (hermeneutics) or bracketing this object from all contextual interpretations (phenomenology), Zen teaches that one's authentic nature can only be discovered once *all* interpretation (desires, preferences, discrimination) is suspended. Once this occurs, the nature of thinking and acting is revealed, and an individual can live and act more fully in each moment. Thus, Buddhism is both negative (suspending one's fixed images of self and others) and positive (realizing the essential unity with life and acting more fully within each moment). From the Zen Buddhist tradition stems the notion of being more fully present in each moment, without need for constant worry of the future or regret from the past—and the corresponding release of self-made suffering and the richness of life that come from engaging more fully in ongoing committed activity.

Existential Philosophy

The study of existentialism arose out of a need to appreciate individual experience rather than a more metaphysical (and less personal) philosophical tradition. Existential writers have ranged from those interested in describing the life *as it is lived* to those concerned with *living more authentically* and richly in everyday life.

Albert Schopenhauer, who taught opposite Hegel at Berlin University in the 1820s, was also adamantly opposed to key elements of Hegel's philosophy. Hegel felt that although ego was inseparable from the Spirit (*Geist*) that unifies all creation, ego was nevertheless the highest form of evolution and, as such, we should attempt both to act in accordance with Spirit and to further Spirit's manifestation in society by enhancing social well-being. Schopenhauer, who was the first Western scholar to study Buddhism, felt that there is an equally strong drive on the part of Spirit to return to its source—that is, the *will* to "deevolve" or release ego back to its unified oneness. Schopenhauer argued that our pursuit should not be one of mere intellectual curiosity but instead a return to the experience of our essential nature. This occurs through accepting the *will* of Spirit to reclaim itself. Only an acceptance of death allow one's spirit to subsequently shine forth in its fullest potential. Schopenhauer (1958) points to mythology as evidence of our search for the eternal from the perspective of our limited ego.

> Now if we keep in view the Idea of man, we see that the Fall of Adam represents man's finite side . . . limitation, sin, suffering, and death. On the other hand, the conduct, teaching, and death of Jesus Christ represent the eternal . . . side, the freedom, the salvation of man. Now, as such . . . every person is Adam as well as Jesus, according as he comprehends himself, and his will thereupon determines him. In consequence of this, he is then damned and abandoned to death, or else saved and attains to eternal life. . . . (p. 628)

Thus, Schopenhauer provides an existential foundation for appreciating the finite limitations of ego and the freedom that occurs once death of the finite self can be accepted.

Søren Kierkegaard (1832/1968) considered the first existentialist, also reacted against aspects of Hegel's respect for society as the purest manifestation of human ego. Whereas Hegel felt that our essential unity with Spirit meant that individuals are fundamentally inseparable from society and can only be fulfilled by returning our goodwill to society, Kierkegaard observed that it was social conventions that led individuals to develop an inauthentic relationship to Spirit (God). In fact, Kierkegaard (1847/1946) believed that it was only when we could entirely remove societies' influences that our authentic nature could manifest with pure freedom. Yet the rejection of social convention comes at a price. When one breaks the habits that are formed from social conditioning and thus social constraints on perception and action, one is left with anxiety that stems from being responsible for forming one's own opinions and choosing one's own actions (1841/1974). By accepting one's anxiety over separation from society and entering into self-responsibility, one also can enter into an authentic relationship with life. The old socially conditioned self "dies" so that the pure self can emerge (1948/1974)—free to choose and free to love with all of one's being. Kierkegaard introduces the notion of acting out of purity of heart rather than living others' agendas. He also introduced the concept of personal responsibility necessary to reject conditioned influences.

Friedrich Nietzsche, although strongly influenced by Schopenhauer, was unaware of Kierkegaard's writings. Yet like Kierkegaard, Nietzsche (1888/1967) also rallied against social conditioning, arguing passionately that freedom to manifest one's full potential in life can only follow freedom from social conditioning. Yet Nietzsche not only advocated distancing oneself from social *institutions* but also advised separating from one's own *thoughts*, which are formed by social convention. Meaning, purpose and value, he argued, are not our own but, rather, given to us by society. In this regard, he introduced phenomenology into existentialism. One's self-image is formed in large measure by society, and therefore only self-death can free one from oneself! Like a phoenix rising out of the ashes, one can then manifest fully, creating a life that is authentically self-generated rather than formed by others, and therefore rich in meaning, purpose, and value (1883/1961). Yet the conditioned self resists change. Nietzsche (1888/1967) reasons that it is only through suffering that one is ready to abandon social convention and arise to one's full potential: "To imagine another, more valuable world is an expression of hatred for a world that makes one suffer" (p. 311). Nietzsche brought to existentialism the need to accept self-death that comes from first examining and then abandoning our inauthentic assumptions of life, along with the will to manifest fully in the authentic life that follows this effort.

Martin Heidegger both drew from and went beyond all the traditions and existentialists discussed previously. Subsequent existential writers have for the most part expounded on Heidegger's ideas. He based his theory on the hermeneutic notion of self as inseparable from society, and the phenomenological proposition that our thoughts and perceptions are conditioned from social experience. Heidegger (1927/1962) therefore argued that, rather than attempting to discover how society is formed from a group of individual selves, we should attempt to understand how the self arises out of society. The notion of "self" as individual and free is an illusion, and our actions are inauthentic when based on this "natural attitude." Thoughts and actions arise out of society. The only way to become free is to suspend our own thoughts. Heidegger was influenced by Zen Buddhism (Heidegger, 1944/1945, 1966; Nishitani, 1982; Zimmerman, 1986) and believed that inauthentic thought and action can only be noticed from a standpoint of nonthought. Only from this background of nothingness (Nichte) can the meaningful interpretations that form our consciousness be noticed. Only from this authentic unconditional perspective can one authentically choose what action to commit oneself to. The thoughts and actions that then arise following this "moment of vision" are still those provided by society. Yet only following their suspension can they be chosen freely, in a way that will bring greatest meaning, purpose, and value to one's life. However, echoing earlier existentialists, we rarely choose the release of social convention. Rather, willingness to abandon the final self occurs following a breakdown of normal assumptions (e.g., diagnosis of cancer). We can try to cover up these breakdowns, fleeing into social convention once again (becoming a "patient," expecting the doctor to effect a cure). But when the breakdown is so severe (diagnosis of recurrent cancer), covering up may become impossible, and we are left watching our assumptions of life crumble. This death of the self leaves one feeling strange (unheimlichkeit). Only when one can accept this perishing of the self, recognizing that all prior assumptions of life have an empty (*Nichte*) basis, can one remanifest authentically, living fully in each moment.

Other existentialists, especially those who have written plays, novels, and poems (Elliott, Rilke, Camus, Sartre, Ionesco, Dostoyevsky, etc.), have contributed to the dissemination of existential ideas. Yet, from the standpoint of defining the tradition that had such an impact on existential psychotherapy, the previously discussed traditions are most central to the existential thesis. This thesis can be summarized as containing five major components (see Table 5.1).

Components of Existentialism

From the sources listed earlier, and especially Martin Heidegger, who went furthest in summarizing the field to date, five distinct aspects of existentialism can be described. These form the basis of interventional approaches to existential psychotherapy for terminally ill patients.

Hermeneutic Basis of Self

Because we are interpretive beings, we are fundamentally unified through the social interpretations given us by society. An individual's expression of his or her meaningful existence can only be understood by appreciating (1) his or her personal experience, and (2) the historical–social context within which the expression of meaning is made (see Figure 5.2).

TABLE 5.1. Essential Elements of Existentialism

1. *Hermeneutic basis of self*
   - Self is formed from and manifests within a social–historical–cultural basis.

2. *Inauthentic assumptions of our world and our self*
   - We incorrectly assume that we are a fixed entity and perceive the world as it is.

3. *Breakdown of inauthentic assumptions*
   - Crisis threatens the stability of our images of self and world.
     a. We attempt to cover up this breakdown by fleeing into social convention.
     b. When covering up is not possible, self breaks down and we experience distress.

4. *Moment of vision*
   - Suspending fixed images of self and world permits authentic vision of one's condition.

5. *Authentic commitment*
   - Once free of habitual limitations, one is free to identify, choose, and fully engage in meaningful activity.

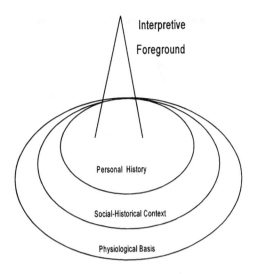

Fundamental Background

FIGURE 5.2. Hermeneutic basis of self as arising from an integrative context.

Inauthentic Assumptions of Our World and Our Self

We do not realize that our self-image and our images of the world are merely mental constructions that are provided to us by society through a lifetime of unconscious conditioning, forming habits, and in turn limiting our perceptions and our freedom of actions. Instead, we assume a "natural attitude" whereby we believe that our impression of life (ourselves and our world) directly matches the "world as it is." We tend to take ourselves as fixed entities that exist in stable form and similarly view our world as fixed and regular. Failing to appreciate that the way we think of self, others, and our world is dictated by social rules that we learn, we do not appreciate that what we think of as free choice in our lives is nothing more than inauthentic constraints of society to large measure dictating what we consider to be our options. Such unconscious assumptions form the basis of suffering and limit freedom to select and fully engage in the most meaningful activity (see Figure 5.3).

Breakdown of Inauthentic Assumptions

Because ego exists to safeguard itself and to perpetuate its stability, it requires an external crisis to shatter our assumptions. There are small everyday breakdowns, such as a mechanism (door knob) not working, which lead to tempo-

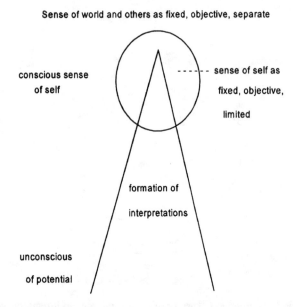

Sense of world and others as fixed, objective, separate

conscious sense
of self

sense of self as
fixed, objective,
limited

formation of

interpretations

unconscious

of potential

FIGURE 5.3. Inauthentic self is based on the interpretation that self is fixed, limited, and independent from a separate objective world.

rary recognition of our assumptions (assume that turning the knob opens the door) until we can find an alternative mechanism to work for us (lock). Whenever possible, we cover up such breakdowns of our habitual assumptions, fleeing into conveniently provided social conventions. Yet there are more serious breakdowns, such as the loss of a loved one or the diagnosis of terminal illness, for which the usual alternative habitual mechanism just simply does not work. When the breakdown is so severe that we cannot simply flee into social convention, we instead experience anxiety (*angst*), where usual everyday activity appears to be absurd and where we feel a sense of dissociated depersonalization (*unheimlicheit*). Such a state occurs because there is no longer a basis for understanding what is occurring. And thus we recognize that what we took for granted has been artificial and inauthentically derived and maintained (see Figure 5.4).

Moment of Vision

When an external crisis facilitates a breakdown and subsequent recognition of assumptions, one experiences a kind of emptiness. The emptiness of an a priori order and meaning to life (*Nichte*) for the first time provides a background against which one can take an authentic look at one's inauthentically

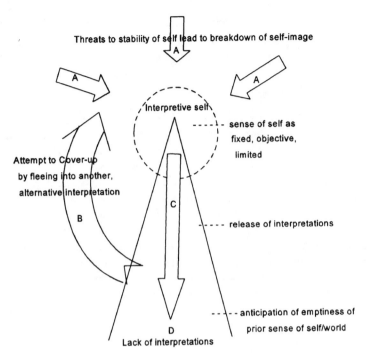

FIGURE 5.4. Breakdown of self-image occurs when (A) an external catastrophe challenges fixed assumptions of self, others and world, leading to (B) an effort to "cover up" this distress, or (C) distress from an inability to flee this breakdown, leading to (D) a realization of the lack of a priori interpretations and a sense of emptiness as one's foundation.

derived and maintained foregrounded assumptions about one's life. The extent to which a breakdown of assumptions cannot be covered up corresponds to the depth of authentic understanding about one's life activities. For instance, if a person assumes his health to be adequate, he will probably give issues of health or longevity little consideration. Yet when he is diagnosed with coronary artery disease followed by a coronary artery bypass graft, he must consciously and seriously address the actual state of his health and the extent to which he can influence it. If a woman breaks up with a man she has dated for several months, she can justify the breakup by blaming him or circumstance. However, if her husband of 40 years dies suddenly of acute myocardial infarction, any amount of rationale or social convention provides little comfort. Occasionally, a person is not only thrust into examining the specific assumption that has been disrupted (health, relationships) but may be further compelled to reconsider the "natural attitude" itself! Once one recognizes that one has been essentially "fooled" by oneself, the potential for consideration of one's unconsciously derived assumptions becomes possible. The more that assumptions break down, the more one is able to recognize one's prior assumptions (see Figure 5.5).

Authentic Commitment

The more one is able to recognize one's prior assumptions, the more one is able to enter into authentic action. If the moment of vision is limited to one element (heart), one's freedom to choose authentically typically is limited to that realm (cardiac rehabilitation). If one's vision extends to recognizing a more general concept (life at risk), then one has the opportunity to reevaluate one's life (in light of the potential of dying soon) and may therefore reevaluate several critical activities to live more meaningfully (in the time remaining). Finally, if one's vision encompasses the general notion that all prior assumptions about one's life have all been largely other-derived and unconsciously maintained, then one has the potential to begin anew to reevaluate all one's life activities and select those that will bring greatest meaning, purpose, and value to one's life (see Figure 5.6).

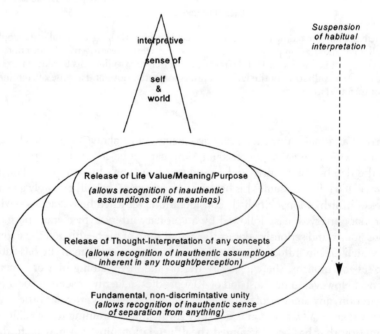

FIGURE 5.5. One's moment of vision (conscious realization of the inauthentic nature of one's previous existence and the potential for authentic action) corresponds to the depth to which one suspends interpretation.

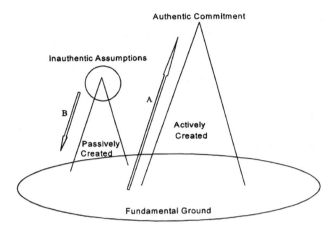

FIGURE 5.6. Authentic commitment to activity that brings greatest personal meaning, purpose, and value (A) stems from a release of passively developed habitual assumptions about self and the world (B).

Existential psychotherapy for seriously ill patients can help facilitate the breakdown (to whatever extent the patient is able to tolerate), avoid the need to cover up one's distress, and facilitate exploration of authentic activities to commit oneself in order to live each moment of one's life to its fullest extent. The following section explores the methods existential psychotherapists have utilized to promote this existential development.

EXISTENTIAL PSYCHOTHERAPY

Existential psychotherapy stands in contrast to other approaches, which tend to cover up the existential cause of distress and facilitate "fleeing into social convention." Such nonexistentially oriented approaches quickly assist with finding specific solutions to specific problems, without regard to patients' more general existential concerns. They assume that quality of life is diminished as a result of a patient's pain or anxiety, and patients' quality of life can be restored by reducing this distress (e.g., through psychopharmacology or relaxation). However, psychotherapy for medically ill patients that exclusively focuses on symptom reduction too often supports the inauthentic existence of patients and misses a valuable opportunity to pursue deep-seated existential concerns. It is not particular psychotherapeutic techniques that operate in contrast to existential considerations but, rather, the paradigm of individual practitioners who wish to dull patients' pain. Yet, in doing so, these therapists may unintentionally dull the opportunity for patients to get the most out of the days remaining to them. Existentially, anxiety and excess suffering stem from the attempt to return to one's prior psychosocial status; when this is clearly impossible, the attempt only *increases* suffering. Ideally, approaches can be found that reduce acute suffering while enhancing the extent to which patients can live life as fully as possible. This is the intent of existential psychotherapy for medically ill patients.

There are three approaches to existential psychotherapy that have emerged over the past century, apparently influenced by hermeneutics, phenomenology, or Buddhism. Existential psychotherapy for the medically ill uses aspects found in all three of these emphases, and a brief review provides a useful context for applications to the terminally ill.

Hermeneutic Influence

The earliest forms of existential psychotherapy put into practice the hermeneutic principles of allowing meaningful expression to be understood from the patient and his or her context. Instead of imposing a deductive theoretical framework on patients by testing them with standard assessments, putting them into preexisting categories, and treating them according to standards appropriate to that category, an effort is made to understand patients inductively, from within their own constructed world.

The conflicts patients subjectively experience are the material used in existential psychotherapy. Karl Jaspers (1913) and Ludwig Binswanger (1945/1958) felt that they best served patients by understanding their existence from a thorough study of the patients' direct experience and the context within which that experience arose. The hermeneutic orientation is constructivist. As Viktor Frankl (1978) pointed out, patients create their own unique sense of order and meaning in the world. Yet our construct of the world may not keep up with the constant changes occurring in the world or ourselves. This gap, between a patients' construct of life and the challenges constantly provided by a changing world, is the basis of neurosis.

The task of the existential psychotherapist, therefore, is to find the gaps in a patient's world order, providing a link to patients' difficulty relating to world events. According to Medard Boss (1958), the role of the therapist is to point out the inconsistencies of the way the world has been created by the patient, and to do so as much as possible from *within the patient's perspective*. Through first understanding and then questioning the patient's created world, the existential psychotherapist provides a setting in which a "lateral perspective" can be gained, viewing life from various perspectives. Moreno (1946) had patients *act out* various archetypal aspects of their meaningful life, therefore bringing their background beliefs and assumptions into the foreground. The way that cognitive therapists Ellis (1962) and Glasser

(1965) challenge patients' belief systems can be seen as operating from within this hermeneutically influenced existential tradition.

Phenomenological Influence

One of the most powerful aspects of existential psychotherapy is that, in the face of crisis, the therapist can (1) facilitate the breakdown of a patient's inauthentic assumptions, (2) help avoid covering up, so that a moment of vision can be obtained, and (3) facilitate authentic commitment to chosen activities that will bring the richest meaning, value, and purpose to the patient's life. The phenomenologically oriented existential psychotherapist attempts to help the patient notice their foregrounded activities from a background of *Nichte* (nothingness). This is usually achieved by having patients consider their living in the face of loss, even death. The old adage, "you don't appreciate something until it is gone," applies here.

The breakdown of normal assumptions that naturally follows a major crisis can be facilitated therapeutically. The therapist should ease the anxiety sufficiently such that the patient can allow the breakdown to occur (rather than immediately fleeing into a comfortable convention) yet in a way that does not cover up the recognition of prior conditioned assumptions that contribute to excessive suffering. It is only when such breakdowns occur that authentic growth can occur—allowing fuller adjustment to the new situation. The reason that adjustment is difficult lies in holding on to a fixed image of the way we considered ourselves and the world to be. The therapist can assist in the release of such old fixed images by first raising these assumptions to conscious awareness and next helping the patient accept that this life is now past and it is best to look to the present. In this way, patients can begin to consider how they *want* to live rather than the way they were living *out of habit*.

Yalom (1980; Yalom & Greaves, 1977) has used existential psychotherapy of this sort with patients facing incurable cancer, as well as with their families. In this approach, patients are encouraged to accept the fact of their illness and eventual death so that they can also fully accept their lives. No effort is made to deny or reject the negative aspects of their lives in favor of concentrating on the positive or the hopeful.

Bugental (1973/1974) has developed a series of exercises to help both therapists and patients appreciate what it means to honestly face death, enabling them to live more authentically and fully in each moment. For example, "*If you had one year to live, what would you do that would bring greatest meaning into your life—that would allow you to live your fullest in that last year of life?*" For medical patients, these types of exercises help facilitate authentic exploration of issues that are current and relevant. For therapists, family members of medically ill patients, or patients with psychosocial dysfunction, such exercises help stimulate existential issues that have been ignored. Exercises of this sort are likely to generate a great deal of authentic discussion in therapy. More of these types of exercises are presented later.below.

Zen Buddhist (Experiential) Influence

Zen Buddhism has influenced a number of experientially based approaches to psychotherapy. Buddhist-influenced approaches to existential psychotherapy stem from a different sort of fundamental background than hermeneutically or phenomenology-oriented approaches. Hermeneutics concerns itself with expression as having meaning only within the context of social meaning. Phenomenology concerns itself with understanding by suspending interpretation and therefore recognizes meaning from a background of nothingness (*nichte*, empty of a priori interpretation and meaning, purpose, value). In contrast, Buddhism emphasizes dissolving the limited self-ego into the fundamental ground of nondiscriminative unity with all existence. The main tenet of Buddhism is that once interpretation has been suspended, a person experiences a sense of oneness. It is from this greater sense of fullness with life (which comes from suspending interpretation, and thus preference and biased discrimination) that a person is able to confront any interpretation, no matter how fearful it once was.

This approach maintains that once a person suspends thinking (interpreting, reflecting), he or she also suspends worry, and only body sensations remain (Zimmerman, 1986, 1989). This physiological sense is generally very comforting. When people cease to regret the past or worry about the future, they are left with a general sense of well-being (Miller, Kodeletz, Schroeder, Mangan, & Sedlacek, 1996; Spira, 1996b). The feeling of the breath and warmth of the body, simple light patterns and sounds, and tastes and smells all combine to afford people the same sense of presence that a young baby experiences after it has had its fill of milk, when it is bundled in its mothers arms or the way a cat or dog feels resting by the fireplace.

This condition is not an altered state of consciousness but, rather, a normal and natural state that exists all the time. Yet this condition can only be fully noticed when one ceases to attend primarily to one's reflection. Thinking about swimming and swimming are very different experiences. To the extent that one thinks about swimming while actually swimming, one detracts from the direct experience of the swim itself.

Of course, reflection can be useful for attempting to improve one's future. Yet the quality of reflection can be only as good as the experiential data the individual has to work with. Therefore, Zen advocates that one think when it is truly necessary and suspend thinking to experience more fully what one is engaged in whenever possible. The practice of meditation is intended to facilitate the ability of a person to be more fully present in the moment, free of socially influenced interpretation and thus in fuller and freer relationship with life. Maslow (1968) refers to this as "peak experiences," after which a person's sense of joy at being in the world increases tremendously. Fritz Perls (1969) knew the value of being totally "in the moment" and "in one's body." He developed techniques around this experience to examine how people attempted to flee moving toward this experience (what they were afraid to let go of). Gendlin (1979) described this presence in the moment as a "felt sense" (*Gefindlikheit*) and, like Perls, uses this as a basis for exploring existential issues. 20In a technique Gendlin calls "focusing," a therapist serves as an active mirror for patients, both being in this felt sense as well as asking them questions that help them notice how they flee from this felt sense and lead them to a feeling of being "integrated" when they allow themselves to operate from this felt sense.

Reich (1942) was probably not directly influenced by Zen. Yet in an experiential approach to psychotherapy, he utilized deep breathing rather than free association in an extension of Freud's efforts to break down resistance to unconscious fears. Through breathing and moving, past fears and their present manifestations become recognized. By discussing these fears while remaining calm, patients are able to work through this neurosis and manifest more freely in their lives. Bugental also bases his psychotherapeutic technique on nonconceptually being in the moment. To reveal patient resistance, the therapist listens to the patient's concerns yet points out nonverbal aspects of the patient's expression (speed of speech, pauses, flippant gestures, etc.). In this way, patients can notice their tendency to cover up their deep-seated concerns, allow authentic feeling to arise, and enter more fully into each moment of their lives.

Reynolds (1980) describes what he calls the quiet therapies, methods of psychotherapy that incorporate silence into their methodology. Developed in Japan, this approach combines Zen meditation with Western psychotherapy. In one of these applications, developed by Shomno Morita (Reynolds, 1976), patients are kept in social and sensory isolation for some time, often in a quiet room or even in bed rest, for 1 week. During this time, their "noise" becomes more apparent to them and can begin to subside. Later phases are geared toward redirecting attention to pragmatic activities (sweeping, eating, etc.) rather than on habitually evoked feeling or thoughts. Therapeutic intervention is geared toward helping patients find that they are able to work despite how they impulsively feel or think. In this way, thoughts, whether negative or positive, no longer deter from the activity in which patients are engaged. In other words, patients habitual patterns of thinking and reacting no longer control them. This approach is continued until the patient is able to engage fully (without distractions from habitual thoughts or feelings) in a variety of activities, including his or her career work.

Zen Meditation

Zen is the most direct, simplest, and perhaps most challenging of any experiential method whatsoever. That is because it challenges the practitioner to suspend complexity (in the way of reflection and reaction) and rest in the most fundamental sense of being that is possible for humans. By becoming completely absorbed in the light that comes to one's eyes, the sound that vibrates one's eardrums, the pressure that touches one's body, one is able to cease attention to interpretation and thus notice the tendency to interpret. With practice, a person can completely suspend interpretive thinking and enter into the natural and fundamental state of *Samadhi*, from which he or she can be said to be "existentially free," and act with complete authenticity. Yet even short of a complete submersion into sensation, *the extent to which one can absorb oneself with all one's attention is the extent to which one can mature existentially.* Thus, any amount of meditation is useful (Spira, 1996a). Although Zen is the most direct method used to gain this insight, other forms of meditation can be helpful as well, including Yoga, Tai Chi Chuan, or even Christian chanting or Jewish davening.

Similar to what Heidegger (1944/1945, 1966) refers to as simply waiting, without awaiting for anything in particular, Zen meditation develops the skill of noninterpretive awareness. The following description of becoming absorbed in a simple sensation such as the breath reflects this emphasis:

> What is important here is that the exhalation be done without anticipation, without end-gaining; there must be no more intention in it. When you give the order to your body to breathe in a certain way, there is intention. But you must free yourself from the intention and be only the perceiving.
>
> When the exhalation is done without anticipation, without end-gaining, without any goal, then it flows in its home ground, in silence. It is very important that the student be completely attended in this moment and wait without waiting for the need of the body to inhale. The inhalation is done in the same way, without anticipation. Be aware of the tendency to push with the exhalation and grasp with the inhalation. Your breathing must be completely smooth and soft, without intention. The first body of all bodies, the Adamic body, is breathing. The posture and the breathing refer to the background, to the silence. Because in reality there is not a posture, there is only silence. (Bodian, 1991, p. 100)

Existential group psychotherapy utilizes all the principles discussed by philosophical existentialists (see Figure 5.1). However, although all existential psychotherapists share many of the principles from hermeneutics, phenomenology, and Zen, various practitioners may tend to emphasize one aspect more than another (see Table 5.2). Yet, in contrast to existential philosophers who have tended to recognize and comment on existential issues arising out of some extreme turn of events, the existentially oriented

TABLE 5.2. Major Approaches to Existential Psychotherapy

1. *Hermeneutic influence*
   World view: Self and world are fundamentally interrelated
   Proponents: Jaspers, Binswanger, Boss
   Approach: Appreciating and working with the patient from the standpoint of their personal–historical and cultural context within which their meaningful world is created. Therapists help patients notice inconsistencies within their world to find alternative ways to view self and others.

2. *Phenomenological influence*
   World view: Self and world are fundamentally empty of a priori meaning
   Proponents: Bugental, Yalom
   Approach: Understanding distress as the fear of and attempt to deny death (demise of fixed interpretations of oneself and one's world). Being able to tolerate this distress means being able to live more authentically and freely.

3. *Experientially based (Zen Buddhist) influence*
   World view: Self and world are fundamentally complete, without imposing meaning
   Proponents: Maslow, Perls, Gendlin, Reynolds
   Approach: All interpretation is simply a mental construction and therefore inauthentic. Only by suspending interpretation and entering fully into the moment with feeling and attention can one break through one's habitual limitations and live authentically in every action one engages in.

psychotherapist goes further, utilizing the therapeutic encounter to *promote* existential maturity. Moreover, the existentially oriented psychotherapy *group* may very well be the best environment within which to explore such issues. Existential group psychotherapy uses many of the methods of the existential psychotherapists described earlier, yet, in many ways, can go further by utilizing the benefits of the *group*. The remainder of this chapter describes these methods in detail.

But first, a caution: Existential psychotherapy can use numerous techniques. However, it is the manner in which techniques are used, rather than the technique itself, that determines its applicability to facilitating existential maturity. For instance, hypnotherapy, often used to dissociate from an unpleasant situation, can also be used to explore existential dimensions (Spira & Spiegel, 1992; Spiegel & Spira, 1992). By teaching them a simple controlled dissociation, patients are able to consider difficult issues in a relaxed state and in a way that bypasses their old habit ways of interpreting the situation. However, hypnosis that merely focuses on comfort and wishful thinking can be used to cover up rather than uncover a patient's existential concerns.

Group therapy, and the numerous techniques that can be utilized within this format, can similarly help or hinder a patient's existential development.

METHODS IN EXISTENTIAL GROUP PSYCHOTHERAPY

How do philosophy and existential psychotherapy traditions translate into existential group therapy for persons with advanced illness? Kierkegaard was concerned that *the group* promoted inauthenticity rather than authentic relationships. Yet if the group is filled with persons for whom inauthentic considerations have begun breaking down and is led by a therapist skilled in existential facilitation, the group can instead be a place where members establish authentic relationships in a way far beyond what is possible in individual therapy.

The Use of the Group in Existential Psychotherapy

The ultimate goal of the I–Thou relation is a loving fusion with the other in which each self realizes itself by being itself with and through the other. . . . *Loving-and-fusing with the other self is a precondition of the vitality, the growth and the wholeness of the individual self.* This loving-and-fusing is the "natural" and normal orientation of the human self. When the individual cannot relate to other human beings in this way, presumably because of some feeling of threat that is so overwhelming that it forces him to build defenses and relate to them as inhuman "its," he does not live to the full, does not grow to the full, and is indeed neurotic; instead, he "plays roles," "presents himself," and in general acts-out his inner problem inauthentically by building defenses against the perceived threats of other selves. (Douglas, 1983, pp. 42–43)

Group therapy has the potential for being an extremely beneficial way for existential psychotherapy to proceed because it contains the three basic factors outlined earlier: hermeneutic–existential appreciation, phenomenological–existential selflessness, and the Buddhist–existential experience of common basis. Groups composed of those suffering from traumatic loss or who face their own loss from illness are even more likely to be benefited by the group environment (Spira, Chapter 1, this volume). Therapeutic groups can be seen as potentially existential in nature for several reasons.

Groups Reveal Patterns

Interaction allows for insight that is difficult to achieve within individual therapy. When authentic expressions and interactions are encouraged within the group, the potential for patients to notice their assumptions and actions increases, not only because patients are encouraged to express them but also because patients can notice how they express themselves more fully through interaction with others in the group struggling with similar issues. Zen Master Joshu Sasaki Roshi (1978) has described neurosis as unmanifested thought. The group offers an environment where neurotic worries can be healthfully expressed. Moreover, manifesting subjective impressions in relationship to others can help to reveal the way in which a patient has maintained his or her "subjective reality," not only to the therapist but to the group as well. By hearing others' realities, patients can begin to put their own worldview into perspective as merely one way of coping with difficulty—and then they become more open to exploring other possibilities.

Groups Manifest Unity

The group can provide an environment that helps reveal both unity and isolation. Groups promoting intimate connections with others during therapy provide a framework for helping patients more easily connect with others in general. The bonding that can occur within a group promotes an intimate I–thou (Ich–du) encounter (Buber, 1958), dissolving the sense of others as separated by a bridge of isolation that can never be breached. Besides pointing out the ability of individuals to suspend a sense of individual separateness in order to enter into unhesitant relationships, such groups also are helpful in pointing out resistance to suspending one's sense of separate self.

Intimacy with others is an example of manifested unity. To enter into an intimate relationship with others in the therapy, patients must first suspend their own concerns for themselves (however temporary and to whatever extent). Such intimacy is seen as the group members mature. Initially, each member speaks of his own concerns and listens politely to the concerns of others. With time, however, as patients become more open to expressing their own issues, they are increasingly able to suspend their own problems and worries temporarily to respond to the needs of the other group members. The Buddhist Vimilakirti Sutra (Thurman, 1976) is an example of commitment to unity and compassion. Vimilakirti states that if one sick being exists, then he, who is not separate from others, must also be sick. He goes on to describe how he will be healthy only when all sentient beings are healthy. This type of empathic commitment to realizing others' pains and attempting to support others in their time of suffering is something that naturally develops in a therapy group focusing on the development of honest intimacy.

Groups Provide Support

Groups provide members with the support they need to examine existential issues that might otherwise be too difficult. This is in stark contrast to Kierkegaard's concerns, who argued that society only distracts from an authentic relationship with life. Although this may be true of the individual operating within society in general (*Dasein*), the therapeutic group supportive of existential maturity can offer patients emotional support that will enable them to pursue difficult areas of experience into which they might not otherwise be able to delve. In other words, groups can offer support helpful in releasing a person's fixed self-image to more fully accept what is transpiring in the moment and consider more authentic alternatives.

When faced with a traumatic event, people show a strong tendency to cover up and flee from the reality that confronts them—especially when they feel isolated and highly distressed. Yet, in the face of a traumatic event that shatters a person's lifelong meanings and assumptions, *covering up* is less likely to succeed, and the reality of the situation rushes in. The diagnosis of recurrent cancer, HIV, or congestive heart failure, and thus imminent death, is one of the most confrontive and life-shattering events that can occur. Even here, however, people frequently attempt to interpret their disease in a socially conventional way ("I'll be strong and lick this thing"; "It's God's will"; "The doctor said I should"; etc.). Still, the diagnosis of a terminal illness occurs with such ferocity as to shatter these socially conventional meanings such that no interpretation can make good sense out of what is happening. It is at times such as these that the power of the group to support the patient becomes apparent.

For example, a cancer patient who is having her breasts removed can be prepared psychologically for the procedure for weeks in advance. There is sufficient literature on the subject and others who have undergone it so that the details of the procedure come as no surprise. But after the operation, the reality of her body's change opens her to a level of honesty beneath which any social interpretation or cognitive image could have prepared her. Just as having a hysterectomy can reveal the finality of never having children, seeing a friend die of the same disease that one has can reveal the fact of one's imminent death more than mere intellectual considerations can hope to. The existentially oriented group can allow such expressions to occur within the presence of others who have gone through a similar experience, buffering the stress of isolation, so that the ability to confront and learn from such experiences is intensified.

Groups Ensure Authentic Commitment

Being involved in an ongoing group means that patients will not fall into the trap of substituting a "socially offered" newfound meaning for the loss of meaning in their life. That is, if people simply replace an old fixed image of themselves with a new fixed image of themselves (positive or negative), they remain inauthentically fleeing their authentic basis—especially if the new image is one conveniently provided to the person's new social "role." Group members can prevent the newly diagnosed person from attaching to a sick-role image, and they can also consider in more depth new thoughts of a person who has suddenly "found religion," whether that religion is a new group, an herbal remedy, or an agency to volunteer with. The group can help the patient see that these options are not poor ones but only poorly chosen when too hastily accepted. Instead, the group can assist the person to evaluate all his or her actions on a continual basis. In this way, Heidegger's admonition to "take back the commitment" from time to time should help keep patients "honest."

General Principles of Existential Group Facilitation

Existentially, patients have greater difficulty living fully in each moment if they cling to images of the way their life was prior to the illness. Engaging in existential group psychotherapy assists in the release of old fixed habit images of oneself and one's world, allowing for greater freedom to engage anew and manifest fully given the situation at hand. From this type of intervention, patients should be better able to cope with the diagnosis and treatment, adjust to living with the illness, and live more fully in the face of dying. But general principles and specific strategies of therapeutic intervention are required for this to occur.

Therapeutic Activity

Therapists do not lecture, nor give advice. Rather, therapists employ a Socratic method of asking questions to lead patients to explore their existential situation. Patients are probed to help them:

1. Recognize their distress and avoidance of it.
2. Achieve a state of safety and comfort within themselves and from the group.
3. Explore and express their concerns authentically without fear of social appropriateness.
4. Interact openly, honestly, and meaningfully with others, offering and receiving support.
5. Explore what they are, at their base, now that the medical crisis has shattered their fixed assumptions of themselves and their world.
6. Determine what brings them greatest meaning, purpose, and value in their life now and in the time they have left.
7. Manifest their understanding into committed action.

Despite their guidance toward these goals, therapists are not the central focus of the group. Therapists only interact as needed to keep patient exploration "on track." When interaction is open and honest between group members, therapists need not intervene at all. Specific areas of emphasis, discussed next, help to describe the process of group therapy utilized with medically ill patients in a way that facilitates existential maturity.

Content

In general, therapists take an inductive approach to therapy with regard to topics of discussion (Spira, Chapter 1, this volume). Rather than presenting a set series of topics or exercises, therapists allow the group to raise whatever issues are important to them that day. Even structured exercises follow the interests or needs of the patients at any given time. If there is a concern regarding some topic yet insight is not forthcoming, or even if there is a lapse in substantial dialogue, specific exercises can be used to stimulate further discussion.

What is discussed in the groups usually takes care of itself, especially with groups of patients dealing with life-threatening illness, who have been together for some time (4 months or longer). Occasionally, however, the therapist needs to bring the discussion back to the reason the group is meeting. Special exercises can also be used to more rapidly move patients to consider important issues. Yet when "directed" to consider such issues, patients invariably have a different experience than if they are tackling such an issue in their lives at that moment. Therefore, the use of special exercises should stem from the patients dealing with a topic, not lead patients to a topic. If patients are lax in generating topics of concern, or if they continue to be distracted by irrelevant or abstract dialogue, therapists have several options. First, therapists might inquire as to why, in a room full of patients who have life-threatening illness, with all the obvious concomitant problems, no one can think of an issue of personal concern. If this question fails to generate discussion, a brief structured exercise may be helpful. Periodically, it is useful for the therapist to briefly summarize a theme being discussed to reveal it more closely and to keep the discussion of it going further. If group members introduce multiple topics, the therapist can point them out, decide to begin with whichever topic appears to be most "pressing" for the group or a group member, and try to get to the others at some point during the group.

Existential Development in Group Psychotherapy

To allow these methods to occur, the therapist must remain clear that the point of the group is to help reveal inauthentic meanings that the patients use to cover up feelings and thoughts about the death of their ordered world. Therapists must continually appreciate that people can live more fully in the face of their dying ("dying" meaning the demise of self-image). In fact, perhaps it is only in the face of death (fundamental emptiness) that a person can authentically engage in activities that are of greatest value. Although this may be clearest for patients with incurable life-threatening illness, it is no less true for others. To flee from dying is to flee from living more fully. Instead, a person must be able to remain open and expressive about his or her situation. In other words, the therapist must assist the patient to tolerate discomfort (*unheimlicheit*)—which means that the therapist must *also* be willing to tolerate discomfort. Only when the distress of broken-down interpretations is fully experienced can patients begin to authentically consider what actions to take. Patients will be able to fully experience such a commitment not for any meaning that others have given to the activity but rather for the meaning that the patients can give to it. The group should also be a format for reflecting about engaging in the committed activity—and the difficulties and rewards of doing so.

Although the group can be an opportunity for those experiencing traumatic loss (of self or other) to confront the inauthentic nature of their existence and to begin to live authentically, progress depends on the quality of the groups and the group leaders. If the therapists can create an atmosphere in which patients feel free to openly and honestly express feelings and thoughts actually occurring for them (rather than what they wish was occurring), the patients can begin to explore the nature of their lives more openly and honestly on their own. Moreover, the group becomes synergistic. Once one person begins addressing these existential issues, others in the group find it easier to follow. Although there are substantial barriers to examining such threatening issues, there is also a strong will (Schopenhauer, 1958) to return to this more authentic state of being. Thus, given the opportunity along with the modeling provided by the group, patients can make relatively rapid progress.

However, therapists must be mindful of the tendency in themselves and others to support patients' prior image of themselves and the way they have constructed their world. In a rapidly changing world for these patients, no fixed image of self or others is correct (Habermas, 1968/1971). Rather, the more patients can abandon the world of yesterday, the better they can enter into the world of today. As long as yesterday "worked" for the patient, there was a reluctance to examine implicit assumptions. However, a crisis can create the context necessary for existential therapy to begin, and a group setting can be an ideal place for that experience to occur.

Specific Methods Useful for Facilitating Existentially Oriented Groups

Both the specific process of group facilitation and selected topics that can be facilitated through structured exercises are presented next.

Process of Group Facilitation

The following guidelines of group facilitation are effective in eliciting authentic exploration of one's life. They allow for personal, specific, affective interaction between group members. They also facilitate ways to take personal responsibility for future actions and lead patients away from fleeing into social convention (keep a "stiff upper lip"), artificial hope ("everything will be all right"), or externalizing control, whether it be blame and benefit ("The doctors didn't notice it in time"; "The doctors are doing all they can").

Before asking a leading question, it is usually a good idea to make a rapport statement. Therapists who rephrase or summarize patients' feelings and topics make sure they themselves understand what has been said and increase the patients' confidence that the therapist truly does understand their concerns. Patients are more likely to follow a therapist's lead if they believe the therapist has been following their feelings and thoughts (Roberts, Cox, Reintgen, Baile, & Gibertini, 1994). Asking a few simple, open-ended questions to help patients express their concerns in more personal, specific, affective ways to others can assist in accessing more authentic intimate personal feelings and also exploring other ways of coping with a problem. Following are some examples of the types of leading questions useful in facilitating authentic expression and further exploring concerns. They are organized by the subject and object of the patient's concern, their affect and approach to coping with a problem, and the style of interaction in which they engage (Spira, in press-a). Adjustment to living in the present moment is also facilitated (Spira, in press-b). Table 5.3 gives a brief overview of these specific interventional emphases.

Subject. When the patient's expression is *externally* focused on a subject other than him- or herself, the therapist should ask the patient a question that will lead him or her to phrase their concerns in more *personal* terms. In general, when the patient is talking about someone or something else, the therapist should ask how the matter affects the patient personally. For example, if a patient says, "My doctor simply is not interested in listening to what options his patients might want. He's pretty sure of himself," the therapist can redirect, "How do you react when you are speaking with him and want him to listen to your concerns, but he doesn't?" An exception to personalizing can be made, however, if one patient is expressing concern for another, as long as it does not go too far.

Object. When the object of the patient's expression is in *general or abstract* terms, the therapist should ask a question that leads the patient to phrase concerns in more *specific and concrete* terms. In general, when the patient is speaking abstractly or vaguely, without reference to specific time and place, the therapist should ask the patient to give a specific example of how

TABLE 5.3. Facilitating Group Therapy Discussion

Lead	Quality of expression		
	From inauthentic	$\longrightarrow$	*To authentic*
Subject	Impersonal/external	$\longrightarrow$	Personal/internal
	("How does that affect you personally?")		
Object	Abstract/general	$\longrightarrow$	Concrete/specific
	("Can you give a specific example of that problem?")		
Affect	Intellectual/repressed	$\longrightarrow$	Emotional expression
	("How does that make you feel?")		
Relationship	Solipsistic/isolated	$\longrightarrow$	Supportive/interactive
	("Has anyone else had that type of experience?")		
Coping	Passive/helpless	$\longrightarrow$	Active/appropriate control
	("What can you do to handle the situation in a way that works better for you?")		
Adjusting	Habitual assumptions	$\longrightarrow$	Living fully in the moment
	("You said you've always trusted doctors to help you, and now nothing is helping. What would happen if the doctors said there was nothing further they could do for you?")		

Note. When needed, therapists ask open-ended questions to elicit more authentic patient expression. For example, in response to "Doctors never care what's going on with you, only what's going on with the tumor!" the therapist might ask one or several of the above questions, depending on the patient's subsequent responses (typically in the order indicated, as required).

he or she has experienced situation. For example, if a patient says, "Doctors are really not interested in listening to what options patients want. They are trained to tell, not to listen," the therapist can redirect, "Has this happened to you? Can you give us an example of an interaction with your doctor when he did not listen to your concerns?" If the patient has no such experiences, this patient was simply engaging in speculative intellectualization and the therapist can ask other group members about their personal experiences in this type of situation.

Affect. When the expression is personal and specific, and of obvious concern to the patient, but is stated *intellectually* or void of emotion, the therapist should probe the patient's *emotional* state. In general, when a patient is talking about a difficult subject in emotionally neutral or even overly positive terms, the therapist should ask what negative feelings that brings up. For example, if a patient states, "I know exactly how I am going to end my life, once it is clear that there is no more hope. I am going to fly to Paris, get a hotel room with a view of Sacre Coeur, and take an overdose of sleeping pills," in an intellectual fashion, void of emotion, as if in casual conversation, the therapist might respond, "This is a *very* major step you are considering. And you seem to be talking about it so lightly. But when you think about getting sicker, there being no hope, and taking your own life, doesn't that bring up a lot of feelings in you?"

Tolerating negative affect is of tremendous value to the patient and the group as a whole. It details the fear associated with loss of self and others and permits open and honest exploration of existential issues. Therefore, staying with negative affect for as long as possible is beneficial. However, it is important for the therapist not to push too hard when eliciting a patient's expression of feelings. Therapists should simply offer an opportunity to explore. They can point to the door, even open it a crack, but they should not drag the patients through. Over-zealousness on the part of the therapist usually results in patients having (1) a rush of feelings that they are unable to cognitively integrate, and thus becoming more distressed than relieved, (2) a feeling that they are being unduly pressured by the therapist or group, or (3) both. Ultimately, it is up to the patient whether and to what extent to explore frightening emotions. Another, more emotionally expressive person in the group can serve as a good model for exploring negative emotions. Eventually, the fear of the "flood gates opening and never closing again" will subside as it becomes clear from observing others in the group that crying which comes freely during expression of concern is usually a positive release, leaving the person feeling better, not worse.

Also, the group as a whole tends to become "informational" when difficult issues and emotions arise, or following an especially emotional session. The therapist must appreciate the emotional threshold of each person and the group as a whole. Part of not "pushing too hard" includes allowing some lightness, even humor to emerge, before returning to difficult topics.

Relationship. One of the benefits of group therapy is that it offers patients the ability both to express emotions about their condition and to give and receive support within a community of persons whose experiences are somewhat close to their own. Therefore, although allowing personal expression is important, therapists should attempt to have the expression directed to another person, the group as a whole, or, if necessary, the therapist. Yet therapists should be wary of turning a group into a series of individual patient expressions or conversations with the therapist. In fact, the therapist is relatively silent in this type of group. When necessary to get a patient or the group "back on track," therapists typically ask one to three questions before turning the focus to another person or opening the discussion to the group as a whole to maintain an interactive discussion among members.

In general, when a patient is expressing but not relating, the therapist has several methods to elicit interaction, among them the following.

1. *The therapist.* It is useful for the therapist to establish a connection with the patient by asking questions (eliciting personal, specific, and affective statements about their distress and ability to cope with it). Following a patient's statement that is external, abstract, or intellectual or is evidence of passive coping, the therapist should probe for more authentic types of expressions in two or three questions, then redirect the next question to the group or to another group member to commence a dialogue between patients (see item 3).

2. *The group.* Therapists should limit their interaction with a group member to just a few questions and responses before asking the group as a whole to get involved. It is useful for the therapist to briefly summarize what the patient has been saying (e.g., "It sounds as if you have been finding it difficult to get your concerns across to your doctor"), followed by statements such as: "Has anyone else had a similar difficulty?" or perhaps "Does anyone who has faced these same difficulties have some advice for [patient]?"

3. *Another member.* Whenever possible, it is useful to facilitate an interaction between two group members. This direct patient interaction is an ideal way to give and get support and establish a more intimate relationship than can be established with the therapist alone or with the group in general. Therefore, following a patient's statement, whether a second patient responds, a second patient responds to a general question addressed to the group as a whole, or the therapist happens to recall that another patient has had a similar experience, the therapist should attempt to establish a two-way conversation for a time before redirecting to the group. For example, "Janet, you told us last week that you were finding ways to tell your doctor your concerns about continuing chemotherapy. Can you offer any suggestions to Sarah that might help her out in her current situation?" Then, after some discussion: "Sarah, do you think the way Janet handled her situation could assist you in your situation?" This approach is especially effective if the therapist can have two patients taking roles that help both of them as well as each other. Consider a group in which one member is very quiet and tends to ask for help and then reject it, while another member is very free in giving advice to others yet rarely discusses his own situation with the group. It would be an ideal situation if the therapist could facilitate a discussion where the "quiet" member is able to use his or her experience to offer advice to the "helper" member who would be encouraged to reflect on this advice.

Typically, therapists find it easier to facilitate interaction in the order just presented (first with the therapist, next the group, and then another member). However, although easier perhaps, these are in reverse order of value to the patients. Interaction with other members of the group is in many ways superior to interaction with the group leader. This is evident when group leaders find that they may give advice at some point yet only when another group member offers similar advice does the patient becomes stimulated enough to act on the suggestion.

Coping. Existentialism emphasizes personal responsibility for current and future actions. When patients discuss problems in a way that implies *helplessness* and lack of control, it is useful to ask a question that leads them to explore ways they can *cope actively* rather than merely give up in despair. Of course, in reality a patient has no control over a great deal of things. Yet patients can always actively participate in something with regard to their problem. They may learn to react in a better way to the crisis, improve communication with others involved in the situation, or, if possible, seek ways to improve the situation itself other than those ways already attempted. In general, when patients say that there is nothing they can do regarding their illness in general, or some aspect of it, therapists can ask questions that lead patients to explore areas over which they in fact *do* have some degree of participation. For instance, if a patient states, "The doctor says that I have to go back for more hyperthermia treatment. But it hurts so much that I just don't think I can take it again," the therapist might ask, "Have you tried discussing this with your radiologist or the technicians?" Or, even better, ask the group (truly a "panel of experts") whether anyone has a suggestion. A patient's focus on guilt because of past actions (I caused my cancer through smoking; I gave myself a heart attack by working too hard) can be redirected to actively coping in the present. Asking, "What have you learned from this experience?" and then, "How can you use this knowledge now to improve your life?" can go far in helping patients bring important personal resources to aid them in living more fully in their current circumstances.

Rather than offering ready-made solutions to patients, it is almost always better to find a way for the patient to actively seek solutions in the group. After all, if the goal is for patients to develop active coping skills, simply giving them advice makes for a poor learning experience. It is usually useful to follow a step wise progression in leading patients to explore active solutions to their problems. The therapist should ask questions that require the patients to find a solution to their own problems ("What can you do to improve the situation?"). If this proves too difficult, it can be helpful to ask questions that bring principles of active coping to light ("How would you rather react to this difficult situation, in a way that would leave you feeling better afterwards?"). If this still does not lead to active exploration on the part of the patient, the therapist can ask for suggestions from the group as a whole. Finally, as a last result, it may be useful to offer an interpretation of what seems to be happening with a patient and then ask the patient or the group to comment on this interpretation ("Sometimes people become more distressed when they feel out of control. I wonder if you are experiencing so much distress because you feel out of control with the treatment? You seem to be rejecting all the help that is being offered to you. Is that because you feel so helpless that you really believe there is nothing you can do to improve your situation?").

Adjusting to the Present Moment. In the face of a changing world, the extent to which an individual clings to an old way of being may correspond to the extent to which that person suffers as a result of an inability to adjust to current circumstances. When patients cling so much to an image of the way they were before becoming ill, so much so that it significantly interferes with their well-being, it is valuable to challenge their habitual assumptions of who they are so that they can better adjust to present circumstances. Before developing bone cancer, a professional dancer insisted on continuing to teach until she froze up with pain in the middle of lesson, causing the students to complain. A woman with cardiomyopathy continued to work full days, preparing all meals, cleaning the house, and bringing in extra income to support her college-age children until she literally collapsed from utter exhaustion. Against medical orders, a "retired" business executive checked himself out of the hospital 3 days following coronary artery bypass surgery to attend a meeting of one of the corporate boards on which he sat. As with many persons, letting go of the self-image these patients had invested so much time and effort in developing was a greater threat than hastening their physical death. After some time in existential group psychotherapy, each of these persons could look back with amazement at how dearly they clung to their former lives—lives they now claimed were in many ways far less fulfilling than their current existence.

In the face of such strong effort to cling to old assumptions about oneself and one's existence, the therapist must find ways to challenge old assumptions and promote examination of life in the present moment. Yet this challenge must be undertaken with caution. If patients can go so far as to destroy their bodies rather than let go of their habitual self-image, directly challenging that image is likely to meet with, at the least, strong resistance. People can use several methods to challenge habitual assumptions about themselves and their world. All the methods entail asking questions that challenge the speakers to examine their lives in new ways, in light of their illness. The questions can be directed toward the speaker or, or if the patient is too resistant, they can be posed to the group as a whole, as our own patterns can often be more successfully recognized when we hear others' experiences. Three methods (influenced by the three aspects of existential psychotherapy) are as follows:

1. *Encourage lateral perspective* (hermeneutic influence). Ask others to discuss various ways they would deal with a situation, and ways they have

grown since the illness. If John says, "My entire life has been geared toward getting to the top. I'm not going to let my heart slow me down now," the therapist might ask the group, "In what ways have you found your lives changing since you've had to let-go of your previous lifestyle. Have any of the changes taught you anything about yourselves you've found useful?"

2. *Imagine that the old self has perished* (phenomenological influence). People often cling to what they know (no matter how unpleasant it becomes) because the unknown can appear to be even more frightening. If Margaret states, "I know I am eligible for 80% disability, since I get so tired and I have to take a lot of breaks all the time. But they need me at work, because I am coordinating this new project. So, except when I need to go in for chemo and radiation, I'm going to keep working full time," the therapist might ask her, "What would it be like to no longer go to work? What would you do? What would you be?" Or, "What was it like for others of you who had to go on disability? What was lost and what was gained?"

3. *Be in the moment* (Zen influence). If the patient is constantly regretting the past and worrying about the future, then valuable time passes during which he or she could be enjoying the richness of each day. If a patient or the group as a whole continually discuss the past (what they should have done differently) and/or the future (what they plan to do), it is helpful to direct their attention back to the moment. Jamie had been traveling around the globe looking for alternative AIDS treatments and was filling in the group on plans for travel to England to try a new protocol. The group wondered how he could do so much traveling when his chief complaint was his fatigue. The therapist asked, "It almost sounds like you've been traveling around so much in order to find ways to live longer so you can travel around some more looking for ways to live longer. Even here, you've been filling us in on where you've been and where you're going. I wonder, how much time do you get just to be where you are?" Or, if the group is spending little time in the present moment, the therapist could mention, "I notice that much of the discussion has focused on what you were like before the illness, and how you are going to end up later on. But there has not been much talk about how you are doing right now, right here? What would it be like to talk about how you are feeling right now in this room, without reminicing about the past or worrying about the future."

Summary. The six approaches to therapist intervention described in this section—eliciting responses from the patient that are personal, specific, emotional, interactive with the group, coping oriented, and based in the present moment—are usually useful when employed in the manner presented above. Once a person is speaking authentically (personalizing, being specific, and with affect) and then interacting with others from this basis, exploring active ways to cope and examining ways to be more fully in the moment are worthy of pursuit.

Heuristic Concerns in Facilitating the Group Process

In addition to the specific methods of facilitation, it is helpful to keep some general guidelines in mind. It is useful to have an existential and experiential focus in the group and to remain a facilitator of process rather than a lecturer.

Mature Focus. Existentially, the concept of maturity can be considered the willingness to rest with one's discomfort. The mature group can facilitate individual maturity. The therapeutic process described earlier allows for authentic examination of existential concerns, without the impression of psychological "games" that are often experienced in deductive or brief coping skills groups. Because issues are patient driven, discussion stays close to the concerns of the group members. Process facilitation by the therapist ensures continued authenticity in patients' quality of expression. In addition, this process can facilitate patients' ability to be more fully "in the moment," rather than lingering in the past or worrying about the future.

Giving Advice. When facilitating discussion, therapists must avoid the trap of answering questions with definitive information. Instead, they can draw on the knowledge of the group, which is a superb source of expertise. In educational groups, therapists are teachers relaying information. But in group discussion, therapists' emphasis should be on facilitating the *process*, not providing *content*. Once the therapist becomes the "expert," it is extremely difficult to return to facilitating the process—the patients simply will not permit the therapist to "shift gears." Avoiding giving advice may be difficult for a therapist with expertise, but it is also very important. The expert therapist should find ways to diffuse the question, such as suggesting that the patient ask his doctor or discuss the subject after the group. This approach focuses the patients on the *group process* rather than the group becoming an informational meeting (and correspondingly void of interaction with each other in personal, specific, and affective terms).

Experiential Emphasis. Therapists can look for situations in which the patients can experience a problem and solution firsthand in the group rather than merely comment about it. Rather than attempting to point out habitual ways of thinking and then asking patients to reflect about their beliefs that formed this way of thinking or to expound on existential theory, therapists can offer the opportunity for the patient to directly experience healthy ways of dealing with a problem (Spiegel & Spira, 1991). If Alice is having difficulty getting her husband to understand some of her needs, the therapist attempting to foster reflection and awareness of personality patterns, might say: "Alice, I notice [or you've said] that you sometimes have difficulty expressing your needs and problems here in the group, as well. Is this a common pattern in your life? In what other situations does this pattern arise? Does this stem from low self-esteem?" Certainly, this line of questioning might be useful in a cognitive-behavioral psychotherapy group, which attempts to make unconscious patterns conscious. In groups facilitating authentic expression and support among terminally ill patients, however, it might be more useful to say: "Sometimes it's hard to let others know what you need. Is there a way you can let those of us in the group know what you need, so that we can better understand what you're going through?" or "Julie, do you know what Alice needs?" or "Alice, can you let Julie know what your needs are?" Thus, rather than stimulating reflection about one's patterns, therapists should *look for an opportunity to have patients directly experience their restrictive way of coping in the group and try out a healthy alternative*. A reflective remark *after* such an experience has far greater impact than when stated alone. When the experience is strong enough, such reflective remarks may be totally unnecessary.

Facilitating the Breakdown in Distressed Patients. Crisis can be an opportunity for growth. For this reason, therapists must allow patients to experience their distress for a time, addressing it as openly and honestly as possible before looking for active solutions. This assists in facilitating the breakdown of prior unconscious assumptions and avoids immediately covering up the inauthenticity of these assumptions. Therapists need to be able to facilitate this development of authentic realization and expression rather than put a band-aid of soothing on every crisis that occurs.

However, if the distress is too great, patients will simply "shut down" and be unable to consider aspects of their existential development. Such patients are in a state of physiological arousal and cognitive overload. Therefore, methods of soothing extreme distress can facilitate openness to existential development. Yet different patients require different types of support. Some patients need to become calmer *physically* before they can cognitively address the issues confronting them. For these persons, methods of relaxation, self-hypnosis, or meditation can be helpful. Thus, therapy groups often begin and end with a few minutes of "soothing" and "quieting." These methods can also be used at any time deemed helpful throughout a meeting. Other patients cannot relax physically until their distress is "worked out" cognitively. Frequently, being able to address these issues in a calm and relaxed manner within the group setting can help put the issues into perspective for patients, reducing the cognitive noise and helping them to reduce their generalized arousal. Other times, simply listening to other group members discuss and work through their concerns can provide a modeling that is helpful for later expression.

Facilitating Discussion of Topics

Topics can be addressed through either (1) *open discussion* (facilitated as described earlier) or (2) *brief structured exercises* meant to help the patient personalize these issues in an experiential format, followed by open discussion.

Typical topics that groups raise for discussion include the following:

- Relationships with medical professionals, friends, coworkers, family, and members of group.
- Medical issues: choosing treatments, impact on quality of life, etc.
- Changes in function and functional relationships at work, with friends, in the family, etc.
- Coping with treatment and psychophysical changes.
- Reprioritizing life activities and reconsidering life meaning, values, and purpose.
- Changes in self-image.
- Dying, death, and leaving others behind.
- Being in the moment, with as much comfort and openness as possible.

These are presented in the order of initial ease and frequency of discussion. Eventually, however, the order of topics reverses, as patients find it easier to address more important areas of their lives.

Examples of exercises intended to assist in the development of existential maturity are presented next. These are merely examples, and they appear in greater depth elsewhere (Spira, 1994a). Structured exercises such as these should be used only when needed to stimulate topics that are of current interest to the group. Many groups may never require structured exercises authentically considering issues of relevance to them.

The following are exercises that help reveal one's inauthentic nature.

Exercise 1: The Changing Self

What goes into our self-image? (Factors may include positive or negative aspects of body image, personality characteristics, beliefs, things you do, people you know, etc.)

1. Write down the 10 most important aspects of your self-image, those things without which you would not have been you.
2. Write down what your self-image was like when you were 20 years old.
3. Write down what your future self-image will be like 6 months before you die.
4. Which is the most accurate? How does self-image affect what you do and how you do it?

Exercise 2: Portrait Exercise

Draw two rectangles.

1a. The left rectangle contains an imaginary portrait that has been drawn of you and your life. Inside the frame use words to describe this "portrait." Write down aspects of yourself that comprise your self-image. These could be positive or negative, personality characteristics, beliefs, things you do, people you know, how you look, etc.

1b. Outside the rectangle list those factors that have contributed to your current self-image. These can include genetics, early family environment, families' socioeconomic status, early schooling, later choice of relationships, work, etc.

1c. Consider how much of your current self-image and activities have been chosen *for you* versus *by you.*

2. Now look at the blank portrait to the right. If you could draw your self-image of the way you would like it to be *1 year from now* (given constraints out of one's control, such as genetics, illness, etc.) how would you *choose* this portrait to be? Inside the rectangles write down the characteristics you would most respect in yourself. Outside, put the activities you would most like to engage in.

3. What is preventing you from becoming more like the triangle on the right, and how can you move more toward that in your life?

The following are exercises that facilitate the breakdown, and prepare one for authentic commitment.

Exercise 3: Beliefs Exercise

There are many beliefs, attitudes, and characteristics we developed early in our lives that are still with us and influence the way we see ourselves, others, and the world and limit the decisions we make. For example, if we believe that others are fundamentally separate from us, and everyone has to fend for himself and get what he can from others, it will be natural to be suspicious of others and to remain vigilant, to become aggressive in protecting our own interests, to be at a greater stage of physiological readiness, and to be especially competitive to secure our position. If, on the other hand, we believe ourselves to be incapable of achieving success, the world to be uncaring and unsupportive, and the future to hold no possibility of improvement, then our thoughts are bound to be depressive and our emotions flat, and we are bound to have low physiological arousal and little motivation to work. Thus, our attitudes about ourselves and our world influence the way we act. Other beliefs include having to be "perfect," believing that we are not good down deep, having to take care of others before ourselves, never showing emotions (e.g., "If I can't work like I did before, then I have no value," etc.).

1. Write down a general belief, characteristic, or attitude you have about yourself, others, or your world that may negatively affect your health or quality of life.
2. When was this belief formed. What were the circumstances at that time.
3. How did this belief serve you well at that time?
4. How does this belief still serve you well?
5. How does this belief limit you now?
6. What alternative belief, attitude, or characteristic would be beneficial to have to complement the old habit belief, so that you could choose to use either one at any time, whichever belief was most useful?

Exercise 4: Orpheus Exercise

(This exercise is based on one described by Bugental, 1973/1974.)

1. Write down the 10 most important aspects of your self-image, those things without which you would not have been you. (These can be positive or negative, and include aspects of body image, personality characteristics, beliefs, things you do, people you know, etc.)
2. Now rank-order these aspects of yourself with 10 being least central and 1 being most central to your self-image.
3. Next, take number 10 in your list, and cross it out. Take a minute to imagine what your life would be like without this aspect of yourself. When you can do that, then do the same with number 9, etc. until you finish with number 1. When all items have been removed, what remains? Can you let go of even this? (When finished, notice that some of the items might have been very difficult to cross off, while others were easy to remove.)
4. Now, turn the page over. Write down the two or three most important characteristics you would like to have if you could now re-create the type of self-image you would like, that would allow you to live as fully as possible in the future. (When finished, how many of these were different from items you had crossed off your first list?)

Exercise 5: One Year to Live

If you had only 1 year to live,

1. What personality characteristics would you like to get rid of?
2. What activities would you want to cease doing?
3. What personality characteristics would you want to have to be able to live your life more fully and enjoyably?
4. What activities would you like to be engaged in that would give your life most meaning and value?
5. What is stopping you from making these changes now?
6. What can you do to overcome these barriers?

The following are exercises that help one reprioritize one's activities and consider manifesting more authentically.

Exercise 6: Priorities Exercise

Draw three columns on your page.

1. In column 1, list the 10 major activities you are engaged in during a typical week.
2. In column 2, prioritize these items in terms of which activity you *spend the most time with* on top and, progressively, the items you spend the least time with on the bottom.
3. In column 3, reprioritize the items again, but this time list the activity that *brings most meaning to you, those items that make life worth living,* on top, and the items of lessening personal value toward the bottom. You may also wish to add new items to the list that you wish you could get to but do not usually have the time.
4. Draw lines between similar items in column 2 and 3. If you have large X's, or if your lines go mostly straight across, what does this mean to you?
5. What can you do to spend more time engaged in those activities that make your life worth living? What "has to go" to bring this more centrally into your life?

Exercise 7: Contrasting Self Exercise

Draw three large figures on the page, a square on the top of the page and two circles on the bottom, side by side.

1. In the top square, describe what your situation will be at some point in the future. What will be your level of health, your level of functioning, the people around you, etc.
2a. In the bottom left circle, describe the self-image you have of yourself now.
2b. Imagine that, although your circumstances are changing, you maintain the same self-image in the future. Given your new situation in the future (different age, activities, level of health), how would your current self-image serve you? How would it limit you?
3a. In the circle at the bottom right, describe how your self-image could change to best support the new circumstances you will be facing in the future. What would you need to let go of, and what would you need to develop further?
4. What do you need to do to begin making these changes?

Finally, there are experiential exercises to facilitate the moment of vision.

Exercise 8: Self-Hypnosis Exercise

Self-hypnosis can be used to increase a sense of personal comfort, reducing physical or mental distress, so that from this comfortable basis an individual can consider issues that would otherwise be too difficult to address. Any topic previously discussed in the group or addressed in one of the previous structured exercises could be facilitated in this state. A typical format would be to induce a light trance and imagining a problem situation on a screen off in the distance. An individual can imagine what it would be like to deal with the problem in the "old, inauthentic way" and then imagine what it would be like to interact with it in the "new, authentic manner." Methods of self-hypnosis for the medically ill patient have been described in detail elsewhere (Spira & Spiegel, 1992). Training and experience are, of course, required to use any form of hypnosis effectively. Once this training has been received, utilizing self-hypnosis at the end of a group can help the members address the issues raised in the group in a way that leaves them feeling calm and integrated and knowing that they have addressed important issues at a deeply honest and open level.

Exercise 9: Meditation

Although longer meditation sessions are not feasible in group therapy, beginning each group with a 5-minute Zen meditation can be helpful in settling down and beginning to recognize important issues. In fact, the inability to dismiss certain concerns from the mind during the meditation can serve as the basis of discussion for that session. Although explicit instructions for Zen meditation are contained elsewhere (Spira, 1994b), a simple breath-oriented meditation (zazen) can be both calming of the mind and comforting to the body.

1. Sit comfortably in your chair, with your back erect, eyes open and looking downward, and your hands resting on your belly. (Note: Eyes are open in order to be more fully present, not to dissociate. Eyes open also helps the practitioner notice when they are creating images rather than attending to the image on their retinas.) Whenever you notice your attention being pulled by thoughts (creating your own visual images, conversations, feelings), just note that distraction, let it go, and gently return your attention to what is right here. Do not control your breath, but instead simply observe its effortless activity.

2. Notice the air flowing into and out of your nose and throat. Notice how the temperature changes from the inhale to the exhale, the different places the air touches, the different qualities of the air against the nose and throat. Count 10 more breaths flowing into and out from your nose.

3. Notice your chest expanding and relaxing. Notice that rib cage moves up and down, forward and back, expands out to the sides, and even expands into your back. Find the point in the middle of your body from which this expansion occurs and to which it releases. Count 10 more times the breath expands from this location and returns to it.

4. Notice your belly gently rocking your hands to and fro. Feel the gentle warmth of your body, and the effortlessness with which it rocks your hands. Count 10 more times that your body rocks your hands forward and back.

5. Finally, experience in silence the breath effortlessly expanding and releasing your body. As you breath in, feel as if you are accepting everything you see, hear, and feel into the center of your breath. With every exhale, feel as if you are giving yourself completely away to what you see, hear, and feel. (Everything else is just noise, distraction from this present moment.)

It is useful to begin and end each group therapy session with one of these experiential exercises. Besides training patients to develop these helpful skills, beginning and ending each group with meditation or self-hypnosis will increase patients' confidence that no matter what arises in the groups, they can always return to this calm, comforting basis.

STRUCTURE OF EXISTENTIAL GROUP PSYCHOTHERAPY

Existential group psychotherapy can best occur in groups specifically designed for this style. However, other styles of therapy can also benefit from some aspect of existential principles of facilitation style.

Existential-Oriented Groups

To address existential issues optimally and promote existential development, long-term, ongoing committed groups are best. In these groups, members can join at any time there is an opening and are asked to commit to attend weekly (unless sick or prior arrangement) for at least 6 months or 1 year. After this commitment, they can recommit for another block of time.

It is also useful to strive toward as homogeneous a group as possible. If the type and stage of disease, gender, age, socioeconomic status, and so on, can be made as consistent as possible, patients can immediately begin to gain support through observing others coping with similar issues. Certainly, a more heterogeneous group can also be effective, as long as the severity of disease is life-threatening. However, the more heterogeneous the group members, the more work the therapist will have in pointing out similarities and permitting for differences. In general, group leaders should strive toward greatest homogeneity and settle for heterogeneity of group members as needed to insure a group can be formed (Spira, Chapter 1, this volume).

The optimal size for facilitating existentially oriented discussion appears to be about 10 to 12 members. More becomes unwieldy, as quieter persons do not get as much opportunity to express as do more extroverted types. The use of co-therapists in groups is helpful because each can cover areas missed by the other. For example, if one therapist is tracking themes and affect among those speaking and remembering to get back to a patient about something he or she began to say, the cotherapist can pay attention to quiet persons, who may benefit from speaking at some point in the meeting.

Unlike typical group psychotherapy, contact outside the group is actually useful because persons with medical illness are not coming to the group due to psychosocial dysfunction. Rather, they can benefit from authentic and supportive relationships developed in the group and carry them into their daily lives. Sometimes the group even meets at a patient's hospital bed or at the patient's home when he or she cannot come to the group, and members are encouraged to attend funerals of other group members.

Employing Existential Principles within Other Group Formats

Although the methodology described previously is optimally used within a long-term, committed group of persons with advanced-stage disease, it is possible to employ aspects of existential psychotherapy within other group formats. At the very least, these existential principles can be helpful as *heuristic* guiding principles because many patients will be confronting such issues. No matter what the structure, therapists who are familiar with existential principles must consciously decide whether they are assisting a patient to cover up distress and flee into old habit patterns or social convention regarding existential issues or to what extent they will support expression of a patient's distress to facilitate a release of old assumptions and develop clarity over the patient's existential condition.

The *algorithmic* method of facilitation described earlier (in the section "Process of Group Facilitation") can also be used in any format during the discussion periods, no matter what style or how brief. Educational or cognitive therapy formats can "shift" to this mode during group discussions. However, once a group begins with a more deductive format, it is usually quite difficult to stop teaching and begin facilitating in the way described here. Still, the effort is worthwhile.

Finally, even in purely educational groups, the existential exercises described may be of some use. At the very least, they can encourage some patients to take a closer look at various aspects of their lives previously taken for granted. However, the more authentic the discussion that can be facilitated (as described), the more impact these structured exercises will have. For, it is not the "idea" that is important to achieve but the "experience" of insight that can be translated into action—and authentic expression of this insight in the group is an excellent first step in manifesting one's existential insight.

Groups for Support Persons

Imminent or recent loss of a loved one can be as powerful a threat to the stability of inauthentic ego as one's own illness. Therefore, groups for support persons can follow the same process as described previously, with most of the same issues applying to the group members. Even psychophysical distress can be dealt with in both groups. Although patients might be concerned more with their own pain, support persons can learn to help the patient with pain management and learn themselves to reduce somatic distress common among support persons as well. Although parallel structures are useful, these groups can also be of benefit even if they meet only once or twice each month.

Training of Therapists

Maturity means being able to rest in anxiety, according to Heidegger. In the same way, therapists must be willing and able to stay with the patients' distress rather than attempting to immediately lead them into inauthentic solutions. This means that therapists must be willing to continually examine their own existential condition and make every effort to mature existentially. It is useful for therapists to do the same (written) exercises as patients to continually reexamine their own assumptions. After all, although a therapist may not correctly have an illness, he or she will die sooner or later, and the sooner he or she examines this fact, the fuller life can be in light of it. At the same time, therapists must make sure not to use the group largely for their own benefit. This is especially true of a therapist who has the same illness as others in the group. Nor should therapists expect the patients to tackle issues at the same rate of willingness as themselves (who, presumably, have been at this style of exploration for some time).

Although both cotherapists should have a criterial depth of existential maturity (being willing to tolerate suffering before assisting patients to search for solutions), they can have very differing talents. Some therapists have more group experience; others more in-depth exploration of existential issues. Cotherapists of differing gender and personalities can also be helpful. Because the existential process is not one of giving answers, therapists certainly need not be experts in the medical disease. In fact, it may be helpful to "plead ignorant" and defer to the patients' physicians in medical matters to keep the group on track existentially. Most important, therapists must maintain an appreciation of patients' resources and experience. Every patient is an expert in his or her life, and therapists can only point to ways for patients to access all their resources more fully and employ them with greater sense of purpose.

GENERALIZATIONS, LIMITATIONS, AND CAUTIONS

Generalizations

Existential group psychotherapy is certainly useful for persons with a terminal illness because they are forced to directly confront existential issues every day of their lives. Yet this approach is also useful for a variety of others facing a loss of some sort. Those who are at high risk for developing a life-threatening illness (genetically or as a result of lifestyle) are frequently motivated to discuss their lives in relationship to this life-threatening illness. Those who are dealing with the imminent loss of a loved one or those in bereavement are usually highly motivated to receive support for coping with these issues. Anyone facing a significant loss of self-image (as a result of accident, termination of a relationship, retirement, etc.) may seek therapy, although in such cases only a few distressed persons typically seek therapy, and mostly to end the suffering by covering it up (rather than using it as a springboard to understand and alter the source of the suffering). Of course, we all face losses every day, as we and our world continually change. Thus, existential group psychotherapy can address issues facing every living person; however, only those who are suffering and cannot find a way to cover up this suffering will be willing to accept the loss of their stable world without immediately attempting to find another stable concept to latch on to. For this reason, those with advanced medical illness or those facing loss of a loved one appear to make the best candidates for this approach.

Limitations

Because of limited resources, briefer structured therapy is frequently called for. Here, existential group psychotherapy can serve as a guide of techniques and principles but only to point to issues that patients can address when they are ready.

There are also instances when individual therapy is indicated, because of personality or truly unique psychosocial issues. In many instances, such patients might benefit from combined individual and group therapies. Yet even in individual therapy, the existential principles and methods described here can guide the therapist in method and direction. However, although more uniquely focused, it is often the sharing among peers in a more diffuse and comforting manner that allows issues to be initially stimulated, explored in a safe way, and finally manifested to others. The individual therapist has to find ways to replace the benefits derived from the group experience.

Existential group psychotherapy is difficult to use when a patient makes a greater effort to cover up than to uncover distress. Whereas medically ill patients have less of an ability to do so, there are persons with advanced illness who refuse to confront their assumptions, as well as healthy persons who are more than willing to examine their beliefs to live more fully. It is the role of the therapist to attempt to (hermeneutically) understand the underlying motivating factors of each patient, and to lead patients (phenomenological-ly) into examining how covering up will not allow them to achieve their underlying positive intentions. Providing a basis of comfort and trust (via meditation) can be helpful and drawing from others in the group who have had such experiences is usually very effective. Still, it is important for therapists to recognize that this approach will not work for everyone, and despite their best efforts, there will be some drop out rate.

Unfortunately, there is little way to tell who will be appropriate for the group beforehand. One way to ensure an appropriate "fit" is through patient self-selection. If the group is advertised accurately and then described in more detail to patients before they join, patients who "just want information" will not be interested. For example, patients can be told that groups will offer support for psychological and physical distress and an opportunity for patients to discuss their distress and reexamine their lives in light of their illness to live as fully as possible. Some therapists use psychological assessments upon intake, such as the Minnesota Multiphasic Personality Inventory (MMPI) or a brief checklist of symptom distress. Typically, moderately elevated MMPI 7/2 scales (indicating depression and worried distress) are associated with good prognosis for psychotherapy of this sort. Although other patterns (elevated 3/1, immature reflection; high 4 or 6 patterns, distrust of others or social institutions) usually are associated with poor therapeutic compliance, special groups can be formed to address these personality issues as part of the existential maturation of the patient (as in groups for post-myocardial infarction Type A personalities).

Cautions

It is important to allow, even to gently encourage, but not to push a patient into examining an issue or process too strongly or too early. Therapeutic pressure added to the pressure patients already carry with them may push them into experiencing undue angst, leading them not to uncover but instead to cover up even more strongly, and further becoming fearful of exploring these issues in the future.

It is also necessary to appreciate the fluctuating nature of existential motivation. Hegel described the tendency to evolve consciousness into ego; Schopenhauer described the tendency to release ego and join a greater Spirit (*Geist*). Buddhism discusses each of these as the most fundamental processes in life (*engi*, the process of forming and emptying). Therefore, there will be moments when a person or group members and engaged in discovering their power in their own ego manifestation, and other times when they are engaged in releasing inauthentic beliefs, which might appear as transient depression. Until patients become fluidly engaged in flowing between these two aspects of life, they may appear to themselves and others as struggling emotionally. The existential process *is* a struggle, one of healthy development. Yet therapists must be ever vigilant for *consistent* avoidance or depression in group members. Allowing for each patient's hermeneutic patterns to present themselves permits therapists to interact with each patient, and the group as a whole, in the way that is most effective for patients.

CONCLUSION

It is not uncommon that patients choose to undergo procedures or seek alternative treatments that hold some promise of *longer* life, even though it may severely impair their *quality* of life. Addressing issues of improving quality of life in light of invasive medical procedures and deteriorating health is highly relevant for existential group psychotherapy. The basic assumption in existential group psychotherapy is that authenticity of perception and expression is required for optimal living. Also, improving quality of life appears to be the best chance for living longer. However, it is not necessarily the case that living longer means living better. The existential psychotherapist argues that it is far better to live this moment as fully as possible than to live in dreams of the past or fantasies of the future for an eternity. After all, what exactly does it mean to "live" or to "die"?

Does one ever really die? The notion of dying is very much a social idea. People cannot conceive of death or dying without imagining it in ways learned from family, religion, scientific study, and past experiences of handling death through social conventions such as funerals, flowers, cards, and so on. Because our awareness of death is therefore a social–conceptual phenomenon, what happens if we are able to release any notion of death or dying? Existentially, dying can be understood as the process of releasing our image of death and dying, of self-image, indeed images all together—permitting for interpretless awareness of the fundamental relationship that exists with the world. Images of life and death are then seen as mere social conveniences rather than a "fact" about the world independent of one's interpretation of this fact.

Indeed, death is a powerful concept. It is a concept that can motivate a person to address existential considerations and enter into a developmental path of authenticity. However, an individual might be said to have achieved the ultimate authenticity when that individual appreciates that once the idea of death is suspended, *he or she can live forever in this very moment—in full open relationship with others and the world.*

The example of Susan can serve to illuminate this point:

COPING WITH LIFE-THREATENING ILLNESS

Susan had just graduated college when she was diagnosed with Hodgkin's lymphoma. She came to group therapy to learn to cope with the treatment better, and to keep her spirits up. Susan wanted to know how to "fight this thing." At first, she impressed all her friends and family with how "well" she was holding up with the diagnosis and treatment. She continued to go to lots of parties (more than ever before), to volunteer for activities, and to look for a job (even though she was comfortably supported by her parents for the time being). She was proud to report how much she impressed her friends, who continually called her a model for them. However, over the course of the year, despite ongoing oncotherapy, the disease eventually metastasized and Susan became more introspective.

Using the methods described earlier, Susan slowly began realizing that her idea of "bucking up, being strong, fighting the cancer" was a social construct but only served to cover up the distress she felt every day and night. She also realized that her constant partying and volunteering (which was driving her to exhaustion) was done to avoid confronting her fears. The group helped her to express this distress, and she began sleeping better, eating better, and coping better with treatment. Eventually, Susan was able to reevaluate her activities and choose which activities and relationships were most meaningful to her. She greatly pared down her schedule and spent more time doing those things that gave her life greatest purpose. In the last few months of her life, Susan claimed that now that she no longer feared dying, she finally "was" living. And although she could laugh with the irony of the situation, she also appreciated how it was because of the illness that she was able to finally live life fully, with an open heart and open mind. At her funeral, her friends and family echoed this growth. One friend said that it took more courage for her to "submit" to her illness than it did to "fight" the illness. For, in submitting to the truth of her feelings, she also was free to share this depth of feelings with others.

REFERENCES

Antoni, M. H., Schneiderman, N., Fletcher, M. A., Goldstein, D. A., Ironson, G., & LaPerriere, A. (1990). Psychoneuroimmunology and HIV-1. *Journal of Consulting and Clinical Psychology, 58*(1), 38–49.

Behler, E. (Ed.). (1987). *Philosophy of German idealism*. New York: Continuum.

Berglund, G., Bolund, C., Gustafsson, U., & Sjoden, P. (1994). A randomized study of a rehabilitation program for cancer patients: The "starting again" group. *Psycho-Oncology, 3*, 109–120.

Berkman, L. F., & Syme, S. L. (1979). Social networks, host resistance, and mortality: A nine-year follow-up study of Alameda County residents. *American Journal of Epidemiology, 109*, 186–204.

Binswanger, L. (1958). The case of Ellen West: An anthropological clinical study. In

R. May, E. Angell, & H. Ellenberger (Eds.), *Existence* (pp. 237–364). New York: Simon & Schuster. (Original work published 1945)

Bodhidharma. (1987). *The Zen teachings of Bodhidharma* (R. Pine, Trans.). Port Townsend, WA: Empty Bowl. (Original work 560 A.D.)

Bodian, S. (1991, October). Non-dual Yoga: An interview with Jean Klein. *Yoga Journal*, p. 100.

Boss, M. (1958). *The analysis of dreams* (A. Pomerans, Trans.). New York: Philosophical Library.

Buber, M. (1958). *Land thou* (2nd ed.). New York: Charles Scribner's Sons.

Bugental, J. (1973/1974). Confronting the existential meaning of "my death" through group exercises. *Interpersonal Development, 4,* 148–163.

Cella, D., Sarafian, B., Snider, P., Yellen, S., & Winicour, P. (1993). Evaluation of a community-based cancer support group. *Psycho-Oncology, 2,* 123–132.

Cohen, S. (in press). Social integration and social ties. In J. Holland (Ed.), *Textbook of psycho-oncology.* New York: Oxford University Press.

Copleston, F. S. J. (1946). *A history of philosophy: Greece and Rome.* New York: Image.

Dewey, J. (1910). A short catechism concerning truth. In *The influence of Darwin on philosophy and other essays* (pp. 154–168). New York: Holt.

Douglas, J. D. (1983). The emergence, security, and growth of the sense of self. In A. Fontana & J. Kotarba (Eds.), *Existential theories of the self* (pp. 38–48). Chicago: University of Chicago Press.

Dunkel-Schetter, C., Feinstein, L. G., & Taylor, S. E. (1992). Patterns of coping with cancer. *Health Psychology, 11(2),* 79–87.

Ellis, A. (1962). *Reason and emotion in psychotherapy.* New York: Lyle Stuart and Citadel Press.

Esterling, B. A., Antoni, M. H., Fletcher, M. A., Margulies, S., & Schneiderman, N. (1994). Emotional disclosure through writing or speaking modulates latent Epstein–Barr virus antibody titers. *Journal of Consulting and Clinical Psychology, 62(1),* 130–140.

Esterling, B. A., Antoni, M. H., Kumar, M., & Schneiderman, N. (1993). Defensiveness, trait anxiety, and Epstein–Barr viral capsid antigen antibody titers in healthy students. *Health Psychology, 12(2),* 132–139.

Fawzy, F. I., Fawzy, N. W., Arndt, L. A., & Pasnau, R. O. (1995). Critical review of psychosocial interventions in cancer care. *Archives of General Psychiatry, 52,* 100–113.

Fawzy, F. I., Fawzy, N. W., & Hyun, C. S. (1994). Short-term psychiatric intervention for patients with malignant melanoma: Effects on psychological state, coping, and the immune system. In C. Lewis et al. (Eds.), *The psychoimmunology of human cancer* (pp. 292–319). New York: Oxford University Press.

Fawzy, F. I., Fawzy, N. W., Hyun, C. S., Elashoff, R., Guthrie, D., Fahey, J. L., & Morton, D. (1993). Malignant melanoma: Effects of an early structured psychiatric intervention, coping, and affective state on recurrence and survival 6 years later. *Archives of General Psychiatry, 50,* 681–689.

Fawzy, F. I., Kemeny, M. E., Fawzy, N., Elashoff, R., Gutherie, D., Morton, D., Cousins, N., & Fahey, J. L. (1990). A structured psychiatric intervention for cancer patients, II: Changes over time in immunological measures. *Archives of General Psychiatry, 47,* 729–735.

Fichte, J. G. (1982). *The science of knowledge* (P. Heath & J. Lachs, Trans.). London: Cambridge University Press. (Original work published 1794)

Forester, B., Kornfelf, D. S., Fleiss, J. L., & Thompson, S. (1993). Group psychotherapy during radiotherapy: Effects on emotional and physical distress. *American Journal of Psychiatry, 150*(11), 1700–1706.

Fox, B. (in press). A critique of psychosocial factors and cancer incidence and mortality. In J. Holland (Ed.), *Textbook of psycho-oncology.* New York: Oxford University Press.

Frankl, V. (1978). *The unheard cry for meaning.* New York: Simon & Schuster.

Frenkel, E. M., & Torem, M. (1981). Management of a dying patient in group therapy. *Group, the Journal of the Eastern Group Psychotherapy Society, 5*(1), 54–61.

Friedman, M., & Rosenman, R. (1974). *Type-A behavior and your heart.* New York: Alfred A. Knopf.

Friedman, M., Thoresen, C. E., Gill, J. J., Ulmer, D., Powell, L. H., Price, V. A., Brown, B., Thompson, L., Rabin, D. D., Breall, W., Broug, W., Levy, R., & Dixon, T. (1986). Alteration of Type A behavior and its effect on cardiac recurrences in postmyocardial infarction patients: Summary results of the recurrent coronary prevention project. *American Heart Journal, 112,* 653–665.

Gadamer, H. (1976). *Philosophical hermeneutics* (D. Linge, Trans.). Berkeley: University of California Press.

Gellert, G. A., Maxwell, R. M., & Siegel, B. S. (1993). Survival of breast cancer patients receiving adjunctive psychosocial support therapy: A 10-year follow-up study. *Journal of Clinical Oncology, 11*(1), 66–69.

Gendlin, E. (1979). Experiential psychotherapy. In R. Corsini (Ed.), *Current psychotherapies* (2dn ed., pp. 340–373). Itasca, IL: F. E. Peacock.

Goldstein, D. A., & Antoni, M. H. (1989). The distribution of repressive coping styles among non-metastatic and metastatic breast cancer patients as compared to non-cancer patients. *Psychology and Health, 3,* 245–258.

Glasser, W. (1965). *Reality therapy.* New York: Harper & Row.

Greer, S. (1991). Psychological response to cancer and survival. *Psychological Medicine, 21,* 43–49.

Greer, S., Morris, T., & Pettingale, K. W. (1979). Psychological response to breast cancer: Effect on outcome. *Lancet, 2,* 785–787.

Greer, S., & Watson, M. (1987). Toward a psychobiological model of cancer: Psychological considerations. *Social Science Medicine, 20,* 773–777.

Habermas, J. (1971). *Knowledge and human interests.* (J. Shapiro, Trans.). Boston: Beacon Press. (Original work published 1968)

Habermas, J. (1976). A review of Gadamer's *Truth and method.* In F. Dllmayr & T. McArthy (Eds.), *Understanding and social inquiry* (pp. 335–361). Notre Dame, IN: University of Notre Dame Press.

Hegel, G. W. F. (1967). *The phenomenology of mind* (J. B. Baillie, Trans.). New York: Harper. (Original work published 1807)

Hegel, G. W. F. (1968). *Lectures on the philosophy of religion* (E. B. Speirs, Trans.). New York: Humanities Press. (Original work published 1832)

Heidegger, M. (1962). *Being and time* (J. Macquarrie & E. Robinson, Trans.). New York: Harper & Row. (Original work published 1927)

Heidegger, M. (1966). Conversations on a country path about thinking. In *Discourse on thinking*. New York: Harper Torchbooks. (Original work published 1944/1945)

Heinrich, R., & Schag, C. (1985). Stress and activity management: Group treatment for cancer patients and spouses. *Journal of Consulting and Clinical Psychology, 33*, 439–446.

House, J. S., Landis, K. R., Umberson, D. (1988). Social relationships and health. *Science, 241*, 540–544.

Husserl, E. (1900). *Logical investigations* (Vols. 1 and 2) (J. N. Findlay, Trans.). Boston: Routledge & Kegan Paul.

Husserl, E. (1931). *Ideas: General introduction to pure phenomenology* (W. E. B. Gibson, Trans.). New York: Collier Books. (Original work published 1913)

Jacobi, F. H. (1987). Open letter to Fichte. In E. Behler (Ed.), *Philosophy of German idealism* (pp. 126–127). New York: Continuum. (Original work published 1799)

James, W. (1890). *The principles of psychology*. New York: Holt & Co.

Jaspers, K. (1913). *Allgemeine psychopathologie*. Berlin: Springer.

Kierkegaard, S. (1946). Works of love. In R. Bretall (Ed.), *A Kierkegaard anthology* (pp. 281–322). Princeton University Press. (Original work published 1847).

Kierkegaard, S. (1974). *Fear and trembling* (W. Lowrie, Trans.). Princeton, NJ: Princeton University Press. (Original work published 1841)

Kierkegaard, S. (1974). *Sickness unto death* (5th ed.) (W. Lowrie, Trans.). Princeton, NJ: Princeton University Press. (Original work published 1848)

Levin, D. M. (1985). *The body's recollection of being: Phenomenological psychology and the deconstruction of nihilism*. Boston: Routledge & Kegan Paul.

Lutgendorf, S. K., Antoni, M. H., Kumar, M., & Schneiderman, N. (1994). Changes in cognitive coping strategies predict EBV antibody titers following disclosure induction. *Journal of Psychosomatic Research, 38*(1), 63–78.

Maslow, A. (1968). *Toward a psychology of being* (2nd ed.). Princeton, NJ: Insight Books.

Mead, G. H. (1938). *The philosophy of the act* (C. W. Morris, Ed.). Chicago: University of Chicago Press.

Merleau-Ponty, M. (1962). *Phenomenology of perception* (C. Smith, Trans.). London: Routledge & Kegan Paul.

Miller, S., Brody, D., & Summerton, J. (1988). Styles of coping with threat: Implications for health. *Journal of Personality and Social Psychology, 54*, 345–353.

Miller, S. M., Rodeletz, M., Schroeder, C. M., Mangan, C. E., & Sedlacek, T. V. (1996). Applications of the monitoring process model to coping with severe long-term medical threats. *Health Psychology, 15*(3), 216–225.

Moreno, J. (1946). *Psychodrama (Vol. I)*. New York: Beacon House.

Mulder, C. L., Antoni, M. H., Emmelkamp, P. M., Veugelers, P. J., Sanfort, T. P., Vijver, F. A., & de Vries, M. J. (1995). Psychosocial group intervention and the rate of decline of immunological parameters in asymptomatic HIV infected gay men. *Psychotherapy and Psychosomatics, 63*(3–4), 185–192.

Mulder, C. L., Emmelkamp, P. M., Antoni, M. H., Mulder, J. W., Sanfort, T. P., & de Vries, M. J. (1994). Cognitive behavioral and experiential group psychotherapy for HIV infected homosexual men: A comparative study. *Psychosomatic Medicine, 56*(5), 423–431.

Nietzsche, F. (1961). *Thus spoke Zarathustra* (R. Hollingsdale, Trans.). New York: Penguin. (Original work completed in 1883)

Nietzsche, F. (1967). *The will to power* (W. Kaufman, Trans.). New York: Vintage. (Original notes completed in 1888)

Nishitani, K. (1982). *Religion and nothingness*. Berkeley: University of California Press.

Orth-Gomer, K., & Unden, A. L. (1990). Type A behavior, social support, and coronary risk: Interaction and significance for mortality in cardiac patients. *Psychosomatic Medicine, 52*(1), 59–72.

Palmer, R. E. (1969). *Hermeneutics*. Evanston, IL: Northwestern University Press.

Passick, S., & Redd, W. (in press). PTSD and dissociative disorders. In J. Holland (Ed.), *Textbook of psycho-oncology*. New York: Oxford University Press.

Peirce, C. S. (1931–1935). *Peirce's collected papers* (Vol. V) (C. Harshorne & P. Weiss, Eds.). Cambridge, MA: Harvard University Press.

Pennebaker, J. W., Kiecolt-Glaser, J. K., & Glaser, R. (1988). Disclosure of traumas and immune function: Health implications for psychotherapy. *Journal of Consulting and Clinical Psychology, 56*, 239–245.

Perls, F. S. (1969). *Gestalt therapy verbatim*. Moab, UT: Real People Press.

Reed, G. M., Kemeny, M. E., Taylor, S. E., Wang, H-Y. W., & Visscher, B. R. (1994). Realistic acceptance as a predictor of reduced survival time in gay men with AIDS. *Health Psychology, 13*, 299–307.

Reed, G., & Stanton, A. (1996). *Group psychotherapy for HIV positive symptomatic gay men: A treatment manual*. Manuscript in preparation.

Reich, W. (1942). *The function of the orgasm* (T. Wolfe, Trans.). New York: Noonday Press.

Reifman, A. (1995). Social relationships, recovery from illness, and survival: A literature review. *Annals of Behavioral Medicine, 17*(2), 124–131.

Reynolds, D. K. (1976). *Morita psychotherapy*. Berkeley: University of California Press.

Reynolds, D. K. (1980). *The quiet therapies: Japanese pathways to personal growth*. Honolulu: University Press of Hawaii.

Ricoeur, P. (1979). Th emodel of the text: Meaningful action considered as text. In P. Rabinow & W. Sullivan (Eds.), *Interpretive social science: A reader* (pp. 73–101). (Original work published 1971)

Rickman, H. P. (1979). *Wilhelm Dilthey: Pioneer of the human studies*. Berkeley: University of California Press.

Roberts, C. S., Cox, C. E., Reintgen, D. S., Baile, W. F., & Gibertini, M. (1994). *Cancer, 74*, 336–341.

Sasaki Roshi, J. (1978). *Lectures on the diamond Sutra*. Presented at the seminars on the Sutras, co-sponsored by UCLA and Mt. Baldy Zen Center, Mt. Baldy, CA.

Shekelle, R. B., Gale, M., Ostfeld, A. M., & Paul, O. (1983). Hostility, risk of coronary heart disease, and mortality. *Psychosomatic Medicine, 45*(2), 109–114.

Schopenhauer, A. (1958). *The world as will and representation* (Vol. II) (E. F. Payne, Trans.). New York: Doubleday.

Siegel, B., Spira, J., & Ulmer, D. (1992, December). *Panel discussion: The effects of group therapy on medically ill patients*. Fourth Mind, Body, and Immunity Conference, sponsored by the Institute for the Clinical Application of Behavioral Medicine, Hilton Head, SC.

Spiegel, D., Bloom, J. R., Kramer, H. C., & Gottheil, E. (1989). Effect of psychosocial treatment on survival of patients with metastatic breast cancer. *Lancet, 2,* 889–891.

Spiegel, D., Bloom, J., & Yalom, I. (1981). Group support for patients with metastatic cancer. *Archives of General Psychiatry, 38,* 527–533.

Spiegel, D., & Spira, J. L. (1991). *Supportive expressive group therapy: A treatment manual of psychosocial intervention for treating women with recurrent breast cancer.* Palo Alto, CA: Department of Psychiatry, Stanford University.

Spiegel, D., & Spira, J. (1992). Hypnosis in the treatment of psychiatric illness. In D. Dunner (Ed.), *Current psychiatric therapy* (pp. 517–523). New York: W. B. Saunders.

Spira, J. (1991). *Educational therapy: Existential, educational, and counseling approaches to behavioral medicine intervention.* Unpublished doctoral dissertation, University of California, Berkeley.

Spira, J. (1993, November). *Dissociation and PTSD in the medically ill.* Paper presented at the meeting of the Academy of Psychosomatic Medicine, New Orleans, LA.

Spira, J. (1994a). *Health psychology workbook.* Durham, NC: Duke University Center for Living.

Spira, J. (1994b). *Tai chi chuan and Zen meditation for medically ill patients* [Videotape and manual]. Durham, NC: Duke University Center for Living.

Spira, J. (1996a). *Meditation in medicine.* Paper presented at the symposium, International Society of Behavioral Medicine, Washington, DC.

Spira, J. (1996b). *The relationship between social support, mood, and ability to be in the moment.* Manuscript in preparation.

Spira, J. (in press-a). Group psychotherapy for persons with cancer. In J. Holland (Ed.), *Textbook of psycho-oncology.* New York: Oxford University Press.

Spira, J. (in press-b). Existential psychotherapy in palliative care. In H. M. Chochinov & W. Breitbart (Eds.), *Psychiatric dimensions of palliative medicine.* New York: Oxford University Press.

Spira, J., & Spiegel, D. (1992). The use of hypnosis and related techniques for managing pain in terminally ill patients. *Hospice Journal, 8*(1/2), 89–119.

Spira, J., & Spiegel, D. (1993). Group psychotherapy for the medically ill. In A. Stoudemire & B. Fogel (Eds.), *Psychiatric care of the medical patient* (2nd ed., pp. 31–50). New York: Oxford University Press.

Spira, J., & Reed. G. (1996). *Group psychotherapy for women with first occurrence breast cancer: A treatment manual for demonstration project by Blue Cross of Massachusetts, Inc. and the American Psychological Association.* Washington, DC: American Psychological Association, Office of the Practice Directorate.

Suzuki, D. T. (1934). *Introduction to Zen Buddhism.* New York: Causeway.

Taylor, S. (1984). Attributions, beliefs about control, and adjustment to breast cancer. *Journal of Personality and Social Psychology, 46*(3), 489–502.

Temoshok, L. (1985). Biopsychosocial studies on cutaneous malignant melanoma: Psychosocial factors associated with prognostic indicators, progression, psychophysiology, and tumor–host response. *Social Science and Medicine, 20,* 833–840.

Thurman, R. A. (Trans.). (1976). *The holy teachings of Vimalakirti.* University Park: Pennsylvania State University Press.

Trijsburg, R. W., van Knippenberg, F. C. I., & Rijpma, S. E. (1992). Effects of psychological treatment on cancer patients: A critical review. *Psychosomatic Medicine*, *54*, 489–517.

Vachon, M. L., Lyall, W. A., Rogers, J., Cochrane, J., & Freeman, S. (1982). The effectiveness of psychosocial support during post-surgical treatment of breast cancer. *International Journal of Psychiatry Medicine*, *11*, 365–372.

Watson, M., & Greer, S. (in press). Psychological and behavioral factors in cancer risk and survival: Personality and coping. In J. Holland (Ed.), *Textbook of psychooncology*. New York: Oxford University Press.

Watson, M., Greer, S., Pruyn, J., & Van Den Borne, B. (1990). Locus of control and mental adjustment to cancer. *Psychological Reports*, *66*, 39–48.

Weisman, A., Worden, J., & Sobel, H. (1980). *Psychosocial screening and intervention with cancer patients: Research report*. Cambridge, MA: Shea.

Wheelwright, P. (1966). *The pre-Socratics*. New York: Odyssey Press.

Winick, L., & Robbins, G. F. (1977). Physical and psychologic readjustment after mastectomy: An evaluation of Memorial Hospitals' PMRG program. *Cancer*, *39*(2), 478–486.

Wood, P. E., Milligan, M., Christ, D., & Liff, D. (1978). Group counseling for cancer patients in a community hospital. *Psychosomatics*, *19*, 555–561.

Yalom, I. D. (1980). *Existential psychotherapy*. New York: Basic Books.

Yalom, I. D. (1985). *The theory and practice of group psychotherapy* (3rd ed.). New York: Basic Books.

Yalom, I. D., & Greaves, C. (1977). Group therapy with the terminally ill. *American Journal of Psychiatry*, *134*, 396–400.

Zimmerman, M. (1986). *Eclipse of the self: The development of Heidegger's concept of authenticity*. Athens: Ohio University Press.

Zimmerman, M. (1989, November). *Heidegger and social ecology*. Talk given at the Applied Heidegger Conference, University of California, Berkeley.

PART IV

TREATING BEHAVIORS THAT INTERFERE WITH HEALTH

Group Psychotherapy for the Treatment of Bulimia Nervosa and Binge Eating Disorder: Research and Clinical Methods

DENISE E. WILFLEY

CARLOS M. GRILO

JUDITH RODIN

Although descriptions of eating disorders date back several centuries (Casper, 1983; Parry-Jones & Parry-Jones, 1991), the last 20 years have witnessed a striking increase in attention to disordered eating. This interest, undoubtedly as a result of the increasing prevalence of dieting, body dissatisfaction, and disordered eating in our culture (Brownell, 1991a, 1991b), is also evidenced by the proliferation of clinical research. That the American Psychiatric Association has demarcated bulimia as a distinct eating disorder in the third edition of the *Diagnostic and Statistical Manual of Mental Disorders* (DSM-III; American Psychiatric Association, 1980) and binge eating disorder as a research category in DSM-IV (American Psychiatric Association, 1994; Wilson & Walsh, 1991) is further evidence of the growing concern with eating disorders.

The goal for the present chapter is to provide an overview of the nature and treatment of eating disorders, with a focus on bulimia nervosa and binge eating disorder (BED). We summarize what is known regarding the etiology and maintenance of these two eating disorders and present an integrative biopsychosocial model. We will then review treatment research, with a selective focus on controlled clinical trials. Finally, we detail two specific group psychotherapy treatments: cognitive-behavioral therapy (CBT) and interpersonal psychotherapy (IPT). These two treatments have emerged from the first generation of controlled clinical trial research as the most promising interventions.

BACKGROUND REVIEW

Eating and Weight Disorders: Classification, Diagnosis, and Clinical Description

Several major types of eating and weight-related problems exist. DSM-IV (American Psychiatric Association, 1994) delineates several disorders characterized by gross disturbances in eating. DSM-IV delineates two reasonably well-established categories of eating disorders—anorexia nervosa (AN) and bulimia nervosa (BN)—and one less well-established, if not imprecise category—eating disorder not otherwise specified (EDNOS). DSM-IV also includes a new research category diagnosis, binge eating disorder. Obesity is not included in the DSM-IV as a psychiatric diagnosis because it encompasses a heterogeneous population and is not consistently associated with any distinct psychological or behavioral syndrome. Rather, obesity is generally considered a physical disorder (Brownell & Fairburn, 1996). See Figure 6.1 for a schematic representation of the eating disorder diagnostic categories in DSM-IV. Although we focus on BN and BED, the methods discussed here have application to other forms of eating disorders. Unfortunately, less is known about effective treatments for anorexia nervosa and atypical eating disorders (see Grilo, Devlin, Cachelin, & Yanovski, 1996).

Bulimia Nervosa

BN is characterized by the following essential features: (1) recurrent episodes of binge eating; (2) a loss of control during these eating binges; (3) use of extreme compensatory behaviors designed to prevent weight gain, such as purging (e.g., self-induced vomiting, laxative abuse), strict dieting or fasting, or vigorous exercise; and (4) a persistent overconcern with body shape and weight (American Psychiatric Association, 1994). DSM-IV also requires that binge eating and inappropriate compensatory behaviors both occur, on average, at least twice a week for 3 months.

Diagnostic Issues. The DSM-IV diagnostic criteria for BN include three significant changes (American Psychiatric Association, 1994; Wilson & Pike, 1993; Wilson & Walsh, 1991). The first major change is the exclusion

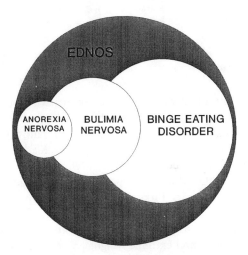

FIGURE 6.1. Schematic representation of the diagnostic categories for eating disorders in DSM-IV. From Spitzer et al. (1992). Copyright 1992 by John Wiley & Sons. Reprinted by permission.

of patients who also meet criteria for AN. This exclusionary criterion was proposed for the following reasons: (1) although BN can be observed across weight categories from anorexic to obese, the majority of persons are within a normal weight range; and (2) low-weight, restricter-type BN has characteristically posed several challenging clinical issues, including the potential need to hospitalize to stabilize weight and more extreme dysfunctional attitudes about shape and weight. Given these similarities to AN patients, a diagnosis of AN appears warranted.

Second, DSM-IV proposes a distinction within BN (without current AN) of two specific types: (1) purging type, which involves the regular use of vomiting, laxatives, and diuretics; and (2) nonpurging type, which involves the use of restrictive dieting, fasting, or excessive exercise to control weight or shape.

Third, following much controversy and discussion regarding what constitutes a binge (Beglin & Fairburn, 1992; Rossiter & Agras, 1988), DSM-IV has stipulated two criteria. First, to be considered a binge, an amount of food that is considered objectively larger than what others would eat in a similar context must be eaten in a discrete period of time defined arbitrarily as 2 hours. Consistent with previous formulations, the person must experience a sense of loss of control over the eating during that particular episode (i.e., an inability to stop or to control the eating). This distinction between objectively large binges and subjective binges (i.e., loss of control but quantity of food not large) remains a subject of debate. Although DSM-IV criteria require the amount of food to be large, there are no published data to support a distinction between large and small amounts. However, some data do suggest that loss of control is a key feature of binge eating (Beglin & Fairburn, 1992; Rossiter & Agras, 1988).

Associated Features. BN frequently co-occurs with other psychological/behavioral problems. Associated psychopathology most frequently includes depression, anxiety, substance abuse, and personality disorders, particularly cluster B (Grilo et al., 1995; Grilo, Levy, Becker, Edell, & McGlashan, 1996; Hatsukami, Mitchell, Eckert, & Pyle, 1986; Higuchi, Suzuki, Yamada, Parrish, & Kono, 1993; Hudson, Pope, Jonas, & Yurgulen-Todd, 1983; Laessle, Wittchen, Fichter, & Pirke, 1989; Powers, Coovert, Brightwell, & Stevens, 1988; Schwalberg, Barlow, Alger, & Howard, 1992). The pervasive preoccupation with body shape and weight (a core feature of BN) coupled with periods of bingeing and extreme weight control practices result in frequent weight fluctuations for many bulimics.

The well-established co-occurrence of BN and affective disorders (Strober & Katz, 1987) has led some researchers to posit that BN is a variant of affective disorder (Hudson et al., 1983). However, the exact nature of the association remains unclear, and more recent research indicates that BN is not simply an expression of affective disorders. For instance, studies have found that the pattern of depressive symptoms in eating-disordered and affective-disordered patients differs and that depressive symptoms often remit when the BN is treated (Laessle et al., 1989; Strober & Katz, 1987).

Epidemiology. The overwhelming majority of patients with BN are female. Although estimates of the prevalence of BN vary widely, rigorous epidemiological studies with strict criteria for BN generally report prevalence rates of roughly 2% of all females (Fairburn & Beglin, 1990; Fairburn, Hay, & Welch, 1993; Kendler et al., 1991). Studies using self-report and questionnaire data have generally reported higher estimates of the prevalence of BN (Fairburn, Hay, & Welch, 1993a; Hsu, 1990a). In fact, some investigators have described BN as nearing epidemic proportions among young females (adolescents and young adults), particularly over the past two decades. However, carefully conducted research using strict operationalization of DSM-III-R (American Psychiatric Association, 1987) criteria with structured clinical interviews and/or case records to verify self-report screenings have generally estimated the prevalence of BN to be less than 3% of females (Drewnowski, Hopkins, & Kessler, 1988; Fairburn & Beglin, 1990; Fairburn, Hay, & Welch, 1993; Kendler et al., 1991; Rand & Kuldau, 1986). Moreover, recent research has suggested that the frequency of problematic eating and dieting behaviors may be leveling off and perhaps declining (Heatherton, Nichols, Mahamedi, & Keel, 1995). It remains unclear whether actual cases of BN have increased in recent years, although some carefully collected data suggest that a cohort shift has occurred (Bushnell, Wells, Hornblow, Oakley Browne, & Joyce, 1990; Kendler et al., 1991; see Fairburn, Hay, & Welch, 1993). For example, females born after 1960 had a higher risk for BN than those born earlier (Kendler et al., 1991).

Epidemiological research has generally documented that BN is most common in Caucasian females of middle to upper social classes in Western cultures (Fairburn & Beglin, 1990; Hsu, 1990a). Recent research, however, suggests that eating-related problems generally, and perhaps BN, may be increasing in non-Caucasian groups, including African Americans (Akan & Grilo, 1995; Gray, Ford, & Kelley, 1987; Langer, Warheit, & Zimmerman, 1991), and in developing non-Western cultures (Hsu, 1990a). High-risk studies have suggested that special populations with heightened weight/shape demands, such as certain athletes (e.g., gymnasts) and dancers, may be more susceptible to BN (Brownell, Rodin, & Wilmore, 1992; Hsu, 1990a). Collectively, research has highlighted the risk factor for disordered eating and BN of being female in a culture (Western) and subcultures (e.g., middle to upper class, certain athletes, or gay/lesbians) in which pressures to conform to a certain ideal body weight/shape may be heightened (e.g., Beren, Hayden, Wilfley, & Grilo, 1996).

More common in the general population are problems of a subthreshold level with binge eating, dieting, and body dissatisfaction (Kendler et al., 1991; Schotte & Stunkard, 1987). Studies documenting the increasing frequency of dieting, eating, and body shape concerns among females in our culture have led some researchers to speak of a phenomenon of "normative discontent" regarding body shape (Rodin, Silberstein, & Striegel-Moore, 1985; Silberstein, Striegel-Moore, & Rodin, 1987; Striegel-Moore, Silberstein, & Rodin, 1986).

Psychosocial Aspects. Significant disturbances in social relatedness and interpersonal deficits among persons with BN have consistently been documented (Herzog, Keller, Lavori, & Ott, 1987; Herzog, Norman, Rigotti, & Prepose, 1986; Johnson & Connors, 1987; Norman & Herzog, 1986; Striegel-Moore et al., 1986). Patients with BN are characterized by difficulties with peers (Pike, 1989), spouses (van Buren & Williamson, 1988), and family members (Dolan, Lieberman, Evans, & Lacy, 1990; Humphrey, 1988, 1989; Pike & Rodin, 1991; Strober & Humphrey, 1987). The degree of social and interpersonal problems has been found to be associated with the severity of BN (Herzog et al., 1986; Herzog et al., 1987). These interpersonal difficulties have been attributed to deficits in ability to experience and tolerate affect and to associated fears of emotional expression and of rejection by others (Johnson & Connors, 1987).

These interpersonal deficits are also manifested in poor coping skills (Cattanach, Malley, & Rodin, 1988; Cattanach & Rodin, 1988), poor social skills, and inadequate social support (Grissett & Norvell, 1992). These social deficits may leave these individuals with a heightened preoccupation how they present themselves and how others perceive them. Indeed, high levels of public self-consciousness and social anxiety are characteristic of BN (Belfer, Crump, & Bradach, 1991; Schwalberg et al., 1992; Striegel-Moore, Silberstein, & Rodin, 1993). Patients with BN are often described as being exquisitely sensitive to certain cues from others and often attempt to guide their own behaviors to obtain approval and prevent rejection. This "false self" or "fraudulence" characteristic has been described by researchers of varied theoretical orientations (Johnson & Connors, 1987; Johnson, Connors, & Tobin, 1987; Striegel-Moore et al., 1993). Because of these social self-deficits coupled with poor self-esteem and a strong desire to be accepted by others, these individuals may be susceptible to societal pressures to diet and to strive for certain shape/weight ideals (Johnson & Connors, 1987; Hsu, 1990a; Polivy & Herman, 1993; Striegel-Moore, 1993). (See Table 6.1 for a summary of biopsychosocial aspects of BN and BED.)

Medical/Biological Aspects. The extreme dietary restriction, bingeing, and purging practices can result in medical complications (Mitchell, Seim, Colon, & Pomeroy, 1987). Dental erosion and periodontal disease are not uncommon (Altshuler, Dechow, Waller, & Hardy, 1980). Electrolyte imbalance can occur (Greenfeld, Mickley, Quinlan, & Roloff, 1995) and may result in serious physical complications such as cardiac arrhythmias. Rare complications include esophageal bleeding, tears, and gastric rupture (Mitchell, 1986). Readers are referred to Kaplan and Garfinkel (1993) and Pomeroy and Mitchell (1989) for detailed discussions of medical problems and management of BN patients.

The metabolic aspects of BN are not well understood (Devlin et al., 1990). Clinically, it is common to hear BN patients speak of their idiosyncratic metabolism. Clinicians tend to view these persistent pleas as either resistance to prescribed nutritional interventions or as symptomatic behavior reflecting their dysfunctional cognitions regarding shape and weight. Biologically oriented research, however, has suggested that dysregulations in the appetite control system may play an important role in disordered eating (Blundell & Hill, 1993). Alterations in caloric utilization, metabolic rate, and energy balance processes may be present in some eating-disordered patients (Kaye et al., 1986; Newman, Halmi, & Marchi, 1987; Gwirtsman et al., 1989; Weltzin, Fernstrom, Hansen, McConaha, & Kaye, 1991). Normal-weight females with BN may have significantly lower metabolic rates than non-BN females (Bennett, Williamson, & Powers, 1989; Devlin et al., 1990; Gwirtsman et al., 1989), a finding that may translate into a difference in energy expenditure of 200 to 300 calories per day in an average-weight female.

The nature of these potential metabolic differences remain unknown

TABLE 6.1. Summary of Biopsychosocial Aspects of BN and BED

Biological aspects

Genetic vulnerability
Biological vulnerability (e.g., comorbidity with affective disorder)
Appetite control dysregulation
Metabolic alterations
Metabolic consequences
  Electrolyte abnormalities
  Dental problems
  Renal complications (e.g., dehydration)
  Gastrointestinal complications (e.g., bleeding, gastric dilation)

BED: excess weight, weight cycling, and associated increased morbidity/mortality

Psychological aspects

Poor self-esteem
Social self-deficits
Interpersonal deficies
Body image dissatisfaction
Poor coping skills
Comorbidity with Cluster B personality disorder
Restricitve dieting
Shame and guilt

Social aspects

Impaired and conflicted social networks
Social isolation

BED: Social stigma associated with overweight

and warrant further investigation. The metabolic differences may reflect either a cause or a consequence of the restrictive dieting and the BN. It is well documented that restrictive dieting is soon followed by decreases (as much as 20%) in resting metabolic rate (McArdle, Katch, & Katch, 1991). Although the cause–effect questions remain unknown, therapists (regardless of theoretical orientation) should be aware of potential metabolic alterations associated with BN and not simply assume that such statements by clients reflect symptomatic behavior. Indeed, excessive dieting produces a decreased resting metabolic rate (McArdle et al., 1991) and may trigger binge eating (Polivy & Herman, 1985, 1993; Keys, Brozek, Henschel, Mickelsen, & Taylor, 1950), a fact therapists should be aware of to provide thorough patient education about the potential hazards of excessive dieting. (For an excellent description of a psychoeducational approach to BN, see Garner, Rockert, Olmsted, Johnson, & Coscina, 1985.)

Assessment Measures. Numerous assessment instruments have been developed relevant to BN (Fairburn & Wilson, 1993). A review is beyond the scope of this chapter but we briefly list and note several instruments that we feel represent state-of-the-art assessments particularly relevant for screening, identification, and outcome research.

Two self-report measures are particularly relevant to BN. The Bulimia Test (BULIT-R; Thelen, Farmer, Wonderlich, & Smith, 1991) is a 28-item, self-report, multiple-choice scale with good psychometric properties. Research has found that the BULIT-R is a reliable and valid instrument by which to identify individuals with BN. Cross-validation work has demonstrated adequate predictive ability. This instrument is based on DSM-III-R BN criteria. The Eating Disorders Inventory—2 (EDI-2; Garner, 1991) is a widely used 64-item, self-report, multiscale instrument that assesses psychological and behavioral features common in AN and BN.

The Eating Disorders Examination (EDE; Cooper & Fairburn, 1987; Fairburn & Cooper, 1993) is a standardized structured investigator-based interview that measures the severity of the characteristic psychopathology of eating disorders and generates diagnoses. The EDE is a present state assessment instrument with an emphasis on the preceding 28 days, except for the DSM-III-R diagnostic items, for which relevant duration criteria are assessed. In addition, the EDE produces four scales of eating-related pathology (dietary restriction, eating concern, shape concern, and weight concern) that are useful for clinical assessment and treatment outcome research. The EDE has shown excellent diagnostic and psychometric properties (Cooper, Cooper, & Fairburn, 1989; Cooper & Fairburn, 1987; Rosen, Vara, Wendt, & Leitenberg, 1990; Wilson & Smith, 1989) and is currently considered the "gold standard" in the assessment of eating disorders. The EDE is used at several leading eating-disorder treatment centers as a psychotherapy process and outcome measure in comparative outcome trials. However, the EDE requires extensive training and supervision, particularly if the user wishes to use the scales for clinical research purposes. In addition, the EDE requires approximately 1 to 1½ hours for administration. The potential user needs to weigh these two factors when considering the benefits of this state-of-the-art interview. As a potential alternative, Fairburn and colleagues have recently developed a self-report version of the EDE—the EDE-Q. Preliminary research using the EDE-Q has demonstrated its utility to identify clinical cases of eating disorders as well as some specific BN features, such as purging frequency (Black & Wilson, 1996; Fairburn & Beglin, 1994; Loeb, Pike, Walsh, & Wilson, 1994; Wilson, Nonas, & Rosenblum, 1993).

Recommended Assessment Measures for Associated Features. We suggest that therapists who wish to assess outcome also consider other relevant assessment instruments. Specifically, the following self-report instruments tap problems frequently associated with BN and are posited to be important in the biopsychosocial model of BN presented here.

We recommend several measures of psychological distress: The Beck Depression Inventory (BDI; Beck, Ward, Mendelson, Mock, & Erbaugh, 1961) is a widely used 21-item multiple-choice self-report instrument that measures severity of depression. The Symptom Checklist 90—Revised (SCL-90-R; Derogatis, 1983) is also a widely used 90-item multiple-choice self-report questionnaire that assesses a wide range of psychiatric symptoms and obtains a global measure of severity. This measure is often useful for initial screening as well as for treatment outcome assessment. The Body Shape Questionnaire (BSQ; Cooper, Taylor, Cooper, & Fairburn, 1987) is a 34-item self-report instrument that assesses attitudinal aspects and level of body dissatisfaction. Body image dissatisfaction is a critical component of BN and is negatively associated with treatment outcome (Keller, Herzog, Lavori, Bradburn, & Mahoney, 1992). The reader is referred to Thompson (1996) for a thorough review of body image assessment.

Several measures of interpersonal and social functioning are posited to play an important role in BN. The Inventory of Interpersonal Problems (IIP; Horowitz, Rosenberg, Baer, Ureno, & Villasner, 1988) is a measure of interpersonal problems and assesses the level of distress associated with interpersonal difficulties. The Social Adjustment Scale (SAS; Weissman & Bothwell, 1976) is a widely used self-report assessment of interpersonal functioning. It is traditionally used in research with IPT and is particularly relevant for outcome research with eating-disorder patients because they often report social difficulties. The Rosenberg Self-Esteem Scale (Rosenberg, 1979) is a widely used 10-item scale measuring general self-esteem. Poor self-esteem plays a key role in etiological models of BN as reflecting one risk factor for heightened sensitivity to societal pressures for thinness. The Self-Consciousness Scale (SCS; Feningstein, Scheier, & Buss, 1975) is a 23-item self-report measure of how persons experience and think about the self. Public self-consciousness and social anxiety, two aspects of the social self, have been linked to body dissatisfaction and bulimia (Striegel-Moore, 1993; Schwalberg et al., 1992).

It is important for clinicians and researchers alike to evaluate the psychosocial aspects of BN in addition to the traditional focus on the behavioral aspects (e.g., bingeing, purging, and restriction) to formulate treatment plans and to assess process and outcome.

Summary: Biopsychosocial Model. BN is a heterogeneous biopsychosocial disorder found primarily in females. BN is typically viewed as a refractory problem often associated with significant comorbidity. Although its etiology remains unknown, research has implicated the potential contributions of genetic, metabolic, developmental, familial, social, cognitive, and behavioral (e.g., restrictive dieting) (Polivy & Herman, 1993) in the development of BN (Kendler et al., 1991; Polivy & Herman, 1993; Striegel-Moore, 1993; Striegel-Moore et al., 1986). Current sociocultural ideals of thinness and fitness and the associated record rates of dieting (Brownell, 1991a, 1991b) undoubtedly represent two factors necessary to account for the normative body weight/shape discontent among females in our culture (Silberstein et al., 1987) in general and, specifically, for the possible increased prevalence of BN (Hsu, 1990a; Kendler et al., 1991; Striegel-Moore et al., 1986). Those individuals with low self-esteem and social self-deficits may be particularly vulnerable to such cultural pressures.

In contrast to our scant knowledge of the etiology of BN, we understand more about its maintenance. Several competing, albeit potentially complementary models, exist (see Fairburn, 1981, 1985; Lowe, 1993; Polivy & Herman, 1993). Integrated biopsychosocial models seem to account best for the available data. Our biopsychosocial model is influenced strongly by contributions from social learning theory, dieting/restraint models, affective–self-/social deficits models, and cognitive views (Fairburn, 1981, 1985; Wilson & Fairburn, 1993).

Chronic restrictive dieting and restraint make certain persons (e.g., those with low self-esteem, social deficits, poor coping skills, and genetic/biological predisposition) vulnerable to dietary disinhibition (Ruderman, 1985) and binge eating (Polivy & Herman, 1985, 1993). Thus, although many individuals may experience body image discontent and begin to diet, the development of extreme dieting, inability to stop dieting, and bingeing are thought to develop only in vulnerable individuals (Polivy & Herman, 1993). BN, once developed, seems to be perpetuated via a vicious cycle of restriction, bingeing, and vomiting (Garner et al., 1985; Polivy & Herman, 1993). The intensification of dieting is coupled with increasingly dysfunctional cognitions about body weight/shape (Fairburn, 1981, 1985). These individuals are cognitively characterized by extreme dichotomous views about eating, dieting, and their bodies (Fairburn, 1981; Zotter & Crowther, 1991). BN patients are exquisitely sensitive to changes in weight/shape and they become *cognitively* preoccupied (e.g., constant thinking about food and weight) and *behaviorally* preoccupied (e.g., frequent weighing or avoidance of weighing). Figure 6.2 summarizes the cyclical model of BN. Each component of the cycle, in turn, is discussed briefly.

Restraint models posit that excessive dietary restraint makes individuals particularly vulnerable to food cues and hence dietary disinhibition and binge eating. Individuals may respond by self-imposing increasingly rigid and restrictive eating guidelines, which inevitably are violated (Zotter & Crowther, 1991). These difficulties with diets coupled with the inability to reshape the body at will (see Brownell, 1991a, 1991b) may contribute to increasingly rigid cognitions about weight/shape which, in turn, trigger the

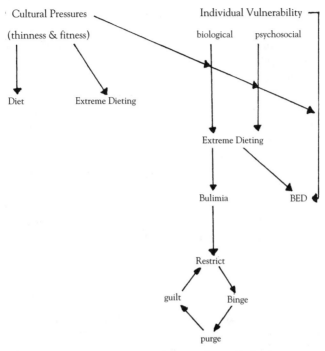

FIGURE 6.2. Schematic representation of the etiology of bulimia nervosa and binge eating disorder. Cultural pressures for thinness create widespread dieting and even extreme dieting in some cases. It is posited that the cultural pressures to diet influence individuals with biopsychosocial vulnerabilities to a greater degree. Extreme dieting in these vulnerable individuals may lead to BN in some cases. Note that BED may develop in some individuals prior to a history of extreme dieting. Once BN develops, it seems to be maintained via a vicious cycle. Excessive dietary restriction sets the stage for binge eating, which often seems to occur in response to food cues, perceived dietary violations, and intra- and interpersonal stress. Bingeing is followed by negative physical and emotional sequelae which trigger purging. Purging is also followed by negative sequelae such as guilt, which lead to a reestablishment of restriction.

reinitiation of dietary restriction. Intrapersonal and interpersonal stressors are experienced by these individuals who are calorie deprived and lacking in coping skill and may also trigger binges (Garner et al., 1985; Heatherton & Polivy, 1992; Hsu, 1990b). Caloric restriction, negative affect, and distorted cognitions about weight/shape have been consistently identified as potent triggers of binges (Davis, Freeman, & Garner, 1988; Fairburn, 1985; Lingswiler, Crowther, & Stephens, 1989a).

Thus, binges can be viewed as both resulting from dietary restraint and deprivation and serving as a coping strategy, albeit a maladaptive one, for distress (Heatherton & Baumeister, 1991). This latter notion, that binge eating represents a coping strategy, is derived from affective regulation models (Heatherton & Baumeister, 1991; Polivy & Herman, 1993). This model may be particularly relevant for those cases of BN and binge eating that do not seem to have been preceded by chronic dieting (Striegel-Moore, 1993; Wilson & Pike, 1993).

Binges are typically followed by physical discomfort coupled with cognitive and emotional distress, which may elicit purging and/or other weight control measures such as laxative abuse or frenzied exercise (Cooper et al., 1988; Garner et al., 1985; Hsu, 1990b; Lingswiler, Crowther, & Stephens, 1989b; Polivy & Herman, 1993). The purging seems to relieve (at least temporarily) some of the negative binge sequelae in some, but not all, BN patients (Cooper et al., 1988). After purging, however, many bulimics, then experience intense guilt and disgust. These purge sequelae, together with the extreme cognitions pertaining to weight/shape, serve to trigger the reinitiation of restrictive dieting.

BN is behaviorally composed of an irregular cycle between dietary restraint (when not binge eating) followed by periods of bingeing and purging and/or restrictive dieting (American Psychiatric Association, 1994; Hsu, 1990b; Hsu, Santhouse, & Chesler, 1991; Polivy & Herman, 1993). Overvalued cognitions regarding weight and shape fuel overly restrictive dieting (Fairburn, 1985). Binges seem to be triggered by dietary restriction (i.e., caloric deprivation), negative affect, dysfunctional cognitions about eating (e.g., all-or-none thinking, perfectionism), and inter- and intrapersonal stressors (Fairburn, 1985; Grilo, Shiffman, & Carter-Campbell, 1994). Negative physical and cognitive–affective reactions following binges are thought to trigger extreme weight control measures and the reinitiation of strict dietary restriction.

Obesity and Obese Binge Eaters

Obesity, generally considered a physical disorder, refers to the surplus of adipose tissue resulting from excess caloric intake relative to expenditure. Overweight, in contrast, refers to weight in excess of an arbitrary standard defined in relation to height (Bray, 1992). Obesity is a heterogeneous, biopsychosocial disorder with multiple etiologies, risk factors, and natural histories (Brownell & Wadden, 1992; Grilo & Pogue-Geile, 1991). Recent years have witnessed a dramatic increase in attention paid to a subgroup of obese persons who regularly binge eat. Identified originally by Stunkard (1959), binge eating in obese persons is now recognized as a prevalent and serious problem. Binge eating is thought to affect 25–30% of those who seek weight loss treatment at university clinic settings (Bruce & Agras, 1992; Hudson et al., 1988; Loro & Orleans, 1981; Marcus, Wing, & Hopkins, 1988; Spitzer et al., 1993; Yanovski, 1993).

Description/Diagnosis. After much debate, the APA Task Force for DSM-IV has included BED as a research diagnosis (Spitzer et al., 1991; Spitzer et al., 1992; Spitzer et al., 1993; Wilson & Walsh, 1991). The research criteria are based in large part on the research efforts of a multisite research trial conducted under the leadership of Spitzer (Spitzer et al., 1991, 1992, 1993; cf. Fairburn, 1992; Fairburn, Welch, & Hay, 1993).

The DSM-IV criteria for BED (Wilson & Walsh, 1991; Spitzer et al., 1993) specify the following:

1. Recurrent episodes of binge eating. It is specified that binges are characterized by the necessary presence of two features: (a) eating, in a discrete period of time (operationalized as 2 hours), an amount of food that is objectively viewed as larger than what most persons would eat in similar circumstances and context, and (b) experiencing a sense of loss of control during that particular episode.
2. Three of the following 5 behavioral indicators suggestive of loss of control must be noted: (a) eating more rapidly than normal, (b) eating to the point of uncomfortable fullness, (c) eating large amounts of food when not feeling physically hungry, (d) eating alone due to social embarrassment regarding the amount of food, and (e) subsequent distress such as disgust, depression, or strong guilt.
3. Marked distress regarding the binge eating.
4. A frequency and duration stipulation that the binge eating occurs, on average, at least 2 days a week for a minimum of 6 months (note that DSM-IV criteria use a different method of determining binge frequency for BED than that used for BN, i.e., number of days binged vs. number of binge episodes, respectively).
5. Exclusionary criteria that BN and AN criteria are not met. The DSM-IV BED criteria have recently been found to be reliable and valid to an acceptable degree (Brody, Walsh, & Devlin, 1994).

Associated Features. Recent research has highlighted the complex clinical problem posed by binge eating in obese persons (Marcus, Wing, & Lamparski, 1985; Marcus et al., 1988; Yanovski, 1993). The prevalence of binge eating increases with increasing adiposity and thus is associated with a subgroup of obese patients at especially high risk for medical complications (Spitzer et al., 1991; Telch, Agras, & Rossiter, 1988). Some treatment outcome studies have found that obese binge eaters appear to fare less well in weight control programs (e.g., lose less weight and have higher attrition and relapse rates) than obese nonbingers (Gormally, Rardin, & Black, 1980; Keefe, Wyshogrod, Weinberger, & Agras, 1984; Marcus et al., 1988; Yanovski, 1993). Moreover, obese binge eaters have been found to experience greater levels of psychopathology (especially depression, anxiety, substance abuse, and personality disorders) than their non-binge eating obese counterparts (Brody et al., 1994; Marcus et al., 1990; Telch & Agras, 1994; Yanovski, Nelson, Dubbert, & Spitzer, 1993). Such differences have lead clinical researchers to conceptualize binge eating as an eating disorder separate from excess weight (Wilson & Walsh, 1991; Spitzer et al., 1992, 1993). To date, these individuals have received the DSM-III-R diagnosis of EDNOS because the majority of obese bingers do not engage in the necessary compensatory and/or purgative weight control practices necessary to meet BN criteria.

In a recent study (Marcus, Smith, Santelli, & Kaye, 1992) that used the EDE to characterize the eating and shape-related pathology of obese bingers, the obese binge eaters showed similar scores on four of the five EDE scales to those reported for normal-weight BN patients in another study (Wilson & Smith, 1989). Obese binge eaters, however, were characterized by lower levels of restraint than the BN patients. More recently, Brody et al. (1994) also found that BED patients are characterized by significantly less dietary restraint than BN patients. Although there are no data available, we speculate that the lower levels of restraint may result from a long-standing history of failed dieting attempts and being unsuccessful at regulating their weight.

Epidemiology.   Obesity is a prevalent public health problem affecting approximately 25% of Americans (34 million persons) (Kuczmarski, 1992). Binge eating is found in a subgroup of obese persons as well as across all weight groups (Devlin, Walsh, Spitzer, & Hasin, 1992). About 30% of obese patients who present to university-based weight control programs report serious problems with binge eating, whereas initial data suggest that in the community, only 2% of women meet BED criteria (Bruce & Agras, 1992; Spitzer et al., 1992). In contrast to AN and BN, preliminary data suggest that BED is common among men. Among patients attending weight loss programs, studies indicate that BED is only slightly more common in women than men (3:2) (e.g., Spitzer et al., 1992, 1993).

Psychosocial Aspects.   Although we do not yet understand the psychosocial aspects of obese binge eaters (Fairburn, Hay, et al., 1993; Wilson & Fairburn, 1993; Striegel-Moore, 1993), obese binge eaters do exhibit similar types of social self deficits (Grilo, Wilfley, Jones, Brownell, & Rodin, 1994; Schwalberg et al., 1992) and perhaps comparable levels of psychopathology as those found in BN patients (Kolotkin, Revis, Kirkley, & Janick, 1987; Marcus et al., 1988; Marcus et al., 1990; Schwalberg et al., 1992; Wilfley, 1989). Obese binge eaters also appear to have heightened body image dissatisfaction compared to nonbingeing obese persons (Cash, 1991; Grilo et al., 1994; Marcus et al., 1990). Available research on the topography of binges among obese binge eaters has implicated negative affect and abstinence violation-type effects (see Grilo & Shiffman, 1994; Marlatt & Gordon, 1985) as salient factors (Arnow, Kenardy, & Agras, 1992). Thus, our working etiological and maintenance formulations for obese binge eaters are guided by those proposed for BN.

Although the prevailing model for the development and maintenance of binge eating is currently guided by that proposed for BN (i.e., chronic dieting and poor affective regulation and coping skills leads to binge eating in certain vulnerable persons), certain aspects of this model may not apply. First, clinical reports and data suggest that binge eating predates dieting in some obese bingers (Spurrell, Wilfley, Tanofsky, & Brownell, in press; Wilson et al., 1993). Second, a major difference between obese bingers and BN concerns dietary restraint. Studies find that BN patients score high on measures of dietary restraint whereas obese bingers do not. Third, the excess weight of obese bingers needs to be considered in any model of binge eating in the obese. Unlike normal-weight bulimics (some of whom have a history of early overweight), many of the obese binge eaters have experienced psychosocial consequences of being overweight (Stunkard & Wadden, 1992; Wadden & Stunkard, 1985).

Medical/Biological Aspects. In addition to the significant risk for morbidity and mortality associated with obesity (Sjostrom, 1992a; 1992b), obese binge eaters may suffer additional medical risk. Preliminary studies have suggested that obese bingers may have histories of considerable weight cycling (Spitzer et al., 1992), a finding associated with increased mortality independent of the excess weight (Lissner et al., 1991). More recent studies, however, have not observed a relationship between binge eating and weight cycling (Kuehnel & Wadden, 1994). One study (Wadden, Foster, Letizia, & Wilk, 1993) found that obese binge eaters and obese non-binge eaters did not differ significantly in resting metabolic rate. The physiological and metabolic correlates of binge eating remain unknown and merit further research. Some studies have reported lowered metabolic rates and body composition changes to be associated with weight cycling whereas others have failed to show such effects (Brownell & Rodin, 1994; Wing, 1992).

Assessment Measures. Several self-report measures of binge eating exist. The Binge Eating Scale (BES; Gormally, Black, Daston, & Rardin, 1982) is a 16-item self-report instrument that measures the behavioral components of binge eating as well as some common triggers for binge eating. The Binge Scale (BS; Hawkins & Clement, 1980) is a nine-item, multiple-choice self-report scale designed to measure binge eating, with a focus on such *behavioral parameters* as frequency, duration, rate of eating, and attitudinal aspects of binge eating and bulimia. While easy to use, a problem with the BS is that it is based on DSM-III criteria. The Compulsive Eating Scale (CES; Dunn & Ondercin, 1981) is a 32-item Likert-type self-report instrument designed to assess *emotional aspects* of binges in addition to behavioral aspects (e.g., frequency, alternation with fasting). The Three-Factor Eating Questionnaire (TFEQ; Stunkard & Messick, 1985) is a self-report measure that comprises three factors: *cognitive restraint*, perceived hunger, and tendency toward dyscontrolled eating.

The EDE (Cooper & Fairburn, 1987), discussed earlier for BN assessment, may represent the best available assessment instrument relevant to BED. However, this investigator-based structured interview needs to be modified slightly if it is to be used to assess BED. Most notably, the duration criteria specified by DSM-IV for BED (i.e., 6 months of twice-weekly binge eating) is not currently assessed by the EDE. The clinical researcher would need to employ a detailed calendar recall method with careful anchoring to determine whether the patient has binged two times a week over the past 6 months.

The Questionnaire on Eating and Weight Patterns—Revised (QEWP-R; Spitzer et al., 1992; see Yanovski, 1993) is the self-report questionnaire that was used in the DSM-IV field trials for BED. The QEWP-R generates the DSM-IV BED diagnosis and assesses for important weight history, weight cycling, and body image variables. A recent study of the QEWP reported good psychometric properties and the utility of their measure to identify BED (Nangle, Johnson, Carr-Nangle, & Engler, 1994).

Summary. Obese binge eaters are a distinct subset of the overweight population. Persons with BED do experience more specific psychopathology (e.g., recurrent binge eating, body image disparagement, weight cycling, and concerns about eating, shape, and weight) and general psychopathology (e.g., depression, anxiety, substance use, and personality disorders) than their non-binge eating counterparts. Whereas studies of obese and normal-weight persons reveal minimal differences in psychological functioning (Stunkard & Wadden, 1992), they reveal robust differences in psychiatric symptomatology between obese binge eaters and obese non-binge eaters (see Yanowski, 1993, for a full review). We suggest comprehensive multidimensional assessment of individuals who suffer from BED. In addition to evaluation of the behavioral and physical aspects of BED, psychosocial evaluation is indicated. We recommend this assessment for clinicians and researchers alike to formulate treatment plans, assess progress, and evaluate process and outcome.

CLINICAL INTERVENTION RESEARCH

Effective Treatments for Bulimia Nervosa

Since BN was first described a decade ago (Russell, 1979), there have been more than 50 studies of its prevalence and more than 20 controlled treatment trials (Fairburn, 1990; Wilson & Fairburn, 1993). A recent comprehensive review of these trials concluded that CBT is found superior to other approaches in treating BN, with the one exception of IPT (Fairburn, Agras, & Wilson, 1992; Wilson & Fairburn, 1993). Each of these two approaches is discussed here.

Cognitive-Behavioral Therapy versus Pharmacological Treatments

Considerable research has been conducted on the efficacy of pharmacotherapy. Controlled trials have found that three major classes of antidepressants (tricyclics, monoamine oxidase inhibitors, selective serotonin reuptake inhibitors) produce outcomes superior to placebo and/or waiting-lists in the roughly 20 trials conducted to date (Fluoxetine Bulimia Nervosa Collaborative Study Group, 1992; Mitchell & Zwaan, 1993; Jimerson, Herzog, & Bratman, 1993). However, it has been questioned whether antidepressants can be recommended as the treatment of choice because high relapse rates are observed once the medication is withdrawn (Craighead & Agras, 1991; Walsh, Hadigan, Devlin, Gladis, & Roose, 1991; for a review, see Fairburn et al., 1992). Pharmacotherapy appears to affect bingeing and purging without affecting other important features of the disorder. For instance, findings suggest that dietary restraint remains high following pharmacological treatment; patients consume few meals or snacks (Mitchell, et al., 1989) and eat a small amount of food outside binges episodes (Rossiter, Agras, & Losch, 1988). In contrast, patients who completed CBT increased the amount of food eaten outside of binge episodes, a behavioral change that likely reflects a decrease in restraint and increase in normalized eating (Rossiter, Agras, & Losch, 1988).

The failure of medication to decrease dietary restraint may be one cause of high relapse rates. In fact, Fairburn et al. (1992) suggest that high relapse is predicted following pharmacotherapy because excessive dietary restraint promotes overeating (Polivy & Herman, 1985, 1993; Charnock, 1989). Generally, research indicates that individuals in CBT drop out less frequently (Agras, 1991; Mitchell et al., 1990) and respond more favorably over the long term than those treated with pharmacotherapy (Fairburn et al., 1992). Several recent studies have compared the relative and/or combined efficacy of pharmacological and CBT treatments (Agras et al., 1992; Fichter et al., 1991; Leitenberg et al., 1994; Mitchell et al., 1990). Collectively, these studies and ongoing studies at Columbia and Toronto universities suggest that CBT is superior to medication alone, combining CBT with medication is superior to medication alone, and a combination of CBT with medication is generally not superior to CBT alone. Thus, CBT emerges as the treatment of choice (Wilson & Fairburn, 1993). These studies, however, have suggested that the combination of CBT and medication could perhaps be useful for certain associated symptoms such as hunger, appetite, and depression.

Cognitive-Behavioral Therapy versus Alternative
Psychological Treatments

The majority of treatment studies have focused on CBT in comparison to waiting-list controls or alternative psychological treatments. CBT is consistently superior to waiting-list control conditions (Agras, Schneider, Arnow, Raeburn, & Telch, 1989; Freeman, Barry, Dunkeld-Turnbull, & Henderson, 1988; Lacey, 1983; Lee & Rush, 1986; Leitenberg, Rosen, Gross, Nudelman, & Vara, 1988). Moreover, CBT has been shown to be superior to various other alternative psychological treatments (for a full review, see Fairburn et al., 1992; Fairburn, 1995). Two studies from Stanford researchers (Agras et al., 1989; Kirkley, Schneider, Agras, & Bachman, 1985) demonstrated superior results for CBT at posttreatment. The first study (Kirkley et al., 1985) found significant reductions in bingeing and vomiting for group CBT condition in comparison to a nondirective group treatment. However, both treatments were comparable by the 3-month follow-up. The second study (Agras et al., 1989) compared CBT with two alternative treatments (nondirective psychotherapy plus self-monitoring and CBT plus response prevention) and a waiting-list control. This study revealed significant change in the CBT condition in comparison to the other three conditions at both posttreatment and 6-month follow-up. At the 6-month follow-up, 59% in CBT abstained from vomiting, which was a higher percentage than that obtained by either the CBT plus response prevention group or the nondirective psychotherapy plus self-monitoring group (20% and 18%, respectively). Thus, the data suggest that CBT is a more effective group treatment than the other two alternative treatments (CBT plus response prevention and nondirective psychotherapy plus self-monitoring). Agras (1993) has speculated that the addition of response prevention to CBT led to a poorer outcome because less time was spent on CBT, the more potent of the two treatments.

CBT has also been found superior to traditional behavior therapy (BT) at posttreatment (Fairburn, Jones, Peveler, O'Connor, & Hope, 1991) and at 4-, 8-, and 12-month follow-ups (Fairburn, Jones, Peveler, Hope, & O'Connor, 1993). At the 1-year follow-up, there were more nonresponders in BT than in CBT (48% and 20%, respectively) and more who met strict criteria for good outcome in CBT than in BT (36% and 20%, respectively). Fairburn, Jones, et al. (1993) conclude that BT cannot be recommended as an alternative to CBT.

In addition, CBT has been found superior to supportive–expressive therapy (SET; Garner et al., 1993). Although posttreatment results were comparable on binge eating, CBT was more effective in reducing purging, dietary restraint, concern with body shape, poor self-esteem, and general psychological distress. These data are important because they suggest that CBT is treating not only the binge eating but also important associated eating-disorder pathology. Moreover, the 1-year follow-up data revealed that almost half the SET patients had to obtain additional treatment in comparison to less than 10% of the CBT patients (D. M. Garner, personal communication, June 1993). Although not all findings are consistent (Freeman et al., 1988) results indicate that CBT is superior to most alternative treatments for BN (Fairburn et al., 1992; Wilson & Fairburn, 1993).

Cognitive-Behavioral Therapy versus Interpersonal Psychotherapy

A focused psychotherapy that seems as effective as CBT is IPT. IPT was developed by Klerman, Weissman, Rounsaville, and Chevron (1984) for the treatment of depressed outpatients and is based on an interpersonal view of the maintenance of depression. Recently, Fairburn et al. (1991) modified IPT for patients with BN and completed a study with 75 BN patients comparing BT, CBT, and IPT. Results showed that IPT and CBT both were significantly more effective than BT at each of the follow-up periods (4 months, 8 months, and 12 months) (Fairburn, Jones, et al., 1993). Although at post-treatment CBT was more effective than IPT on secondary measures of eating pathology (e.g., dietary restraint and attitudes toward shape and weight), these differences dissipated by the 4-month follow-up. Participants in CBT remained the same throughout all follow-up assessments whereas participants in IPT continued to improve (Fairburn, Jones, et al., 1993b). In fact, at the 4-, 8-, and 12-month follow-ups, there were no differences between CBT and IPT on any measures of eating pathology (e.g., binge eating, dietary restraint, and attitudes toward weight and shape). The results of Fairburn, Jones, et al. (1993) suggest that IPT (like CBT) is a specific and effective treatment for bulimia nervosa.

These comparable results between CBT and IPT for BN are notable because IPT does not directly address dietary issues or body weight and shape. Thus, these findings suggest that treatment does not have to focus on eating, weight, or shape to decrease binge eating or associated eating pathology. Consequently, many questions emerge surrounding these two very different models of symptom maintenance: (1) What are the mechanisms leading to change in IPT as there is not a focus on eating, shape, or weight? (2) Is the CBT model sufficient for understanding BN or are there equally important interpersonal problems that contribute to the maintenance of the disorder? and (3) Will some individuals respond differentially to the two treatments? For instance, do those with more distorted attitudes toward shape and weight fare better in CBT and those with more interpersonal problems respond better to IPT? The follow-up data of Fairburn, Jones, et al. (1993) with BN patients and Wilfley et al. (1993) with overweight binge eaters offer preliminary answers to these questions. Their data and the CBT and IPT models of symptom maintenance are discussed next in more detail.

Two Models of Symptom Maintenance

Figure 6.3 offers a schematic comparison of the CBT and IPT models of symptom maintenance.

Cognitive-Behavioral Therapy. The CBT model of BN assumes that eliminating excessive dietary restriction, increasing the intake of a wider variety of foods, and decreasing cognitive distortions are necessary for treatment effectiveness (Fairburn, 1985; Wilson & Fairburn, 1993). This model is based on the cognitive view of binge eating that societal pressure for thinness leads some individuals to develop dysfunctional attitudes toward eating, shape, and weight. In turn, these distorted attitudes lead to excessive dietary restraint and eventually to binge eating. Accordingly, CBT should be particularly effective in lessening concerns about eating, shape, and weight and in decreasing dietary restraint, with resultant improvements in binge eating behavior. CBT has been shown to increase overall caloric intake outside of binge episodes (Rossiter, Agras, Losch, & Telch, 1988) and to decrease distorted attitudes to eating, shape, and weight (Fairburn et al., 1991; Fairburn, Jones, et al., 1993). See Figure 6.3 for a schematic representation of the CBT model of binge eating.

Interpersonal Psychotherapy. The IPT model of BN assumes that improvement of current social roles and adaptation to interpersonal situations

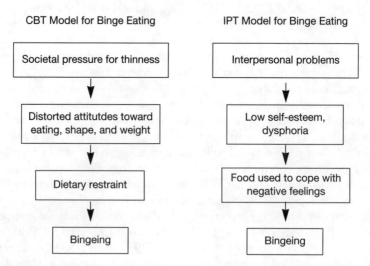

FIGURE 6.3. Schematic representation of the CBT and IPT models of symptom maintenance. Adapted from Agras (1991). Copyright 1991 by the Physicians Postgraduate Press. Adapted by permission.

are necessary for treatment effectiveness because of the interrelationship between interpersonal functioning, low self-esteem, negative mood, and eating behavior (Fairburn, 1981). Evidence suggests that the IPT model may be well suited for women with BN and binge eating. During a laboratory study, researchers documented that women with disordered eating reported an increased desire to binge after exposure to stressors of an interpersonal and social nature (Cattanach et al., 1988). This reactivity seems to stem from profound social impairment (Herzog et al., 1987; Norman, & Herzog, 1986; Spitzer et al., 1992) including disturbed relationships (Van Buren, & Williamson, 1988; Wilfley, 1989), social anxiety (Gross, & Rosen, 1988; Striegel-Moore et al., 1993), and public self-consciousness (Heatherton, & Baumeister, 1991; Striegel-Moore et al., 1993). IPT is posited to work by improving social functioning with consequent increases in self-esteem and positive mood which, in turn, lead to reductions in binge eating. These positive changes are posited to decrease concerns about eating, shape, and weight and to result in a decreased tendency to diet excessively (Fairburn, 1993). See Figure 6.3 for a schematic representation of the IPT model of binge eating.

In a preliminary study, Wilfley et al. (1993) used group forms of CBT and IPT to test these models with overweight binge eaters. This study is presented following a discussion of two trials that also examined treatments for overweight binge eaters.

Controlled Treatment Studies of Binge Eating among the Overweight

Although binge eating was first described in 1959 (Stunkard, 1959), little is known about effective treatments for this subset of the overweight population. To date, most binge eaters have been treated in traditional weight loss programs with minimal success (Yanovski, 1993). Recent studies have examined whether treatments that focus on binge eating rather than weight loss would be effective in treating overweight binge eaters. Studies have shown that obese binge eaters (nonpurging bulimics) respond similarly to treatments used with BN patients: antidepressant medication (McCann & Agras, 1990), group CBT (Smith, Marcus, & Kaye, 1992; Telch, Agras, Rossiter, Wilfley, & Kenardy, 1990; Wilfley et al., 1993), and group ITP (Wilfley et al., 1993). The comparable effects of these treatments across disorders suggest that a similar mechanism may underlie the binge eating syndrome in normal-weight bulimics and overweight binge eaters, and that similar treatments may be used with both.

Although antidepressants significantly decreased binge eating by the end of treatment, participants relapsed and were back to pretreatment levels of bingeing within 4 weeks after the drug was discontinued (McCann & Agras, 1990). These findings parallel those obtained when using pharmacological treatment for normal-weight BN patients (Fairburn, 1992). That is, initial positive effects were followed by significant relapse once the medication was discontinued. A second controlled treatment outcome study conducted by Stanford researchers found that group CBT was superior to a waiting-list control group (Telch et al., 1990) for reducing binge eating in overweight patients. Although there was some relapse at the 10-week follow-up, the frequency of bingeing remained substantially improved compared with baseline levels.

Given the promising results from the prior study (Telch et al., 1990), a comparative psychotherapy trial with overweight binge eaters was conducted by Stanford researchers. This study was designed to assess both treatment effectiveness and models of symptom maintenance (Wilfley et al., 1993). Fifty-six women with nonpurging bulimia (binge eaters) were randomly assigned to one of three groups: CBT, IPT, or waiting-list (WL) control. Treatment was administered in small groups that met for 16 weeks. At posttreatment, both group CBT and group IPT showed significant improvements in reducing binge eating while the WL did not (see Figure 6.4). Furthermore, both group CBT and group IPT maintained reductions in binge eating at the 6-month and 1-year follow-up (Wilfley et al., 1993). Group CBT and group IPT were equally effective at reducing the frequency of binge eating at all time points (posttreatment, 6-month follow-up, 12-month follow-up). These results are similar to those of Fairburn et al. (1991, 1993b) with BN and demonstrate that the positive effects of CBT and IPT may be extended to obese binge eaters.

Next, this study examined these two very different models of symptom maintenance, because each model has different implications regarding the nature and treatment of bulimia and binge eating. To understand these models, secondary measures were included because of their hypothesized sensitivity to CBT and IPT. For CBT, the TFEQ (Stunkard & Messick, 1985) was selected because the CBT model posits that by eliminating dietary restraint, hunger will be reduced, followed by a decreased likelihood for disinhibition. The TFEQ is composed of three subscales: cognitive restraint, tendency toward disinhibition, and perceived hunger. For IPT, the measures of self-esteem, mood, and interpersonal distress were selected because the IPT model posits that improvements in these areas will lead to reductions in binge eating behavior. All measures were administered to both treatment groups (group CBT and group IPT) at pretreatment and posttreatment.

In IPT, only trends for IPT affected the measures hypothesized to be the mechanisms of change. The small sample size may have limited the investigators' ability to find significant differences. Furthermore, in this study, Wilfley et al. (1993) chose to examine the effects of treatment at posttreatment; it may well be that specific effects occurred earlier (e.g., midtreatment) or later (e.g. after treatment or during follow-ups). In future studies, it will be important to measure changes in mood, self-esteem, and interpersonal func-

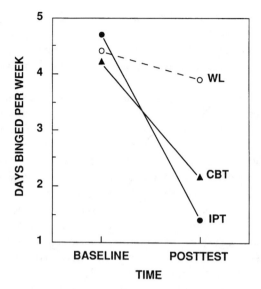

FIGURE 6.4. Self-reported number of days binged per week at baseline and posttreatment (16 weeks) for group CBT (*n* = 18), group IPT (*n* = 18), and waiting list (*n* = 20). From Wilfley et al. (1993). Copyright 1993 by the American Psychological Association. Reprinted by permission.

tioning at more time points (e.g., midway and at follow-ups rather than only at posttreatment).

CBT produced no consistent effects on measures related to its theoretical origin. However, these results are difficult to interpret because the TFEQ has been found to be invalid to measure eating-disorder pathology (Lowe & Caputo, 1991). The EDE interview measures the rigid, irrational beliefs characteristic of eating-disorder patients, while the TFEQ cognitive restraint scale measures temperate, rationale attitudes (Lowe & Caputo, 1991). When using the EDE to assess the effects of a CBT intervention on the core psychopathology of BN (Fairburn et al., 1991; Fairburn, Jones, et al., 1993) and BED (Smith et al., 1992), investigators found that at posttreatment CBT patients experienced significantly fewer eating, shape, and weight concerns. Thus, the EDE interview may be more sensitive to changes in the attitudinal components of eating, shape, and weight concerns than a self-report questionnaire such as the TFEQ. In fact, the EDE is superior to self-report measures in discriminating BN patients from restrained eaters on dysfunctional attitudes toward eating, shape, and weight (Wilson & Smith, 1989). Hence, in future comparative psychotherapy trials the EDE would be a useful instrument to assess the effects of group CBT and group IPT on attitudes toward eating, shape, and weight in obese binge eaters.

More recently, Marcus, Wing, and Fairburn (1995) completed a comparative clinical trial of individual treatment for BED. Subjects who received CBT and BT improved significantly. Binge eating, eating/shape concerns, and depression all improved substantially and those improvements were well sustained over an 18-month period. In addition, the BT condition produced weight loss.

In sum, although we are still in the early stages of identifying effective psychosocial treatments for BED, several approaches have shown promise. In particular, cognitive-behavioral (CBT), interpersonal (IPT), and behavioral (BT) approaches have been empirically validated. Studies investigating CBT and IPT (e.g., Wilfley et al., 1993) have tended to focus treatment on resolving the eating disorder whereas BT treatment has tended to focus on weight loss (Marcus et al., 1995). It is our clinical impression that the goals of resolving the eating disorder and developing more effective weight regulation strategies are not incompatible—if approached in a sensible manner. Moreover, because most BED patients do suffer from two problems (an eating disorder and excess weight), treatment approaches have to be flexible (albeit focused) enough to address both concerns.

Few data are available to suggest whether the treatments should be sequential or combined (Agras et al., 1995). This complex issue represents a pressing research need (Grilo, Devlin, et al., 1996). In general, we believe that the focus of treatment should be on resolving the eating disorder versus weight loss per se (by using CBT, or IPT modified for BED) with the hope that amelioration of the eating disorder will aid the individual in effective weight management. We explain to patients that neither CBT nor IPT is a weight loss treatment, but either one can help them eliminate their problems with binge eating, which, in turn, can help them stabilize their weight and prevent further weight gain. For example, patients are informed that binge eating is negatively correlated with weight regulation while preliminary data suggest that refraining from binge eating is associated with modest weight loss. Moreover, patients are told that as they resolve their eating disorder and begin to feel better about themselves, it is likely that they will be more able to implement lifestyle behaviors compatible with reasonable weight loss and weight maintenance (e.g., heart-healthy eating and moderate exercise). Finally, we counsel patients to focus on losing small amounts of weight (i.e., 5% to 10% of thier body weight) as modest weight losses will be more readily maintained.

Time Course and Specificity of Therapeutic Effects

Whether or not CBT or IPT achieves its results in BN and BED through different or shared mechanisms is presently unknown. It may be that CBT and IPT have the same outcome but operate through different mechanisms (Hollon, DeRubeis, & Evans, 1987). For example, Wilfley et al. (1993) showed that CBT and IPT were equally effective at all time points for reducing binge eating among overweight binge eaters. Fairburn, Jones, et al. (1993) found similar results with BN patients. Other measures, however, revealed a differential pattern of change over time (Fairburn, Jones, et al., 1993). IPT subjects initially improved on bingeing and psychosocial adjustment as rapidly as CBT; however, not until the 4-month follow-up did IPT show changes in other important aspects of the disorder (lessened concern with shape and weight, decreased dietary restraint). Therefore, the results of Fairburn, Jones, et al. (1993) suggest that eating pathology changes more rapidly with CBT than IPT. Fairburn et al. (1995) hypothesize that with IPT, interpersonal functioning changed first because eating-related measures changed gradually (yet significantly) over the course of the 1-year follow-up.

Figure 6.5 was adapted from Fairburn (1993) to depict the hypothesized time course of change in group CBT and group IPT. Currently, Wilfley and colleagues are testing two main predictions in a comparative psychotherapy trial of group CBT and group IPT. First, in group CBT, they hypothesize that changes in dietary restraint and attitudes toward eating, shape, and weight will occur before a secondary effect on interpersonal functioning occurs. This sequence of change fits with the CBT model and suggests that decreasing the eating pathology will positively influence self-esteem and interpersonal functioning. Indeed, it is known that each dieting attempt not only results in more bingeing but also brings social isolation and decreased self-esteem

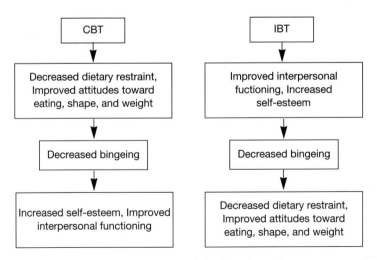

FIGURE 6.5. Schematic representation of the hypothesized time course of group CBT and group IPT. Adapted from Fairburn (1993). Copyright 1993 by the American Psychiatric Association. Adapted by permission.

(Heatherton & Polivy, 1992). Thus, decreasing eating pathology should affect self-esteem and interpersonal functioning. Second, in group IPT, they hypothesize that interpersonal functioning and self-esteem will change faster than attitudes toward eating, shape, or weight. This result would be consistent with the findings of Fairburn, Jones, et al. (1993) because IPT was slower to work on important aspects of the disorder (concerns regarding shape and weight, dietary restraint) and takes longer to be established than in CBT.

Predictors of Treatment Outcome

Since CBT and IPT appear beneficial for both BN patients (Fairburn et al., 1991) and overweight binge eaters (Wilfley et al., 1993), the question becomes whether particular types of patients may respond differentially to the two treatments. Certain patient characteristics have been shown to predict differential outcome in CBT trials for BN. One study revealed that high cluster B scores of bulimic women (consisting of antisocial, borderline, histrionic, and narcissistic features) predicted poor outcome at 16 weeks in CBT, pharmacological, and combined conditions (Rossiter, Agras, Telch, & Schneider, 1993). Another study demonstrated that self-esteem is a significant predictor of treatment outcome (Fairburn, Kirk, O'Connor, Anastasiades, & Cooper, 1987).

Perhaps binge eaters who struggle with more affective lability, low self-esteem, and interpersonal distress (e.g., patients with personality disorders—Axis II of the DSM-III-R) may have a better response to IPT because IPT directly focuses on these areas whereas CBT does not. IPT may lead to reductions in binge eating by helping such patients control the intense affective instability, low self-esteem, and interpersonal conflicts that plague them.

Summary of Treatment Research

Results suggest that binge eaters can be treated effectively with interventions used for BN patients. Two of these treatments seem especially promising: group CBT and group IPT. Given that both CBT and IPT have been shown to be equally effective with both BN patients and BED patients, the remainder of the chapter focuses on group CBT and group IPT intervention protocols.

WHY GROUP THERAPY VERSUS INDIVIDUAL THERAPY?

Recently, Fairburn (1992) noted that more studies are needed to investigate group psychotherapy as a treatment modality for eating disorders. CBT treatment has been conducted in either group or individual formats whereas IPT been adapted to a group format only recently (IPT-G; Wilfley et al., 1993). A recent review by Gotestam and Agras (1989) revealed that studies using Fairburn's cognitive-behavioral therapy in an individual therapy format have led to reductions in bingeing by nearly 90% and that between 50% and 60% of individuals will cease bingeing by the end of treatment. A recent group treatment study showed comparable reductions in bingeing (90%) and a similar number of abstainers (50%) (Mitchell et al., 1990). In general, controlled group treatments (Gray & Hoage, 1990; Kirkley et al., 1985; Telch et al., 1990; Liedtke et al., 1991; Mitchell et al., 1990; Wilfley et al., 1993; Huon & Brown, 1985) and individual trials (Fairburn et al., 1992; Mitchell et al., 1990) reveal comparable percentage reductions on binge eating. Only future research will determine the possible advantages and disadvantages of group CBT versus individual CBT (Wilson & Fairburn, 1993) or group IPT versus individual IPT. Nonetheless, data suggest that both individual and group are viable formats for CBT (Agras, 1991) and IPT (Fairburn et al., 1991; Fairburn, Jones, et al., 1993; Wilfley et al., 1993).

Although a group format allows less time for intensive individualized attention, it has some distinct advantages. First, the sharing common experiences with other patients is helpful to counter some of the shame associated with BN and BED. Second, the use of the group as a laboratory or forum for applying and practicing some of the CBT interventions (discussed in the CBT protocol) may be a strength. Third, conducting IPT in a group setting may facilitate treatment. Wilfley et al. (1993) found that the most common interpersonal problem for binge eaters was interpersonal deficits, which include a long-standing history of social isolation, low self-esteem, and an inability to form or maintain intimate relationships. According to the IPT model (Klerman et al., 1984), interpersonal deficits are treated best in an interpersonal milieu such as the therapist–patient relationship or in this case the group context. Thus, group IPT provides an opportunity for members to work on the relationship difficulties they experience in their outside social life. Given the number and different types of interpersonal interactions in a group setting, the interpersonal skills that are developed may be more transferable to their outside social life than the relationship patterns that are addressed in a one-to-one setting (individual therapy).

Within the last 5 years, many of the leading health and behavior research groups have implemented controlled trials using group treatment as the primary psychosocial intervention for the medically ill (Spira & Spiegel, 1993). Both cognitive-behavioral and social–support groups have been found effective in buffering the immunological system (Antoni et al., 1991; Fawzy et al., 1990) and altering Type A behavior (Thoresen, Friedman, Powell, Gill, & Ulmer, 1985). Moreover, Spiegel, Bloom, Kraemer, and Gottheil (1989) have found that a group intervention actually prolonged the lives of women with breast cancer.

On a practical level, group therapy has been found to be four times more affordable for patients and such institutions such as health maintenance organizations (Hellman, Budd, Borysenko, McClelland, & Benson, 1990). Group treatment may, therefore, allow patients to benefit from a therapy they could not otherwise afford. Hence, group therapy is a treatment modality that merits further investigation.

GROUP COGNITIVE-BEHAVIORAL THERAPY AND GROUP INTERPERSONAL PSYCHOTHERAPY PROTOCOLS

Given that IPT has only recently been adapted to a group format, we describe group IPT in more detail than group CBT. Several other sources are available for more detailed CBT treatment protocols (i.e. Fairburn, Marcus, & Wilson, 1993; Telch & Agras, 1992; Wilson & Pike 1993).

Cognitive-Behavioral Therapy

Therapists

Because therapists must have specific knowledge of biopsychosocial aspects of eating disorders, therapists with specific experience and supervised training with eating-disordered patients are preferred to generalist clinicians who adapt techniques across patients. We also recommend that therapists thoroughly familiarize themselves with more general CBT descriptions and procedures, such as those developed initially for depression and anxiety (e.g., Beck, Rush, Shaw, & Emery, 1979; Fennel, 1989; McMullin, 1986; Persons, 1989; Young & Beck, 1982). These eloquent descriptions of the principles and techniques of cognitive therapy are richly detailed and provide excellent grounding. In addition, specific knowledge of the biopsychosocial aspects of BN, in general, and of the CBT model of treatment for BN, specifically, is essential.

Initial Assessment and Preparation of Patients

Initially, the clinician completes a thorough biopsychosocial evaluation. Differential diagnosis of the eating disorder is necessary as we find that eating-patients do not respond well in a mixed-group composition because of their varied needs and weights. Diagnosis of AXIS I, II, and III pathology also determines whether further consultation is indicated (e.g., pharmacological consultation if significant major depression is present or internal medicine consultation if low weight or excessive purging is present) and appropriate treatment recommendation (e.g., inpatient treatment if at dangerous low weight or alternative treatment if active substance dependence is present). Findings from this individualized evaluation determine whether the patient is appropriate for the group therapies described next.

Prior to the start of treatment, the therapist describes the treatment rationale during an individual session with each prospective group member. The primary rationale (following the biopsychosocial model presented previously) is that societal pressure for thinness leads *some* women to develop dysfunctional attitudes toward body shape and weight. These attitudes, in turn, lead to excessive dieting and dietary restraint. Binge eating is conceptualized as a response to the repeated restrictive dieting and the associated dysfunctional thoughts. The purging and excessive dietary restraint that follow binges are also viewed as resulting from the distorted views regarding shape and weight in addition to representing attempts to counteract the physical, cognitive, and affective consequences of the binges.

Thus, clients are informed that when they reduce dietary restraint, they can gradually break the binge cycle. Clients are informed that CBT involves active participation and that treatment procedures include self-monitoring of food intake and identifying triggers of binge eating. One major emphasis in CBT is the establishment of a regular, healthy eating pattern, including three meals a day, scheduled snacks, healthy foods choices, and decreased avoidance of specific foods. CBT also examines the cognitive and emotional contributions to binge eating. Clients are informed that the group will serve as an opportunity to learn from each other by identifying together more healthy eating patterns and alternative coping strategies to their binge eating. The group will also serve as a milieu to challenge their dysfunctional attitudes toward shape and weight.

Positive Therapeutic Alliance

A positive therapeutic alliance is essential for CBT with BN patients in the same way as with CBT for other problems, or for successful therapy of any nature (Jacobson, 1989; O'Leary & Wilson, 1987; Wilson, 1984). Thus, therapists need to pay careful attention and exert effort toward establishing a positive relationship from the initial individual evaluation meetings through the entire course of treatment. Core therapy skills such as genuineness and empathy cannot be discarded simply because of the structured and active therapy process. Establishment of trust is particularly critical because CBT for BN involves the prescription of behaviors that can be distressing to patients. In fact, the early behavioral interventions of eating three meals a day represent a frightening endeavor for a patient with intense fears of gaining weight and losing further control.

Successful CBT with BN also necessitates that the therapist adeptly combine firm structure with genuine concern. Firmness and consistency around particular issues, most notably homework and any other contingencies that may need to be set (e.g., around weight limits, need for medical consults, and destructive or self-injurious behaviors) are essential for successful treatment to progress. To be successful, CBT therapists must also stay with a consistent and focused agenda.

Treatment Protocol

This chapter describes CBT for patients with BN. This treatment is a modified version of the protocol developed initially by Fairburn (1981, 1985; Fairburn, Marcus, et al., 1993) and is representative of cognitive-behavioral treatments for BN at several major centers (Agras et al., 1989; Wilson & Fairburn, 1993; Wilson & Pike, 1993). The therapeutic interventions are also relevant to the treatment of obese binge eaters. Necessary adaptations to this CBT protocol for use with obese bingers are detailed following its description for BN. The modifications of the CBT protocol for use with obese bingers are based on those initially developed at Stanford (Telch et al., 1990) and are representative of CBT treatments at several major sites (Fairburn, Marcus, et al., 1993; Wilfley et al., 1993).

CBT is a semistructured, problem-focused approach with a present and future orientation. CBT is delivered in three stages with no attention paid to developmental or psychodynamic issues. Attention is paid to dysfunctional interpersonal patterns only to the extent that dysfunctional cognitions are triggered which in turn serve to trigger binge eating or other symptomatic behaviors. The treatment involves an active collaborative process with the responsibility for behavior change resting with each group member.

All sessions contain the following: (1) brief overview of the agenda, (2) review of homework, (3) active collaborative work on the agenda items, (4) group feedback, and (4) assignment of homework. Careful pacing and timing are essential to ensure that these components receive adequate attention every session.

Stage 1 (Sessions 1–8). A major goal of the first few weeks is to establish a positive collaborative alliance between the therapist and the patients. Strengthening this alliance should be viewed as a continuation of the efforts initiated during the initial evaluation meetings and preparatory individual session. It is also critical to enlist the group members in a collaborative effort.

The first stage of treatment has several components. First, the cognitive-behavioral view of the maintenance of the eating disorder is presented. The relationship of the patient's current difficulties to the eating disorder is discussed. The structure and goals of treatment (originally discussed individually with each patient prior to the start of the program) are now carefully delineated within the group. Patients are informed about ways they presently maintain their eating disorder. Information about healthy nutrition and weight regulation is provided.

Patients are encouraged to eat three well-balanced meals a day (and one or two snacks if necessary). This key behavioral prescription is intended to decrease the level of dietary restraint and frequency of binge eating. Therapists introduce self-monitoring of eating behaviors as a tool to increase awareness of restrictive eating patterns and of triggers for binge eating. Once patients use self-monitoring, the therapist introduces a rationale for cognitive restructuring procedures.

Sessions 1–2. Sessions 1 and 2 can be viewed as a group review of the individualized meetings held prior to treatment. Details regarding the group structure are provided. Sessions are 90 minutes long and occur for 20 consecutive weeks. Attendance is essential and therapists need to clarify procedures for missed sessions (calling to cancel, billing, etc.). The therapists should explicitly state that treatment requires full commitment and must represent a priority in the person's life. The responsibility of each person to him- or herself and to the group is discussed. The therapist should stress the need for active in-group participation and between-group (homework) commitment.

The second step is to allow the group members to introduce themselves and to briefly review their reasons for treatment and expectations for the group. The therapist presents the psychosocial model of BN using specific aspects of the group members' statements to illustrate key points. The therapist restates the rationale for CBT and estalishes the agenda for the treatment. Therapists need to foster reasonable expectations about the course of treatment and outcome.

Therapists need to explain that they will give homework each week and that this work, a critical aspect of treatment, will be reviewed at the start of each session following the brief introductory comments regarding the agenda for the session. The initial homework assignments include the commitment to begin establishing regular meals and to eliminate skipping meals. Therapists then introduce the principle of self-monitoring. Self-monitoring, a key component of CBT, is intended to track eating patterns and to help patients identify such problems as excessive restraint (e.g., skipped meals or inadequate meals) and the occurrence of bingeing and purging. Patients are given self-monitoring forms and specific instructions are provided on how and when to complete these forms (see Figure 6.6). Therapists should stress to patients that self-monitoring needs to be completed as close in time as possible to the actual events. (For a detailed description of effective self-monitoring, see Wilson, 1993.)

Session 2 represents the first opportunity to establish that the proposed structure and agenda for treatment will be followed. Therapists need to review the homework needs to be reviewed carefully. If certain participants do not complete the homework, it is essential to determine what prevented them from doing the homework. Sensitivity to the difficult task of monitor-

Name _____

Day _____ Date _____

Time eating began/time eating ended	Food eaten: Type and quantity (please provide as much detail as possible, e.g., ingredients of combination dishes)	Meal (M), snack (S), or binge (B)	With whom and location of eating	Activity while eating	Eating speed (0–10): 1 = very slow, 10 = very fast	Other eating-style behaviors

Exercise:

FIGURE 6.6. Daily Food Record Sheet to be used for self-monitoring in CBT. From Telch and Agras (1992). Reprinted by permission of the authors.

ing their eating (which can produce distress and strong feelings of shame and embarrassment) must be combined with gentle firmness regarding the importance and nonnegotiable requirement for self-monitoring.

Patients are asked to review their self-monitoring forms. The therapist should integrate these reports into the biopsychosocial model. The most useful feedback is specific in nature. Detailed and specific feedback regarding monitoring is likely to increase the utility of this key intervention. The therapist needs to reinforce the efforts of patients as well as the interactive aspects of the group. The early feedback style of the therapist guides the group interactions—which represent a key therapeutic function. When patients do not self-monitor, we recommend verbally reviewing a specific day with them and jointly completing a self-monitoring form in the session using input from all the group members. We find this to be very helpful to the patient and enhances compliance.

Sessions 3–6. Sessions 3 through 6 involve more detailed discussions of the prescribed normalized eating, self-monitoring, and the patients' increased awareness of their patterns. It is critical to foster increased group activity focused on identifying maladaptive eating patterns. The therapists are slowly helping clients establish a regular, healthy eating pattern. Clients are encouraged to notice how eating more regularly (i.e., three meals a day and a variety of foods) helps control excessive hunger and decrease binge eating.

Sessions 7–8. Self-monitoring continues with an increased emphasis on identifying triggers for binge eating (see Figure 6.7 for Binge Triggers Form). The self-monitoring focuses on identifying situations that lead to binge eating. The major emphasis is on the antecedent feelings and thoughts. This intervention is essential to help patients begin to recognize the sequence of events that precipitate binge eating. This reconstruction shows that certain events can trigger feelings and thoughts, which, in turn, may trigger binge eating. Initially, it is helpful to have patients provide actual examples in the group and to illustrate how the forms are to be completed. The group members can then begin to discuss how certain feelings tend to be associated with certain types of thoughts about the events.

Patients are told that this process requires considerable effort and is harder to do than it sounds. Patients are also told that although identifying thoughts and feelings may be uncomfortable at first, they will soon feel more (not less) in control when they are able to do so. Homework assignments need to be reviewed carefully in each subsequent group. Again, the type of feedback that is most helpful is generally specific in nature.

Stage 2 (Sessions 9–15). The second stage of treatment becomes increasingly cognitively focused. Self-monitoring continues to be a key ingredient to continue to monitor for and to identify dysfunctional eating patterns and to identify triggers to binge eating. Patients continue to focus on identifying cir-

Name _____   Day _____ Date _____

Binge circumstances	Events prior to binge	Mood prior to binge	Thoughts prior to binge	Coping alternatives used and degree of success
Example: Tues. night at home alone while trying to work at kitchen table, ate 4 slices of pizza.	Boss ordered a report done by tommorow. Had to cancel plans with friend.	Angry, guilty	I must be unimportant or my boss would treat me with more respect. I'm sure my friend will be angry at me for canceling.	Asserted self w/ boss explaining limits on work hours. Checked out with friend rather than mindread. Very successful.
1.				
2.				
3.				
4.				
5.				

FIGURE 6.7. Binge Triggers Form to be used during the early stages of self-monitoring. This record is used to help patients identify triggers for binges with a focus on antecedent events, feeling, and thoughts. From Telch and Agras (1992). Reprinted by permission of the author.

258

cumstances surrounding urges to binge, triggers for bingeing, antecedent thoughts and feelings, and sequelae (cognitive–affective reactions such as abstinence violation effects, purging, reinitiation of caloric restriction).

Attention is now paid to the identification of maladaptive or dysfunctional cognitions. Cognitive restructuring is used to challenge these dysfunctional cognitions and beliefs. The cognitive restructuring can also focus on specific reactions triggered by troublesome intrapersonal and interpersonal problems. Patients are taught to question their interpretations of events, to consider evidence in favor and against their interpretations, and to consider alternative interpretations. The group becomes a forum for learning how to be increasingly aware of the occurrence of dysfunctional cognitions, for addressing them and for generating possible alternatives. Figure 6.8 shows a cognitive restructuring sheet that can be used to guide the process.

During this stage, the group is also used as a forum for generating problem-solving and coping strategies. The self-monitoring and cognitive restructuring interventions help patients to evaluate troublesome events more effectively and thereby set the stage for more effective problem solving. The development of alternative coping skills continues to represent a key therapeutic task.

The same philosophy and approaches from the first stage are continued in the second stage. Cognitive change is not effectively achieved by a didactic approach. Rather, patients are encouraged to engage in "brainstorming" of alternative perspectives and "behavioral experiments" designed to test their dysfunctional attitudes.

During the latter part of this stage (i.e., sessions 12–15), the restructuring is focused on the dysfunctional thinking about body weight and shape. Helping patients set reasonable goals is critical. Although total comfort and acceptance of body shape and weight are unlikely, patients are gently encouraged to identify the sources of body distress and to begin restructuring work around establishing the importance of other attributes in their self-concept (see Wilson, in press-a).

Stage 3 (Sessions 16–20). The third stage of treatment is concerned with the maintenance of change following treatment and especially with the consolidation of the normalized eating and coping skills. Progress is reviewed and the continued use of realistic goal setting is stressed. In particular, patients are encouraged to continue to follow heart-healthy eating patterns and to avoid restrictive dieting. Relapse prevention strategies occupy a central role in this final stage (Marlatt & Gordon, 1985). Therapists continue to emphasize problem solving and coping skills for high-risk situations, urges to binge, and possible setbacks (lapses can include any symptomatic behaviors such as restrictive dieting, binging, purging, or the use of any other extreme weight control measures).

Situation	Feeling(s)	Automatic thought(s)	Evidence for thought(s)	Evidence against thought(s)	Outcome
Describe the event that led to the unpleasant feeling(s).	(1) Specify sad, anxious, angry, etc. (2) Rate degree of feeling, 1–100%.	Write the automatic thought(s) that accompany the feeling(s).			Options, plans, rate feeling(s), etc.
		Restructured thoughts: Is there any other way of looking at this?			

FIGURE 6.8. Cognitive restructuring sheet to be used to identify maladaptive ("automatic") thoughts associated with specific events and feelings. Patients are instructed how to identify thoughts, how to evaluate them, and how to restructure them if necessary.

Modifications for Binge Eating Disorder

The presentation of the CBT rationale to the obese binge eaters represents a considerable challenge to the clinician. Our CBT model is that treatment will focus on the binge eating and the associated dysfunctional cognitions, which need to be addressed prior to consideration of traditional weight loss methods. We emphasize to clients that we view binge eating as a serious problem in its own right because left untreated it appears to contribute to continued escalation of weight. We also emphasize that binge eating is associated with considerable emotional distress. Therefore, the primary aim of the treatment is to eliminate the binge eating, which, in and of itself, should decrease emotional distress and markedly decrease continued weight gain. Thus, the potential physical and psychological benefits derived from binge abstinence define treatment success.

The therapist must empathically discuss the nature of the patient's concerns regarding excess weight. It is critical, however, that the therapist confidently present the biopsychosocial model and rationale for treatment. Excessive weight control measures are to be discussed as a contributing problem to the binge eating rather than a potential solution. It is made clear that reasonable weight loss and weight control strategies will be discussed when the patients binge eating is under control (see stage 3).

Following clear presentation of the rationale and goals for treatment, we recommend that the therapists negotiate with the patient a plan so that he or she will not attempt any excessive forms of weight control during the program. We also recommend that no concurrent weight loss program be sought. If a patient is not willing to follow this critical stepped approach, we recommend that the therapist not offer the group therapy. (For discussion of issues and findings pertaining to more traditional weight loss treatment of obese binge eaters, see Yanovski, 1993; Telch & Agras, 1993.)

Stage 1. Modification. Modifications include the prescription of heart-healthy eating patterns. Whereas normalization of eating for BN often necessitates increased eating, in the case of the obese binger, clearer demarcation of meal times is indicated. In contrast to the BN patient for whom decreased restraint is a goal of treatment, increased restraint is a focus for the obese binger. Excessive restraint is, of course to be avoided, but normalization of eating and elimination of "grazing" and bingeing are necessary.

Stage 2. No changes.

Stage 3. Modification. As in the treatment of BN, patients are encouraged to continue heart-healthy eating practices and to avoid restrictive dieting. This prescription represents a sensitive and complex issue. In some cases, although patients achieve healthy eating and eliminate binge eating, weight loss has not occurred. Some patients are satisfied with their progress (elimination of binge eating, healthy eating, and enhanced psychological well-being) and are no longer interested in dieting to lose weight. In some cases, these changes can be associated with decreased risk for morbidity and mortality. In other cases, however, the excess weight still represents heightened risk for medical problems, and lifestyle weight management programs may then be discussed.

Data support that patients who continue to binge eat, even if at reduced levels, generally continue to gain weight. In contrast, data from the few treatment studies of BED suggest that only those patients who abstain from binge eating successfully lose weight (Agras et al., 1994; Smith et al., 1992). Thus, we recommend that for those individuals who are continuing to binge eat, continued treatment be aimed at further decreasing the bingeing. For those individuals who are abstinent, weight loss approaches can be discussed.

With those patients who abstain from binge eating and who still wish to lose weight, several steps might be indicated. Patients should be encouraged to identify how excessive dietary restrictive created problems for them prior to treatment. Determining reasonable weight goals is also critical (see Brownell & Wadden, 1992). Progress should be reviewed in detail to highlight important principles for healthy change (e.g., reasonable goals, lifestyle change, and increased importance of non-body-related attributes) and successful techniques to help achieve those changes (e.g., goal-setting, self-monitoring, cognitive restructuring, problem solving, and coping skills; Wilson, in press). Patients are encouraged to do honest self-assessments periodically to determine whether old patterns (e.g., restrictive dieting and food avoidance) are gradually reemerging.

Interpersonal Psychotherapy

IPT was developed for the treatment of depression (Klerman et al., 1984). Fairburn et al. (1991) modified IPT for patients with BN. Wilfley et al. (1993) used Fairburn and colleagues' approach, making adjustments for a group format and BED. This treatment protocol focuses on using IPT-G for obese binge eaters. The reader can easily adapt this group treatment protocol for BN patients because the focus is on the interpersonal problems and not the eating disorder per se.

IPT-G was developed from two primary sources: Klerman et al. (1984) and Fairburn (1993). These two sources have been used and adapted to a group format for patients who suffer from BED (Wilfley, Frank, Welch, Spurrell, & Rounsaville, in press). It is assumed that therapists who intend to use this treatment protocol are familiar with both resources; this treatment protocol is designed to be a supplement to these resources. The purpose of this protocol is to indicate how IPT is applied to BED patients in a group format. Repeated references are made to the aforementioned resources.

Rationale

Recent descriptive studies of obese binge eaters indicate that as a population they are underassertive, plagued by negative emotions, low in self-esteem, and deficient in basic coping, problem-solving, and interpersonal skills (Marcus et al., 1988; Prather, & Williamson, 1988; Wilfley, 1989; Yanovski et al., 1993; Schwalberg, 1990). These data corroborate clinical reports that suggest that binge eating is frequently accompanied by interpersonal and social deficits as well as low self-esteem. These results are comparable to studies of bulimic patients which suggest that as a group they are socially isolated, withdrawn and sensitive to rejection; have difficulty expressing emotions; and are unassertive and unable to handle conflict constructively (Van Buren, & Williamson, 1988). In fact, in several descriptive studies, bulimics and binge eaters were alike in these domains and significantly different from controls (Hudson et al., 1988; Schwalberg, 1990; Wilfley, Kunce, & Welch, 1992).

IPT-G is a short-term, time-limited therapy that emphasizes the current interpersonal relations of the overweight binge eater. The rationale is that there is an interrelationship between negative mood, low self-esteem, traumatic life events, interpersonal functioning, and the patient's eating behavior. Central to the treatment is the notion that the eating problems are a maladaptive solution for "underlying interpersonal difficulties" (Fairburn, 1993). Major therapeutic tools are techniques such as clarification of emotional states, improvement of interpersonal communication, reassurance, and testing of perceptions and performance through interpersonal contact. Group IPT concentrates on current disputes, frustrations, anxieties, and wishes as defined in the interpersonal context. The influence of early childhood experiences is recognized as significant but is *not* emphasized in the therapy. Rather, the work focuses on the *"here and now"* (Klerman et al., 1984).

Outline of the Treatment

IPT-G focused IPT treatment that progresses through three stages (initial, middle, late) in a time-limited (20 sessions over 20 weeks) manner with an almost exclusive focus on interpersonal problems and their relationship to binge eating symptoms. The aim is to encourage mastery of current social roles and adaptation to interpersonal situations with the assumption that improvements in these areas will lead to the amelioration of binge eating symptoms.

Once the patient is assigned to IPT-G, an initial individual intake session is conducted to inform the patient of the rationale for IPT-G. In addition, this initial session is used for identification of "major problem areas" that form the interpersonal basis of the patient's current difficulties. These problem areas are identified using three different procedures: (1) a review of the patient's past interpersonal functioning (e.g., family, school, and social), (2) an examination of his or her current interpersonal functioning (e.g., family, work, social), and (3) an identification of the interpersonal precipitants of episodes of binge eating.

By the end of this initial individual intake session, the therapists and patient agrees on the interpersonal problem areas and goals. Treatment goals evolve from the four main interpersonal problem areas as specified by Klerman et al. (1984): "(1) *grief*; (2) *interpersonal disputes* with spouse, lover, children, other family members, friends, co-workers; (3) *role transitions*—a new job, leaving one's home, going away to school, relocation in a new home or area, divorce, economic or other family changes; and (4) *interpersonal deficits*—loneliness and social isolation" (p. 88).

These identified problems and resultant goals serve as the basis for the patient's focus on interpersonal issues in IPT-G. During the initial stages of IPT-G the patients learn how to use the group format to work on goals. The "work" on the goals is the focus of the middle stage of IPT-G. The Late phase of IPT-G concentrates on goal evaluation and termination. During this last stage, the goal is to move the patient toward recognition of his or her independent competence.

A. Establish a sound therapeutic relationship.

B. Discuss binge eating.
   1. *Review binge eating symptoms.* Therapists will discuss the nature of the patient's binge eating behavior with them.
   2. *Give the syndrome a name.* Inform patients that binge eating disorder (BED) is a newly described condition that probably affects millions of Americans. Individuals with BED experience frequent episodes of eating large amounts of food while feeling a loss of control.
   3. *Explain binge eating disorder.* Patients are provided information about BED. The therapists explain that most people with serious binge eating problems experience the following:
      • Frequent episodes of eating what other people would consider a large amount of food.
      • The episodes of overeating are accompanied by the feeling that they cannot control what or how much they are eating.
      • The behavior causes them considerable distress.

- The binges are accompanied by a least three of the following:
  —Eating much more rapidly than usual.
  —Eating until they are uncomfortably full.
  —Eating large amounts of food, even when they are not physically hungry.
  —Eating alone out of embarrassment about how much they are eating.
  —Feelings of disgust, depression, or guilt after overeating.
- They do not regularly purge after binge eating through vomiting or the use of diuretics (water pills) or laxatives, and they do not frequently fast (eat nothing at all for at least 24 hours) or exercise for more than 1 hour specifically to lose weight or avoid gaining weight after a binge.

C. Identify the patient's major problem areas to establish a treatment contract.
  1. *Determine which relationship or aspect of a relationship is related to the binge eating and what might change in it.*
     a. *Obtain a detailed review of the patient's past.* The goal is to gain an understanding of the context in which the binge eating developed and is maintained. As recommended by Fairburn (1993), the following topics are assessed one-by-one:
        1. The history of the binge eating (and changes in weight).
        2. The patient's interpersonal functioning prior to and since the development of the binge eating.
        3. The occurrence of major life events.
        4. Problems with self-esteem and depression.
     b. The goal is to identify connections between interpersonal functioning, self-esteem, and mood; the occurrence of life events; and the onset and maintenance of the eating problem. A thorough review of these areas will reveal the relationship between these four areas.
     c. Review current and past interpersonal relationships as they relate to current binge eating symptoms. Have the patient describe:
        1. The nature of interaction (frequency of contact, intimacy, reciprocity) with significant persons (partner, confidants, family, friends, people at work, children).
        2. His or her expectations of these close relationships and whether these were or are fulfilled.
        3. The satisfying and unsatisfying aspects of the relationships.
        4. The changes the patient wants in his or her relationships.
     d. *Identify the interpersonal and emotional precipitant of individual episodes of overeating.* The context in which the patient binges is relevant for the identification of problem areas. Particular emphasis is placed

on any interpersonal events that are precipitants to binge episodes. Aside from these inquiries during the assessment phase, it is not a goal of IPT-G to discuss eating, weight, or shape concerns. However, when this topic is initiated by group members, therapists encourage members to discuss how this is related to their interpersonal problems.

2. *Determine the interpersonal problem area related to current binge eating and set the treatment goals.* The interpersonal assessment culminates in the identification of major problem areas. It should be made clear that the focus of treatment will be on the identified problem areas as they currently affect the patient. Previous work (Wilfley et al., 1993) has found considerable overlap in the problem areas identified by binge eaters. The most common primary problem area was interpersonal deficits (e.g., social isolation and low self-esteem) which were present in 55% of the subjects. Interpersonal disputes (e.g., marital conflict) were found in 28% of the cases and was the next most common problem. The two other IPT problem areas (grief and role transitions) were encountered less often. In three cases (17%) grief was the major unresolved issue. In these cases, the subjects identified bingeing as a response they used to cope with the loss of significant others. Difficulties with role transitions were only encountered as a secondary problem in two cases (one had recently retired and the other was now her mother's caretaker). Both of these individuals linked their bingeing with these significant role transitions.

D. Explain the IPT concepts and contract
   1. *Outline therapists' understanding of the problem and encourage the patient to discuss his or her understanding of the problem.* The stated rationale is that binge eating occurs as a response to interpersonal disturbances (e.g. social isolation and fears of rejection) and consequent negative moods. After the assessment is conducted, therapists can individualize their discussion of the problem to the patient's particular interpersonal history.
   2. *Agree on treatment goals* (which problem area(s) will be the focus).
   3. *Describe procedures of IPT*: present focus, need for patient to discuss important concerns; review of current interpersonal relations; discussion of practical aspects of treatment—length, frequency, times, and policy for missed appointments.
      a. *Setting of the group.* A circular seating arrangement is necessary as all group members must be able to see one another.
      b. *Size of the group.* An ideal size for a group is 7 or 8 members, and certainly no more than 10. For our research purposes, we begin the groups at 9 members.

  c. *Duration of the meeting*. We recommend that groups meet for 90
     minutes.
  d. *Procedure for group preparation*. Group member preparation for
     group IPT is conducted during an initial 2-hour session with both
     group therapists. The patient is informed about the time, location,
     composition, procedure, and goals of the group during this session.
     The interpersonal model of bingeing is presented.
     • Therapists help the patient translate his or her interpersonal
       goals into specific ways they may be manifested in the group mi-
       lieu. For instance, if a member struggles with interpersonal
       deficits it is likely that he or she will have a difficult time con-
       necting with group members and may assume that others do not
       like him or her. Predicting these difficulties is often the first step
       in helping a patient work toward change.
     • Therapists inform the patients that the group will be a place to
       work on their identified interpersonal problem areas. Subjects
       are be told that this interpersonal laboratory provides a unique
       opportunity to: (a) work on the relationship difficulties they ex-
       perience in their social life; (b) recognize and accept their feel-
       ings, opinions, and needs; and (c) transfer newly learned inter-
       personal skills to their outside social life.
  e. *Likely outcome*. Patients are informed that on the basis of our pre-
     vious findings they should expect to improve their binge eating
     and to maintain their improvements. However, Fairburn (1993)
     suggests that two qualifications be provided: (1) patients will typ-
     ically still have some problems with binge eating at the end of
     treatment, but often there is continued improvement over the 1-
     year follow-up period as new patterns of interpersonal behavior are
     being established; and (2) patients should view binge eating as a
     way they have coped with stress for most of their adult life and
     thus, it may remain their first reaction under stress, but between
     such times it will often be much less of a problem. However, they
     may expect to be more sensitive than the average person about
     eating, shape, and weight.

Three Phases of Group Interpersonal Psychotherapy

*Phase 1: Establishing a Contract and Identifying Key Interpersonal Prob-
lem Areas.* The *initial* sessions (1–5) are spent formulating an interpersonal
focus to binge eating, emphasizing the affect associated with the interpersonal difficulties, and identifying interpersonal problem areas. The two most
common interpersonal problem areas for overweight binge eaters are interpersonal deficits (i.e., long-standing history of social isolation, low self-es-

teem, and an inability to form or maintain intimate relationships) and role disputes (e.g., difficulties with spouse) (Wilfley et al., 1993).

Phase 2: Addressing the Problem Areas. The middle sessions (6–15), the "work" stage, are used to focus on the interpersonal problem areas identified in phase one. A key premise in using IPT-G for binge eating is that binge eating plays a role in the patient's attempt to cope with problems in social relationships. When IPT is used for treating depression, the therapist attempts to focus interventions on resolving interpersonal problems of four types: interpersonal role disputes, interpersonal deficits, grief, and role transitions. In our experience, the issues addressed in each of these problem types are also found among binge eaters and strategies devised for managing these issues in depressives can be adapted to the treatment of binge eaters. Given that the techniques for addressing the four problem areas are provided by Klerman et al. (1984), this protocol only provides an outline of the goals and strategies for the four problem areas. This outline is adapted with permission from Klerman et al. (1984).[1] Because interpersonal deficits and interpersonal role disputes are the most common problems for binge eaters (more 80% of binge eaters identify these two areas as the most problematic), references are made throughout this protocol about how these two problem areas are addressed in IPT-G.

A. *Interpersonal deficits.* Binge eaters have profound and persistent disturbances in social relationships. Such patients are often quite socially isolated or involved with others in such a superficial manner that the relationships are chronically unfulfilling. Relationships are typified by a lack of emotional expression, avoidance of conflict, fears of rejection, and a lack of perceived support. Hence, binge eating may be a coping mechanism that is inextricably linked with problems in interpersonal and social relationships. *When the binge eating is used to reduce feelings of failure from social problems, the therapists' strategies are to help the patient focus on the interpersonal difficulties and help him or her devise more successful strategies for handling them.* In helping the patient reduce his or her social isolation, the therapists can review past relationships with the aim of helping to discover the social behaviors that have led to past failures. The IPT-G is an ideal setting for identifying *in vivo* the social difficulties with which the patient struggles and identifying ways to improve his or her social skills in the context of a therapeutic social milieu.

---

[1]The following outline was adapted for BED from Klerman et al. (1984, pp.73–76). Copyright 1984 by G. L. Klerman, M. M. Weissman, B. J. Rounsaville, and E. S. Chevron. Adapted by permission.

Goals
1. Reduce the patient's social isolation.
2. Encourage formation of new relationships.

Strategies
1. Review binge eating symptoms.
2. Relate binge eating symptoms to problems of social isolation or unfulfillment.
3. Review past significant relationships including their negative and positive aspects.
4. Explore repetitive patterns in relationships.
5. Discuss patient's positive and negative reactions toward both the therapists and group members and seek parallels in other relationships.

B. *Interpersonal role disputes.* An interpersonal role dispute is identified when the patient and at least one significant other have nonreciprocal role expectations about the roles they should play in the relationship. Binge eating can be initiated or continued as an attempt to resolve a wide range of disputes. When binge eating is related to the role disputes, the goal of treatment is to help the patient clearly identify the dispute and to begin to resolve it through renegotiation of the relationship with the significant other. The IPT-G provides a context for the patient to discuss and to understand the dispute while also developing ways to manage and resolve disagreements.

Goals
1. Identify dispute.
2. Choose plan of action.
3. Modify expectations or faulty communication to bring about a satisfactory resolution.

Strategies
1. Review binge eating symptoms.
2. Relate onset of symptoms' to overt or covert dispute with significant other with whom patient is currently involved.
3. Determine stage of dispute:
   a. Renegotiation (calm down participants to facilitate resolution);
   b. Impasse (increase disharmony in order to reopen negotiation);
   c. Dissolution (assist mourning the loss of the relationship).
4. Understand how nonreciprocal role expectations relate to dispute:
   a. What are the issues in the dispute?
   b. What are differences in expectations and values?
   c. What are the options?
   d. What is the likelihood of finding alternatives?

    e. What resources are available to bring about change in the relation-
      ship?
  5. Identify parallels in the other relationships:
    a. What is the patient gaining?
    b. What unspoken assumptions lie behind the patient's behavior?
  6. Examine how the dispute is perpetuated.

C. *Grief and loss.* It is common for depressive symptoms to follow the loss of a
loved one for up to 1-year after the death of the significant other. However, some individuals suffer from prolonged grief reactions in which dysphoric symptoms do not remit, and others, who are seemingly functioning
well, may have hidden or distorted grief reactions that they have not consciously linked to the loss. Binge eating may begin or become exacerbated
in the context of prolonged or distorted grief reactions in which the patient uses binge eating as a means to avoid painful feelings associated with
the loss. Careful review of important life events can be helpful in recognizing the role of grief in the patient's binge eating behavior. In some cases, binge eaters report that when faced with a loss, they use food to cope
with their feelings. They note that they feel numb and do not remember
feeling sad or upset. If the link between the grief and bingeing is established, the therapists' aims are to help the patient go through a more
healthy mourning process and to help him or her find ways of filling the
space left by the loss. A key premise related to pathological grief is that
the patient has not been able to grieve because of fears of being unable to
tolerate the painful affect associated with the loss. A supportive relationship with the therapists and group members makes the process more bear-
able. When the patient can tolerate and work through the feelings associated with the loss, binge eating is often reduced.

Goals
1. Facilitate the mourning process.
2. Help the patient reestablish interest and relationships to substitute for
   what has been lost.

Strategies
1. Review binge eating symptoms.
2. Relate symptom onset to death of significant other.
3. Reconstruct the patient's relationship with the deceased.
4. Describe the sequence and consequences of events just prior to, during, and after the death.
5. Explore availability and use of social supports around the mourning.
6. Explore associated feelings (negative as well as positive).
7. Consider possible ways of becoming involved with others.

D. *Role transitions.* As binge eaters are often over 40 when they present for treatment, they may experience role transitions difficulties related to middle or late adulthood (e.g., making retirement plans, becoming a parent's caretaker, taking a new job, having a child, and getting a divorce). Binge eating may be used to cope with difficult role transitions by soothing dysphoric affect associated with the role change. When binge eating performs a function in managing role transition difficulties, the therapists' goals are to help guide the patient through the phase without relying on food. In many cases, role transitions may result in more interpersonal disputes with significant others. Binge eating becomes a way to manage negative feelings. Oftentimes, managing a role transition (e.g., retirement) involves the fear of losing one's identity, and the therapists and group members may aid the patient in this process by helping him or her focus on ways of expressing him- or herself in these new circumstances.

Goals
1. Mourn and accept the loss of the old role.
2. Restore self-esteem by developing a sense of mastery regarding demands of new roles.

Strategies
1. Review binge eating symptoms.
2. Relate binge eating symptoms to difficulty in coping with some recent life change.
3. Review positive and negative aspects of old and new roles.
4. Explore feelings about what is lost.
5. Explore feelings about the change itself.
6. Explore opportunities in new role.
7. Evaluate realistically what is lost.
8. Encourage appropriate expression of affect.
9. Encourage development of social support system and of new skills called for in new role.

Throughout Phases 2 and 3. When the topic of eating, weight, or shape concerns is raised, the therapists acknowledge the importance of these concerns. Given the patients' extensive histories of failed dieting attempts and strong desires to lose weight, it is important for the therapist to normalize these concerns yet keep the patients focused on their interpersonal goals. The patients should be reminded that as they continue to work on their interpersonal goals, they will reduce and/or elimate their binge eating and be better prepared to successfully regulate their weight. However, the primary focus of IPT-G is on the patients' current interpersonal problems involved in the development and or maintenance of their binge eating

Phase 3: Termination and Preparation for the Future. During this phase of treatment, the IPT manual (Klerman et al., 1984) is closely followed. The *final* sessions (16–20) are spent evaluating problem areas, exploring the meaning of termination, and outlining remaining work. Patients are informed that as they develop more satisfying relationships, their eating habits will continue to improve. Time is spent reflecting on the changes participants have made in their social functioning and identifying ways to continue developing more satisfying relationships. Termination is used as an opportunity to discuss, explore, and handle feelings of loss.

A. *Discuss termination explicitly.* With at least four or five sessions to go, the therapists should raise the topic of termination and encourage the group members to express their reactions and feelings about the end of the group.

B. *Acknowledge the end of treatment as a time of grieving.* Many patients are unaware of having any feelings about the end of treatment or may be hesitant to acknowledge that they value the treatment and the opportunity to get together as a group. Because patients may actually experience a slight worsening as termination approaches, they are told that toward the end of treatment it is usual for patients to have feelings of sadness, fears of regressing, and so on. However, they are also told that the appearance of these feelings or symptoms does not mean that they have not improved, nor that they will not continue to improve. Patients may also express disappointment or anger at not having met all their goals by the end of treatment. The therapists openly encourage discussion of these feelings, while also pointing out that change often continues to occur after treatment has ended. This is especially true because the individuals will have time to put the knowledge and social skills learned in treatment into practice.

C. *Foster feelings of competence and accomplishment by reviewing with the patient the course of treatment and his or her progress in group therapy.* The therapists encourage patients to identify the changes that they have made and encourage group members to give one another feedback about the changes which they have observed. The therapists systematically call attention to each patient's independent successes throughout treatment. The therapists also emphasize how each patient has worked toward changing his or her own difficulties. Crediting each patient for his or her changes is important because he or she may want to attribute positive changes to the therapists. Misplaced credit may erode the patient's confidence in his or her own ability for continued success and improvement without treatment. These interventions serve to increase the patients self-efficacy.

D. *Future areas of difficulties and ways of handling them.* In the last few sessions, the therapists bolster patients' confidence to handle future problems by

reviewing with them areas in which they might anticipate future interpersonal difficulties and guiding them through an exploration of how to
handle social problems. They are encouraged to identify early warning
signs (including self-criticism, negative mood, and overeating) and to
identify plans of action. Patients are also encouraged to view their eating
problem as a vulnerability or an "Achilles heel" (Fairburn, in press). This
understanding helps foster more realistic expectations about their eating
behavior. Specifically, it is important for patients to realize that when
they are having social or emotional difficulties, eating may be one of the
first ways that they attempt to cope with their difficulties. However, once
they recognize that eating is a sign of distress, and they develop alternative ways to cope with upsetting feelings, they may be less likely to turn
one overeating episode into a pattern of binge eating.

Group Stages and Techniques

It is important for the IPT-G therapist to understand both group stages and
group techniques to maximize the therapeutic benefits achieved with a group
form of IPT. The "relationship-centeredness" of Yalom's (1985) interactive
approach, with its emphasis on fostering direct communication between
members, is compatible with the overall goals of IPT. Most importantly,
Yalom's (1985) approach provides a framework for facilitating interaction
among group members. It emphasizes establishing a safe environment where
patients can receive feedback on how they are perceived by others and can
experiment with new and risky interactional styles. This kind of experimentation can lead to increased social and emotional development.

A unique feature of the interactional approach is the in vivo demonstration of characteristic problems in relating. Yalom's (1985) notion of "social
microcosm" applies here. Skills that patients learn while participating in an
interactive group setting (such as communicating clearly, tolerating interpersonal differences, and resolving conflicts with one another) can be applied to
realtionships in their outside lives. Moreover, the IPT technique of communication analysis is well-suited for an interactional group approach. Therapists can ask a patient struggling with a role dispute to recall (in great detail)
a recent interaction or argument they had with a significant other. Difficulties in communication can be identified and solutions to the problematic interaction generated. Therapists can also ask group memebers if they have noticed similar problematic patterns between the patient and other members of
the group, a question that often generates immediate feedback applicable to
the patient's outside social life.

Interactional techniques are particularly useful for members who are
struggling with interpersonal deficits (long history of social isolation, low

self-esteem, and an inability to form or maintain intimate relationships) which are treated best in an interpersonal milieu as the therapist–patient relationship or, in this case, the group context. In an IPT-G milieu, members develop the social skills necessary to improve their outside social lives.

Written Summaries

A concise and straightforward description of the group session is developed by the therapists and mailed after each session to all group participants (a method adapted from Yalom, 1985). The summary focuses on the transactions that occurred during the session and their implications for each participant's interpersonal goals. From our experience, the group summaries are deemed invaluable by the group members. The written summaries are one way for them to link the work they are doing in the group to their interpersonal goals and outside social lives.

General Guidelines for Therapists

1. *Phrase comments positively.* Therapists create a safe working atmosphere by consistently phrasing comments, confrontations, and clarifications in relatively positive terms. Participation in group therapy is very public and associated with considerable anxiety and fears of negative evaluation. Binge eaters are often sensitive to perceived rejection and/or criticism. Thus, therapists offer feedback in a *descriptive* versus *interpretive* fashion, and feedback focuses on something that is *clearly within the members power to change.* After giving feedback, the therapist asks the patient what he or she heard the therapist say and how it felt to receive the feedback. Asking for the patient's reactions provides an opportunity to clarify any feedback that was heard in a critical and negative way.

2. *Offer a helpful relationship.* IPT-G therapists are nonjudgmental and communicate warmth and unconditional positive regard. In keeping with this stance, the therapists convey an optimistic and hopeful attitude about the patients' ability to recover from binge eating.

3. *Avoid allying with any group member.* The therapists must work to avoid becoming allied with certain members while excluding others. Avoiding an exclusive alliance with group members is critical because members often attempt to develop a special relationship. For example, binge eaters struggle desperately to feel liked and accepted and, thus, often work to gain favor. One way of handling this situation is by asking for other members' reactions to this type of interchange. That is, if a member is trying to engage in a personal relationship with either therapist, it is important to ask for other members' reactions, thoughts, and feelings. If a member calls between ses-

sions to talk with the therapists, he or she must be asked to share this with the group during the next session.

4. *Focus content on targeted problems.* The therapists are responsible for keeping the group members focused on topics relevant to their targeted interpersonal goals. Goals are not left unformulated and sessions do not pass without reference to them or to the specific subgoals that are derived from the primary treatment goals. Vague, unfocused discussions are interrupted to refocus members on specific and personal accounts of the problems being addressed. Tangential discussions are also interrupted or related to the central themes and goals of treatment. Therapists attempt to keep discussions focused on topics of emotional importance to the members while avoiding an abstract, technical, or intellectualized discussion.

5. *Encourage members to accept responsibility.* Therapists are alert to patients' disavowal of their responsibility to change. One general rule for the IPT-G therapist is to avoid asking questions that may elicit a general or passive response. For instance, instead of asking, "How are you doing?" ask members, "How have you been working on your goals this week?"

6. *Monitor communication.* Therapists are responsible for monitoring the communication throughout all group sessions to ensure that it is clear and productive. When the communication is indirect or vague, or when "mind reading" occurs, the therapists directly intervene to discuss the problem or point out the problem in an attempt to encourage the members to correct it themselves. In either case, it is imperative that the group's communication be clear and productive to restore members' hope that discussing their problems can be useful. This restoration of hope is especially important for members who are struggling with interpersonal deficits or interpersonal disputes. Some common communication difficulties and ways to intervene include the following:

  a. *Point out ambiguous, indirect, mixed nonverbal or verbal communication.* Oftentimes, binge eaters use ambiguous and indirect verbal and nonverbal communications in place of open communication. These difficulties contribute to their interpersonal deficits and role disputes. The IPT-G therapists note when the communication has been indirect or ambiguous and ask the communicator to clarify. Another option is waiting for the recipient (group member) to respond, and then ask, "Did you understand what Judy just said? . . . Well, I also had trouble because. . . ." Another important technique is pointing out inconsistences between verbal and nonverbal behavior. For example, "you say that you are angry, yet you are smiling and laughing."

  b. *Identify incorrect assumptions.* Binge eaters tend to assume that others are thinking poorly of them or judging them. This "mind reading" often leads members to anticipate rejection when others may really like them. Therapists should listen for times when members assume they are being judged and encourage them to "check this out" with the other group members.

c. *Discourage silence–closing off communication.* Some members choose to emotionally withdraw when they are upset. These individuals may be unaware of the negative consequences of closing off communication and may use it because they do not feel able to resolve difficulties in relationships. Pointing out the negative aspects of this type of communication is helpful for patients. The therapists can then encourage the member to let other members know when they are beginning to feel shut down or are beginning to close off. This openness about their closing off helps to break this dysfunctional communication pattern.

Encouragement of Affect

Encouragement of affect involves a number of therapeutic techniques intended to help the patient express, understand, and manage affect. In developing new social skills, the understanding of affect may help the patient decide on priorities and help him or her strive toward emotionally meaningful goals.

Depending on the nature of the affect and the patient, IPT therapists may use two general strategies to help the patient: (1) acknowledge and accept painful affects and (2) use his or her affective experience to bring about desired interpersonal changes.

1. *Encourage acceptance of painful affect.* The group provides an arena to experience and express feelings versus using food to cope with feelings. As the feelings are expressed, it is important for the IPT-G therapist to help the patient accept them. It is often helpful to have other members share times that they have felt similarly.

2. *Teach how to use affect in interpersonal relationships.* Although the expression of strong feelings in the group session is seen as an important starting point for much therapeutic work, the expression of feelings outside the session is not a goal in and of itself. The goal is to help the patient act more constructively in interpersonal relationships, which may involve either expressing or suppressing affects, depending on the circumstances. A goal for the patient in IPT-G is to learn when his or her needs are met by expressing affect and when they are better met by suppressing affect. However, a primary goal is helping patients to identify, understand, and acknowledge their feelings whether or not they choose to verbalize them to others.

3. *Help group members experience suppressed affect.* Many binge eaters are emotionally constricted in situations in which strong emotions are normally felt. An example may be group members who are unassertive and do not feel

anger when their rights are violated. On the other hand, they may feel anger but may lack the courage to express it in an assertive manner. Sometimes members will deny being upset when it is clear that an upsetting interaction has just occurred. The therapists might say, "Although you said you were not upset, it appears that you have shut down since Mary said that to you." The therapists do attempt to draw out affect when it is suppressed.

Specific Therapist Techniques

1. *Exploratory*. To facilitate a relatively free discussion of material, general, open-ended questions should be used, especially in the initial phases of a session. Even when completing the interpersonal inventory, open-ended questions should precede more detailed inquiry. For example, "Tell me about your relationship with your family," would be followed by progressively more specific questioning.

2. *Clarification*. The short-goal of this technique is to make the patient more aware of what he or she has actually communicated. Some examples of clarification techniques include the following:

   a. Asking a group member to repeat or rephrase what has been said. This is particularly useful if a group member has said something in an unusual way or contradicted previous statements.

   b. Calling attention to contradictions in the presentation of material. Contradictions may be noted between the member's affect expression and his or her verbal discussion. Discrepancies can also be noted when the same material is discussed in a manner that contradicts earlier material that was presented. For example, "Mary, please help me understand that you said . . . when previously you had said. . . ."

3. *Communication analysis*. This technique is used to identify communication difficulties and to help the patient learn to communicate more effectively. Therapists ask a patient to recall (in great detail) a recent interaction or argument they had with a significant other. Difficulties in communication can be identified and the IPT-G therapists can ask group members whether they have noticed similar patterns between the patient and other members of the group.

4. *Use of therapeutic relationship*. In this technique "the patient's feelings about the therapist and/or therapy become the focus of discussion. Thoughts, feelings, expectations, and behavior in the therapeutic relationship are examined insofar as they represent a model of the patient's characteristic way of feeling and/or behaving in other relationships" (Klerman et al., 1984, p. 149). The premise behind this technique is that people have characteristic ways of interacting with people. This technique is especially helpful for binge eaters because treatment is often focused on interpersonal deficits (the patient develops a relationship with the therapist as a model for other relation-

ships) and interpersonal disputes (the patient receives feedback on how she comes across and, thereby, has the opportunity to understand the nature of his or her difficulties in relating with others).

Therapist Role

1. *Patient advocate, not neutral.* Therapists can help the patients to feel comfortable and safe enough to work on their identified problem areas by fostering a helpful and supportive working relationship.

2. *Active, not passive.* The therapists in IPT are always keeping in mind the focus and goals of treatment and take action at the earliest opportunity to help the patient reach them. The therapists do not wait for the patient to bring in issues related to treatment goals at the patient's own pace but attempt to redirect the focus of the treatment when sessions are not focused on members' interpersonal problem areas.

Summary of Group Interpersonal Psychotherapy

IPT-G is designed to help overweight binge eaters improve their current interpersonal relationships, their ability to cope with negative emotions, and decrease their reliance on bingeing as a means of coping. The primary goals of the IPT-G therapists are to identify, challenge, and alter maladaptive patterns of interpersonal relationships both within and outside the group. The group setting provides an opportunity to explore and to understand ways in which members relate to one another and approach or avoid intimacy and confrontation (interpersonal learning). Although group members are likely to re-create significant experiences with family and friends within the context of any group, IPT-G therapists actively encourage and allow for exploration of how these experiences occur within the here and now of the group (reenactment of significant relationships, e.g., family and marital). The therapists facilitate these tasks by modeling; questioning; clarifying; reinforcing (or not reinforcing); reflecting feelings; making process comments at the intrapersonal, interpersonal, and group level; linking; summarizing; confronting; and giving feedback. Overall, the IPT-G therapists work to achieve a focus on each patient's current interpersonal problems as manifested in the group and his or her outside social life.

Modifications for Bulimia Nervosa

The IPT-G protocol can be easily adapted for BN patients because the focus is on the interpersonal problems and not the eating disorder per se. However, several issues are important to consider. BN patients tend to present for treatment at a much earlier age than BED patients. This age difference may be one reason that the primary interpersonal problems for the BN patients tend to be somewhat different than those of the BED patient. For instance, Fairburn (1993) found that the most common problem for BN was interpersonal role disputes (64%; 16/25 patients) with the majority being marital disputes. BED patients also experienced role disputes but only in 28% of the cases; although BED patients were similar to BN patients in that all of the disputes were marital. The second most common problem for BN patients was difficulties with role transitions (36%, 9/25) which typically took the form of problems separating from parents and adjusting to living away from home. BED patients reported fewer difficulties with role transitions and the two women who did experience that problem were facing late adulthood transitions (i.e., retirement and caring for an elderly mother). Finally, BN patients encountered the most common problem for BED patients (interpersonal deficits) much less often.

THE INTEGRATION OF COGNITIVE-BEHAVIORAL THERAPY AND INTERPERSONAL PSYCHOTHERAPY?

The first question that many clinicians and researchers ask is whether CBT and IPT should be combined. To date, there are no empirical data to answer this question one way or another. However, there are many issues to consider prior to reaching an answer to this question. First, CBT and IPT are derived from different theoretical frameworks, assume different models of symptom maintenance, and involve different intervention strategies. See Table 6.2 for the distinctive features of group CBT and group IPT. This distinctiveness may preclude combining them as the combination may dilute the effect of ei-

TABLE 6.2. Distinctive Features of Group Cognitive-Behavioral Therapy and Group Interpersonal Psychotherapy

Group cognitive-behavioral therapy	Group interpersonal psychotherapy
Cognitive formulation of bulimia	Interpersonal formulation of bulimia
Introduction of a pattern of regular eating	Idenification of problem areas
Graded introduction to avoided food	Focus on current interpersonal problems
Self-monitoring	Group summaries to track progress
Focus on cognitive distortions (attitudes to shape and weight)	Development of more adaptive ways of relating
Identification of binge triggers	Exploration of feelings (negative and positive)
Relapse prevention procedures	Emphasis on termination as separation and loss

Note. From Wilfley et al. (1993). Copyright 1993 by the American Psychological Association. Reprinted by permission.

ther treatment and result in an intervention less potent than either CBT or IPT alone (Fairburn, 1993). We feel this is especially true for a brief psychotherapy (e.g., 20 weeks or less). In a brief psychotherapy (such as what is typically applied with clinical intervention research) it is critical to have a clear framework for treatment. Of course, if clinicians are not involved in a research protocol, there is more leeway to discuss eating habits and attitudes in IPT and interpersonal and social functioning in CBT. Second, there are many unknown answers that ultimately guide us in generating a response to this question. We are currently in need of further research (Grilo, Devlin, et al., 1996) to identify the active ingredients of treatment, the predictors of response to treatment, and the potential role of sequencing of treatments (e.g., Agras et al., 1994, 1995). There are data to suggest that for those BN patients who do not respond to CBT, IPT is an efficacious alternative (Peveler, Fairburn, Boller, & Dunger, 1993). Future research is needed to determine whether there is a role for combining CBT and IPT. A sequential ordering of treatments for nonresponders may be the most judicious approach.

CONCLUSION

Both BN and BED are heterogeneous, biopsychosocial disorders often associated with significant medical and psychiatric comorbidity. The overwhelming majority of individuals who develop BN are adolescent girls or young adult women. In contrast, BED not only is found among young women but also occurs in men and older adult women.

Although the etiology of both BN and BED remain unknown, progress has been made in understanding the maintenance and treatment of BN and BED. Assessment of BN and BED patients must include the behavioral aspects (e.g., binge eating and purging), associated core eating-disorder psychopathology (e.g., dietary restraint and distorted attitudes toward eating, shape, and weight), and psychosocial aspects. This multidimensional assessment is essential to formulate effective treatment plans, assess progress, and evaluate psychotherapy process and outcome.

Two psychosocial treatments have emerged as particularly promising treatment interventions for BN and BED: CBT and IPT. CBT and IPT can be administered in either an individual or a group format. Which format is most effective needs to be empirically tested using controlled treatment trials. However, in the absence of data to suggest that one format is superior to the other, we have offered several reasons that group may be particularly useful for BN and BED. For instance, sharing common experiences with other patients is helpful to counter some of the shame, social isolation, and guilt associated with binge eating.

Although CBT and IPT appear to be equally effective in treating BN and BED, little is known about the mechanisms by which they achieve their effects or the predictors of treatment outcome. Identifying mechanisms will ultimately lead to more effective treatments whereas identifying predictors of treatment outcome will provide information about matching of BN and BED patients to the most effective treatment. Further research is needed to identify the active ingredients of treatment, the predictors of response to treatment, and the potential role of sequencing of treatments (Grilo, Devlin, et al., 1996).

Additional research is also needed to determine how best to help those patients who do not respond to the currently validated CBT and IPT treatments, as well as how to intervene best in those cases complicated by medical and/or psychiatric comorbidities (Grilo, Devlin, et al., 1996). Wilson (1996) presents a number of potential behavioral strategies that might potentially augment existing CBT treatments. Stepped care models, which suggest that treatment nonresponders be given more intensive treatments such as day treatment or inpatient programs (Levendusky, Willis, & Ghinassi, 1994) could also be considered.

ACKNOWLEDGMENTS

Preparation of this chapter was provided in part by funding from the MacArthur Foundation on the Determinants and Consequences of Health Promoting and Health Damaging Behavior. The support of the Jenny Craig Foundation for the Fellowship Program of the Yale Center for Eating and Weight Disorders is also gratefully acknowledged. We are grateful to Robinson Welch, Ph.D., Adele Jones, M.Ed., and Angela Ryan, B.A., for their assistance with the preparation of the manuscript.

REFERENCES

Agras, W. S. (1991). Nonpharmacologic treatments of bulimia nervosa. *Journal of Clinical Psychiatry, 52*, 29–33.

Agras, W. S. (1993, March). *State of the science: Eating disorders*. Lecture presented at the 14th annual Society of Behavioral Medicine Scientific Sessions, San Francisco, CA.

Agras, W. S., Rossiter, E. M., Arnow, B., Schneider, J. A., Telch, C. F., Raeburn, S. D., Bruce, B., Perl, M., & Koran, L. M. (1992). Pharmacologic and cognitive–behavioral treatment for bulimia nervosa: A controlled comparison. *American Journal of Psychiatry, 149*(1), 82–87.

Agras, W. S., Schneider, J. A., Arnow, B., Raeburn, S. D., & Telch, C.F. (1989). Cognitive–behavioral and response–prevention treatments for bulimia nervosa. *Journal of Consulting and Clinical Psychology, 57*, 215–221.

Agras, W. S., Telch, C. F., Arnow, B., Eldredge, K., Detzer, M. J., Henderson, J., & Marnell, M. (1995). Does interpersonal therapy help patients with binge eating disorder who fail to respond toe cognitive-behavioral therapy? *Journal of Consulting and Clinical Psychology, 63*, 356–360.

Agras, W. S., Telch, C. F., Arnow, B., Eldredge, K., Wilfley, D. E., Raeburn, S. D., Henderson, J., & Marnell, M. (1994). Weight loss, cognitive-behaviroal, and desipramine treatments in binge eating disorder: An additive design. *Behavior Therapy, 25*, 225–238.

Akan, G. E., & Grilo, C. M. (1995). Sociocultural influences on eating attitudes and behaviors, body image, and psychological functioning: A comparison of African-American, Asian-American, and Caucasian college women. *International Journal of Eating Disorders, 18*, 181–187.

Altshuler, B. D., Dechow, P. C., Waller, D. A., & Hardy, B. (1990). An investigation of the oral pathologies occuring in bulimia nervosa. *International Journal of Eating Disorders, 9*, 191–199.

American Psychiatric Association. (1980). *Diagnostic and statistical manual of mental disorders* (3rd ed.). Washington, DC: Author.

American Psychiatric Association. (1987). *Diagnostic and statistical manual of mental disorders* (3rd ed., rev.). Washington, DC: Author.

American Psychiatric Association (1994). *Diagnostic and statistical manual of mental disorders* (4th ed.). Washington, DC: Author.

Antoni, M. H., Baggett, L., Ironson, G., LaPerriere, A., August, S., Klimas, N., Schneiderman, N., & Fletcher, M. A. (1991). Cognitive-behavioral stress management intervention buffers distress responses and immunologic changes following notification of HIV–1 seropositivity. *Journal of Consulting and Clinical Psychology, 59:6*, 1–8.

Arnow, B., Kenardy, J., & Agras, W.S. (1992). Binge eating among the obese: A descriptive Study. *Journal of Behavioral Medicine,15,155-170*

Beck, A. T. (1976). *Cognitive therapy and the emotional disorders.* New York: International Universities Press.

Beck, A. T., Rush, A. J., Shaw, B. F., & Emery, G. (1979). *Cognitive therapy of depression.* New York: Guilford Press.

Beck, A. T., Ward, C. H., Mendelson, M., Mock, J., & Erbaugh, J. (1961). An inventory for measuring depression. *Archives of General Psychiatry, 4*, 561–571.

Beglin, S. J., & Fairburn, C. G. (1992). What is mean by the term "binge"? *American Journal of Psychiatry, 149*, 123–124.

Belfer, P. L., Crump, S., & Bradach, K. M. (1991). *Body awareness and self-consciousness in eating and anxiety disordered individuals.* Unpublished manuscript.

Bennett, S. M., Williamson, D. A., & Powers, S. K. (1989). Bulimia nervosa nd resting metabolic rate. *International Journal of Eating Disorders, 8*, 417–424.

Beren, S. E., Hayden, H. A., Wilfley, D. E., & Grilo, C. M. (1996). The influence of sexual orientation on body dissatisfaction in adult men and women. *International Journal of Eating Disorders, 20*, 135–141.

Black, C. M. D., & Wilson, G. T. (1996). Assessment of eating disorders: Interview versus questionnaire. *International Journal of Eating Disorders, 20*, 43–50.

Blundell, J. E., & Hill, A. J. (1993). Binge eating: Psychobiological mechanisms. In C. G. Fairburn & G. T. Wilson (Eds.), *Binge eating: Nature, assessment and treatment.* (pp. 206–224). New York: Guilford Press.

Bray, G. A. (1992). Pathophysiology of obesity. *American Journal of Clinical Nutrition,*

55, 488s.

Brody, M. L., Walsh, B. T., & Devlin, M. J. (1994). Binge eating disorder: Reliability and validity of a new diagnostic category. *Journal of Consulting and Clinical Psychology, 62,* 381-386.

Brownell, K. D. (1991a). Dieting and the search for the perfect body: Where physiology and culture collide. *Behavior Therapy, 22,* 1–12.

Brownell, K. D. (1991b). Personal responsibility and control over our health: When expectation exceeds reality. *Health Psychology, 10,* 303–310.

Brownell, K. D., & Fairburn, C. G. (Eds.). (1996). *Eating disorders and obesity: A comprehensive handbook.* New York: Guilford Press.

Brownell, K. D., & Rodin, J. (1994). Medical, matabolic, and psychological effects of weight cycling. *Archives of Internal Medicine, 154,* 1325–1330.

Brownell, K. D., Rodin, J., & Wilmore, J. H. (1992). *Eating, body weight, and performance in athletes.* Philadelphia: Lea & Febiger.

Brownell, K. D., & Wadden, T. A. (1992). Etiology and treatment of obesity: Toward understanding a serious, prevalent, and refractory disorder. *Journal of Consulting and Clinical Psychology, 60,* 505–517.

Bruce, B., & Agras, W. S. (1992). Binge eating in females: A population based investigation. *International Journal of Eating Disorders, 12,* 365-373.

Bushnell, J. A., Wells, J. E., Hornblow, A. R., Oakley Browne, M. A., & Joyce, P. (1990). Prevalence of three bulimia syndromes in the general population. *Psychological Medicine, 20,* 671–680.

Cash, T. F. (1991). Binge-eating and body images among the obese: A further evaluation. *Journal of Social Behavior and Personality, 6,* 367-376.

Casper, R. C. (1983). On the emergence of bulimia nervosa as a syndrome: A historical view. *International Journal of Eating Disorders, 2,* 3-16.

Cattanach, L., Malley, R., & Rodin, J. (1988). Psychologic and physiologic reactivity to stressors in eating disordered individuals. *Psychosomatic Medicine, 50,* 591–599.

Cattanach, L., & Rodin, J. (1988). Psychosocial components of the stress process in bulimia. *International Journal of Eating Disorders, 7,* 75–88.

Charnock, D. J. K. (1989). A comment on the role of dietary restraint in the development of bulimia nervosa. *British Journal of Clinical Psychology, 28,* 329–340.

Cooper, J. L., Morrison, T. L., Bigman, O. L., Abramowitz, S. I., Levin, S., & Krener, P. (1988). Mood changes and affective disorder in the bulimic binge-purge cycle. *International Journal of Eating Disorders, 7,* 469-474.

Cooper, P. J., Taylor, M. J., Cooper, Z., & Fairburn, C. G. (1987). The development and validation of the Body Shape Questionnaire. *International Journal of Eating Disorders, 6,* 485–494.

Cooper, Z., Cooper, P. J., & Fairburn, C. G. (1989). The validity of the eating disorder examination and its subscales. *British Journal of Psychiatry, 154,* 807–812.

Cooper, Z., & Fairburn, C.G. (1987). The Eating Disorder Examination: A semistructured interview for the assessment of the specific psychopathology of eating disorders. *International Journal of Eating Disorders, 6,* 1–8.

Craighead, L. W., & Agras, W. S. (1991). Mechanisms of action in cognitive-behavioral and pharmacological interventions for obesity and bulimia nervosa. *Journal of Consulting and Clinical Psychology, 59,* 115–125.

Davis, R., Freeman, R. J., & Garner, D. M. (1988). A naturalistic investigation of eating behavior in bulimia nervosa. *Journal of Consulting and Clinical Psychology, 56,* 273–279.

Derogatis, L. R. (1983). *SCL-90-R: Administration manual—II for the revised version.* Towson, MD: Clinical Psychometric Research.

Devlin, M. J., Walsh, B. T., Kral, J. G., Heymsfield, S. B., Pi-Sunyer, F. X., & Dantzic, S. (1990). Metabolic abnormalities in bulimia nervosa: A semistarvation model. *Archives of General Psychiatry, 47,* 144–148.

Devlin, M. J., Walsh, B. T., Spitzer, R. L., & Hasin, D. (1992). Is there another binge eating disorder?: A review of the literature on overeating in the absence of bulimia. *International Journal of Eating Disorders, 11,* 333–340.

Dolan, B. M., Lieberman, S., Evans, C., & Lacey, J. H. (1990). Family features associated with normal body weight bulimia. *International Journal of Eating Disorders, 9,* 639–647.

Drewnowski, A., Hopkins, S. A., & Kessler, R. C. (1988). The prevalence of bulimia nervosa in the US college student population. *American Journal of Public Health, 78,* 1322–1325.

Dunn, P. K., & Ondercin, P. (1981). Personality variables related to compulsive eating in college women. *Journal of Clinical Psychology, 1,* 43–49.

Fairburn, C. G. (1981). A cognitive behavioral approach to the treatment of bulimia. *Psychological Medicine, 11,* 707–711.

Fairburn, C. G. (1985). Cognitive–behavioral treatment for bulimia. In D. M. Garner & P. E. Garfinkel (Eds.), *Handbook of psychotherapy for anorexia nervosa and bulimia* (pp. 160–192). New York: Guilford Press.

Fairburn, C. G. (1987). The definition of bulimia nervosa: Guidelines for clinicians and research workers. *Annals of Behavioral Medicine, 9,* 3–7.

Fairburn, C. G. (1990). Bulimia nervosa. *British Medical Journal, 300,* 485–487.

Fairburn, C. G. (1992, April). *How are we doing? Retrospective/perspective.* Paper presented at the 5th International Conference on Eating Disorders, New York, NY.

Fairburn, C. G. Interpersonal psychotherapy for bulimia nervosa. (1993). In G. L. Klerman, & M. M. Weissman (Eds.), *New applications of interpersonal psychotherapy* Washington, DC: American Psychiatric Press.

Fairburn, C.G. (1995). *Overcoming binge eating.* New York: Guilford Press.

Fairburn, C. G., Agras, W. S., & Wilson, G. T. (1992). The research on the treatment of bulimia nervosa: practical and theoretical implications. In G. H. Anderson & S. H. Kennedy (Eds.), *The biology of feast and famine: Relevance to eating disorders* (pp. 317–340). New York: Academic Press.

Fairburn, C. G., & Beglin, S. J. (1990). Studies of the epidemiology of bulimia nervosa. *American Journal of Psychiatry, 147,* 401–408.

Fairburn, C. G., & Beglin, S. J. (1994). Assessment of eating disorders: Interview of-self-report questionnaire? *International Journal of Eating Disorders, 16,* 363–370.

Fairburn, C. G., & Cooper, Z. (1993). The schedule of the Eating Disorder Examination. In C. G. Fairburn & G. T. Wilson (Eds.), *Binge eating: Nature, assessment, and treatment* (pp. 317–360). New York: Guilford Press.

Fairburn, C. G., Hay, P. J., & Welch, S. L. (1993). Binge eating and bulimia nervosa: Distribution and determinants. In C. G. Fairburn & G. T. Wilson (Eds.), *Binge eating: Nature, assessment and treatment* (pp.123–143). Guilford Press: New York.

Fairburn, C. G., Jones, R., Peveler, R. C., Hope, R. A., & O'Connor, M. (1993). *Psy-*

chotherapy and bulimia nervosa: The long-term effects of interpersonal psychotherapy. Archives of General Psychiatry, 50, 419–428.

Fairburn, C. G., Jones, R., Peveler, R. C., O'Connor, M. E., & Hope, R.A. (1991). Three psychological treatments for bulimia nervosa: A comparative trial. Archives of General Psychiatry, 48, 463–469.

Fairburn, C. G., Kirk, J., O'Connor, M., Anastasiades, P., & Cooper, P. J. (1987). Prognostic factors in bulimia nervosa. Journal of Clinical Psychology, 26, 223–224.

Fairburn, C. G., Marcus, M. D., & Wilson, G. T. (1993). Cognitive behavior therapy for binge eating and bulimia nervosa: A comprehensive treatment manual. In C. G. Fairburn & G. T. Wilson (Eds.), Binge eating: Nature, assessment, and treatment (pp. 361–404). New York: Guilford Press.

Fairburn, C. G., Norman, D. A., Welch, S. L., O'Connor, M. E., Doll, H. A., & Peveler, R. C. (1995). A prospective study of outcome in bulimia nervosa and the long-term effects of three psychological treatments. Archives of General Psychiatry, 52, 304–312.

Fairburn, C. G., Welch, S. L., & Hay, P. J. (1993). The classification of recurrent overeating: The "binge eating disorder" proposal. International Journal of Eating Disorders, 12, 155–159.

Fairburn, C. G., & Wilson, G. T. (Eds.). (1993). Binge eating: Nature, assessment, and treatment. New York: Guilford Press.

Fawzy, F., Kemeny, M., Fawzy, W., Elashoff, R., Morton, D., Cousins, N., & Fahey, J. (1990). A structured psychiatric intervention for cancer patients:II. Changes over time in immunological measures. Archives of General Psychiatry, 47, 729–735.

Fenigstein, A., Scheier, M. F., & Buss, A. H. (1975). Public and private self-consciousness: Assessment and theory. Journal of Consulting and Clinical Psychology, 43, 522–527.

Fennell, M. J. V. (1989). Depression. In K. Hawton, P. M. Salkovskis, J. Kirk, & D. M. Clark (Eds.). Cognitive behavior therapy for psychiatric problems: A practical guide. (pp. 169–234). New York: Oxford University Press.

Fichter, M. M., Leibl, K., Rief, W., Brunner, E., Schmidt-Auberger, S., & Engel, R. R. (1991). Flouxetine versus placebo: A double-blind study with bulimic inpatients undergoing intensive psychotherapy. Pharmacopsychiatry, 24, 1–7.

Fluoxetine Bulimia Nervosa Collaborative Study Group (1992). Flouxetine in the treatment of bulimia nervosa: A multicenter, placebo controlled, double-blind trial. Archives of General Psychiatry, 49, 139–147.

Freeman, C. P. L., Barry, F., Dunkeld-Turnbull, J., & Henderson, A. (1988). Controlled trial of psychotherapy for bulimia nervosa. British Medical Journal, 296, 521–525.

Garner, D. M. (1991). Eating Disorders Inventory–2. Odessa, FL: Psychological Assessment Resources.

Garner, D.M., Olmstead, M.E., & Polivy, J. (1983). Development and validation of a multidimensional eating disorder inventory for anorexia nervosa and bulimia. International Journal of Eating Disorders, 2, 15–34.

Garner, D. M., Rockert, W., Davis R., Garner M. V., Olmsted, M. P., & Eagle, M. (1993). Comparison of cognitive-behavioral and supportive–expressive therapy for bulimia nervosa. American Journal of Psychiatry, 150, 37–46.

Garner, D. M., Rockert, W., Olmstead, M. P., Johnson, C. L., & Coscina, D. V. (1985). Psychoeducational principles in the treatment of bulimia and anorexia nervosa. In D. M. Garner, & P. E. Garfinkel (Eds.), *Handbook of psychotherapy for anorexia nervosa and bulimia* (pp. 513–572). New York: Guilford Press.

Gormally, J., Black, S., Daston, S., & Rardin, D. (1982). The assessment of binge eating severity among obese persons. *Addictive Behaviors, 7*, 47–55.

Gormally, J., Rardin, D., & Black, S. (1980). Correlates of successful response to a behavioral weight control clinic. *Journal of Counseling Psychology, 27*, 179–191.

Gotestam, K. G., & Agras, W. S. (1989). Bulimia nervosa: Pharmacologic and psychologic approaches to treatment. *Nordic Journal of Psychiatry, 43*, 543–551.

Gray, J. J., Ford, K., & Kelly, L. M. (1987). The prevalence of bulimia in a black college population. *International Journal of Eating Disorders, 9*, 501–512.

Gray, J. J., & Hoage, C. M. (1990). Bulimia nervosa: Group behavior therapy with exposure plus response prevention. *Psychological Reports, 66*, 667–674.

Greenfeld, D., Mickley, D., Quinlan, D. M., & Roloff, P. (1995). Hypokalemia in outpatients with eating disorders. *American Journal of Psychiatry, 152*, 60–63.

Grilo, C. M., Becker, D. F., Levy, K., Walker, M., Edell, W. S., & McGlashan, T. H. (1995). Eating disorders with and without substance use disorders: A comparative study of inpatients. *Comprehensive Psychiatry, 36*, 312–317.

Grilo, C. M., Devlin, M. J., Cachelin, F. M., & Yanovski, S. Z. (1996). *Report of the NIH Workshop on the Development of Research Priorities in Eating Disorders*. Manuscript submitted for publication.

Grilo, C. M., Levy, K. N., Becker, D. F., Edell, W. S., & McGlashan, T. H. (1996). DSM-III-R Axis I and Axis II comorbidity in patients with eating disorders. *Psychiatric Services, 47*, 426–429.

Grilo, C. M., & Pogue-Geile, M. F. (1991). The nature of environmental influences on weight and obesity: A behavior genetic analysis. *Psychological Bulletin, 110*, 520–537.

Grilo, C. M., & Shiffman, S. (1994). Longitudinal investigation of the abstinence violation effect in binge eaters. *Journal of Consulting and Clinical Psychology, 62*, 611–619.

Grilo, C. M., Shiffman, S., & Carter-Campbell, J. T. (1994). Binge eting antecedents in normal-weight non-purging females: Is ther consistency? *International Journal of Eating Disorders, 16*, 239–249.

Grilo, C. M., Wilfley, D. E., Jones, A., Brownell, K. D., & Rodin, J. (1994). The social self, body dissatisfaction, and binge eating. *Obesity Research, 2*, 24–27.

Grissett, N. I, & Norvell, N. K. (1992). Perceived social support, social skills, and quality of relationships in bulimic women. *Journal of Consulting and Clinical Psychology, 60*, 293–299.

Gross, J., & Rosen, J.C. (1988). Bulimia in adolescents: Prevalence and psychosocial correlates. *International Journal of Eating Disorders, 7*, 51–61.

Gwirtsman, H. E., Kaye, W. H., Obarzanek, E., George, D. T., Jimerson, D. C., & Ebert, M. H. (1989). Decreased caloric intake in normal-weight patients with bulimia: Comparison with female volunteers. *American Journal of Clinical Nutrition, 49*, 86–92.

Hatsukami, D., Mitchell, J. E., Eckert, E. D., & Pyle, R. (1986). Characteristics of patients with bulimia only, bulimia with affective disorder, and bulimia with substance abuse problems. *Addictive Behaviors, 11*, 399–406.

Hawkins, R. C., & Clement, P. F. (1980). Development and construct validation of a self-report measure of binge eating tendencies. *Addictive Behaviors, 5*, 219–226.

Heatherton, T. F., & Baumeister, R. F. (1991). Binge eating as an escape from self-awareness. *Psychological Bulletin, 110*, 86–108.

Heatherton, T. F., Nichols, P., Mahameid, F., & Keel, P. (1995). Body weight, dieting, and eating disorder symptoms among college students, 1982 to 1992. *American Journal of Psychiatry, 152*, 1623–1629.

Heatherton, T. F. , & Polivy, J. (1992). Chronic dieting and eating disorders: A spiral model. In S. E. Hobfall, M. A. P. Stevens, D. L. Tennenbaum, & J. H. Crowther (Eds.), *The etiology of bulimia: The individual and familial context* (pp. 133–155). Washington, DC: Hemisphere.

Hellman, C. J., Budd, M., Borysenko, J., McClelland, D., & Benson, H. (1990). A study of the effectiveness of two group behavioral medicine interventions for patients with psychosomatic complaints. *Behavioral Medicine, 16 (4)*, 165–173.

Herzog, D. B., Keller, M. B., Lavori, P. W., & Ott, I. L. (1987). Social impairment in bulimia. *International Journal of Eating Disorders, 6*, 741–747.

Herzog, D. B., Norman, D. K., Rigotti, N. A., & Prepose, M. (1986). Frequency of bulimic behaviors and associated social maladjustment in female graduate students. *Journal of Psychiatric Research, 20*, 355–361.

Higuchi, S., Suzuki, K., Yamada, K., Parrish, K., & Kono, H. (1993). Alcoholics with eating disorders: Prevalence and clinical course: a study from Japan. *British Journal of Psychiatry, 162*, 403–406.

Hollon, S. D., DeRubeis, R. J., & Evans, M. D. (1987). Causal mediation of change in treatment for depression: Discriminating between nonspecificity and noncausality. *Psychological Bulletin, 102*, 139–149.

Horowitz, L. M., Rosenberg, S.E., Baer, B.A., Ureno, G., & Villasner, V.S. (1988). Inventory of interpersonal problems: Psychometric properties and clinical applications. *Journal of Consulting and Clinical Psychology, 56*, 885–892.

Hsu, L. K. G. (1990a). *Eating disorders*. New York: Guilford Press.

Hsu, L. K. G. (1990b). The experiential aspects of bulimia nervosa: Implications for cognitive-behavior therapy. *Behavior Modification, 14*, 50–65.

Hsu, L. K. G., Santhouse, R., & Chesler, B. E. (1991). Individual cognitive behavioral therapy for bulimia nervosa: The description of a program. *International Journal of Eating Disorders, 10*, 273–283.

Hudson, J. I., Pope, H. G. J., Jonas, J. M., & Yurgelun-Todd, D. (1983). Phenomenologic relationship of eating disorders to major affective disorder. *Psychiatry Research, 9*, 345–354.

Hudson, J. I., Pope, H. G., Wurtman, J., Yurgelun-Todd, D., Mark, S., & Rosenthal, N. E. (1988). Bulimia in obese individuals: Relationship to normal-weight bulimia. *Journal of Nervous and Mental Disease, 176*, 144–152.

Humphrey, L. L. (1986). Structural analysis of parent–child relationships in eating disorders. *Journal of Abnormal Psychology, 95*, 395–402.

Humphrey, L. L. (1988). Relationships within subtypes of anorexic, bulimic, and normal families using structural analysis of social behavior. *Journal of the American Academy of Child and Adolescent Psychiatry, 27,* 544–551.

Humphrey, L. L. (1989). Is there a causal link between disturbed family processes and eating disorders?. In W. G. Johnson (Ed.), *Bulimia nervosa: Perspectives on clinical research and therapy* (pp. 119–135). New York: JAI Press.

Huon, G. F., & Brown, L. B. (1985). Evaluating a group treatment for bulimia. *Journal of Psychiatric Research, 19,* 479–483.

Jacobson, N. S. (1989). The therapist–client relationship in cognitive behavior therapy: Implications for treating depression. *Journal of Cognitive Psychotherapy, 3,* 85-96.

Jimerson, D. C., Herzog, D. B., & Brotman, A. W. (1993). Pharmacologic approaches in the treatment of eating disorders. *Harvard Review of Psychiatry, 1,* 82–93.

Johnson, C., & Connors, M. E. (1987). *The etiology and treatment of bulimia nervosa.* New York: Basic Books.

Johnson, C., Connors, M. E., & Tobin, D. L. (1987). Symptom management of bulimia. *Journal of Consulting and Clinical Psychology, 55,* 668–676.

Johnson, C., Tobin, D. L., & Dennis, A. (1990). Differences in treatment outcome between borderline and nonborderline bulimics at one-year follow-up. *International Journal of Eating Disorders, 9,* 617–627.

Kaplan, A. S., & Garfinkel, P. E. (Eds.). (1993). *Medical issues and the eating disorders.* New York: Brunner/Mazel.

Kaye, W. H., Gwirtsman, H. E., Obarzanek, E., George, T., Jimerson, D. C., & Ebert, M. H. (1986). Caloric intake necessary for weight maintenance in anorexia nervosa: Nonbulimics require greater caloric intake than bulimics. *American Journal of Clinical Nutrition, 44,* 435–443.

Keefe, P. H., Wyshogrod, D., Weinberger, E., & Agras, W. S. (1984). Binge eating and outcome of behavioral treatment of obesity: A preliminary report. *Behavior Research and Therapy, 22,* 319–321.

Keller, M. B., Herzog, D. B., Lavori, P. W., Bradburn, I. S., & Mahoney, E. M. (1992). The naturalistic history of bulimia nervosa. Extraordinarily high rates of chronicity, relapse, recurrence, and psychosocial morbidity. *International Journal of Eating Disorders, 12,* 1–9.

Keller, M. B., Herzog, D. B., Lavori, P. M., Ott, I. L., Bradburn, I. S., & Mahoney, E. M. (1989). High rates of chronicity and rapidity of relapse in patients with bulimia nervosa and depression [Letter]. *Archives of General Psychiatry, 46,* 480–481.

Kendler, K. S., Maclean, C., Neale, M., Kessler, R., Heath, A., & Eaves, L. (1991). The genetic epidemiology of bulimia nervosa. *American Journal of Psychiatry, 148,* 1627–1637.

Keuhnel, R. H., & Wadden, T. A. (1994). Binge eating disorder, weight cycling, and psychopathology. *International Journal of Eating Disorders, 15,* 321–329.

Keys, A., Brozek, J., Henschel, A., Mickelsen, F., & Taylor, H. L. (1950). *The biology of human starvation.* Minneapolis: University of Minnesota Press.

Kirkley, B. G., Schneider, J. A., Agras, W.S., & Bachman, J. A. (1985). Comparison of two group treatments for bulimia. *Journal of Consulting and Clinical Psychology, 53,* 43–48.

Klerman, G. L., Weissman, M. M., Rounsaville, B. J., & Chevron, E. S. (1984). *Interpersonal psychotherapy of depression.* New York: Basic Books.

Kolotkin, R. L., Revis, E. S., Kirkley, B. G., & Janick, L. (1987). Binge eating in obesity: Associated MMPI characteristics. *Journal of Consulting and Clinical Psychology*, 55, 872–876.

Kuczmarski, R. J. (1992). Prevalence of overweight and weight gain in the United States. *American Journal of Clinical Nutrition*, 55, 495S–502S.

Lacey, J. H. (1983). Bulimia nervosa, binge eating, and psychogenic vomiting: A controlled treatment study and long term outcome. *British Medical Journal*, 286, 1609–1613.

Laessle, R. G., Wittchen, H. U., Fichter, M. M., & Pirke, K. M. (1989). The significance of subgroups of bulimia and anorexia nervosa: Lifetime frequency of psychiatric disorders. *International Journal of Eating Disorders*, 8, 569–574.

Langer, L. M., Warheit, G. J., & Zimmerman, R. S. (1991). Epidemiological study of problem eating behaviors and related attitudes in the general population. *Addictive Behaviors*, 16, 167-173.

Lee, N. F., & Rush, A. J. (1986). Cognitive–behavioral group therapy for bulimia. *International Journal of Eating Disorders*, 5, 599–615.

Leitenberg, H., Rosen, J. C., Gross, J., Nudelman, S., & Vara, L. S. (1988). Exposure plus response prevention in the treatment of bulimia nervosa: A controlled evaluation. *Journal of Consulting and Clinical Psychology*, 56, 535–541.

Leitenberg, H., Rosen, J. C., Wolf, J., Vara, L. S., Detzer, M. J., & Srebnik, D. (1994). Comparison of cognitive-behavior therapy and desipramine in the treatment of bulimia nervosa. *Behavior Research and Therapy*, 32, 37–46.

Levendusky, P. G., Willis, B. S., & Ghinassi, F. A. (1994). The therapeutic contracting program: A comprehensive continuum of care model. *Psychiatric Quarterly*, 65, 189–208.

Liedtke, R., Jager, B., Lempa, W., Kunsebeck, H., Grone, M., & Freyberger, H. (1991). Therapy outcome of two treatment models for bulimia nervosa: Preliminary results of a controlled study. *Psychotherapy and Psychosomatics*, 56, 56–63.

Lingswiler, V. M., Crowther, J. H., & Stephens, M. A. P. (1989a). Affective and cognitive antecedents to eating episodes in bulimia and binge eating. *International Journal of Eating Disorders*, 8, 533–539.

Lingswiler, V. M., Crowther, J. H., & Stephens, M. A. P. (1989b). Emotional and somatic consequences of binge episodes. *Addictive Behaviors*, 14, 503–511.

Lissner, L., Odell, P. M., D'Agostino, R. B., Stokes, J., Kreger, B. E., Belanger, A. J., & Brownell, K. D. (1991). Variability of body weight and health outcomes in the Framingham population. *New England Journal of Medicine*, 324, 1839–1844.

Loeb, K. L., Pike, K. M., Walsh, B. T., & Wilson, G. T. (1994). Assessment of diagnostic features of bulimia nervosa: Interview versus self-report format. *International Journal of Eating Disorders*, 16, 75–81.

Loro, A. D., & Orleans, C. S. (1981). Binge eating in obesity: Preliminary findings and guidelines for behavioral analyses and treatment. *Addictive Behaviors*, 6, 155–166.

Lowe, M. (1993). The effects of dieting on eating behavior: A three-factor model. *Psychological Bulletin*, 114; 100–121.

Lowe, M. R., & Caputo, G. C. (1991). Binge eating in obesity: Toward the specification of predictors. *International Journal of Eating Disorders*, 10, 49–55.

Marcus, M. D., Smith, D., Santelli, R., & Kaye, W. (1992). Characterization of eating disordered behavior in obese binge eaters. *International Journal of Eating Disorders, 12*, 249–255.

Marcus, M. D., Wing, R. R., Ewing, L., Keern, E., Gooding, W., & McDermott, M. (1990). Psychiatric disorders among obese binge eaters. *International Journal of Eating Disorders, 9*, 69–77.

Marcus, M. D., Wing, R. R., & Fairburn, C. G. (1995). Cognitive treatment of binge eating versus behavioral weight control in the treatment of binge eating disorder. *Annals of Behavioral Medicine, 17*, SO90.

Marcus, M. D., Wing, R. R., & Hopkins, J. (1988). Obese binge eaters: affect, cognitions, and response to behavioral weight control. *Journal of Consulting and Clinical Psychology, 56*, 433–439.

Marcus, M. D., Wing, R. R., & Lamparski, D. M. (1985). Binge eating and dietary restraint in obese patients. *Addictive Behaviors, 10*, 163–168.

Marlatt, G. A., & Gordon, J. R. (Eds.). (1985). *Relapse prevention: Maintenance strategies in the treatment of addictive behaviors.* New York: Guilford Press.

McArdle, W. D., Katch, F. I., & Katch, V. L. (1991). *Exercise physiology: Energy, nutrition, and human performance.* Lea & Febiger.

McCann, U. D., & Agras, W. S. (1990). Successful treatment of nonpurging bulimia nervosa with desipramine: A double-blind, placebo-controlled study. *American Journal of Psychiatry, 147*, 1509–1513.

McMullin, R. E. (1986). *Handbook of cognitive therapy techniques.* New York: Norton.

Mitchell, J. E. (1986). Bulimia: Medical and physiological aspects. In K. D. Brownell, & J. P. Foreyt (Eds.), *Handbook of eating disorders* (pp. 379–388). New York: Basic Books.

Mitchell, J. E., Fletcher, L., Pyle, R. L., Eckert, E. D., Hatsukami, D. K., & Pomeroy, C. (1989). The impact of treatment on meal patterns in patients with bulimia nervosa. *International Journal of Eating Disorders, 8*, 167–172.

Mitchell, J. E., Pyle, R. L., Eckert, E. D., Hatsukami, D., Pomeroy, C., & Zimmerman, R. (1990). A comparison study of antidepressants and structured group psychotherapy in the treatment of bulimia nervosa. *Archives of General Psychiatry, 47*, 149–157.

Mitchell, J. E., Seim, H. C., Colon, E., & Pomeroy, C. (1987). Medical complications and medical management of bulimia. *Annals of Internal Medicine, 107*, 71–77.

Mitchell, J. E., & Zwaan, M. (1993). Pharmacological treatments of binge eating. In C. G. Fairburn & G. T. Wilson (Eds.), *Binge eating: Nature, assessment, and treatment.* (pp. 250–269). New York: Guilford Press.

Nangle, D. W., Johnson, W. G., Carr-Nangle, R. E., & Engler, L. B. (1994). Binge eating disorder and the proposed DSM-IV criteria: Psychometric analysis of the questionnaire of eating and weight patterns. *International Journal of Eating Disorders, 16*, 147–157.

Newman, M. M., Halmi, K. A., & Marchi, P. (1987). Relationship of clinical factors to caloric requirements in subtypes of eating disorders. *Biological Psychiatry, 22*, 1253–1263.

Norman, D. K., & Herzog, D. B. (1986). A 3-year outcome study of normal-weight bulimia: Assessment of psychosocial functioning and eating attitudes. *Psychiatry Research, 19*, 199–205.

O'Leary, K. D., & Wilson, G. T. (1987). *Behavior therapy: Application and outcome* (2nd ed.). Englewood Cliffs, NJ: Prentice Hall.

Parry-Jones, B., & Parry-Jones, W. L. (1991). Bulimia: An archival review of its history in psychosomatic medicine. *International Journal of Eating Disorders, 10,* 129–143.

Persons, J. B. (1989). *Cognitive therapy in practice: A case formulation approach.* New York: Norton.

Peveler, R. C., Fairburn, C. G., Boller, I., & Duniger, D. (1993). Eating disorders in adolescents with insulin-dependent diabetes mellitus: A controlled study. *Diabetes Care, 15,* 1356–1360.

Pike, K. M. (1989). *Family, peer, and personality variables associated with disordered eating in high school girls.* Unpublished manuscript.

Pike, K. M., & Rodin, J. (1991). Mothers, daughters, and disordered eating. *Journal of Abnormal Psychology, 100,* 198–204.

Polivy, J. M., & Herman, C. P. (1985). Dieting and binging: A causal analysis. *American Psychologist, 40,* 193–201.

Polivy, J., & Herman, C. P. (1993). Etiology of binge eating: Psychological mechanisms. In C. G. Fairburn & G. T. Wilson (Eds.), *Binge eating: Nature, assessment, and treatment.* New York: Guilford Press.

Pomeroy, C., & Mitchell, J. (1989). Medical complications and management of eating disorders. *Psychiatric Annals, 19,* 488–493.

Powers, P. S., Coovert, D. L., Brightwell, D. R., & Stevens, B. A. (1988). Other psychiatric disorders among bulimic patients. *Comprehensive Psychiatry, 29,* 503–508.

Prather, R. C., & Williamson, D. A. (1988). Psychopathology associated with bulimia, binge eating, and obesity. *International Journal of Eating Disorders, 7,* 177–184.

Rand, C. S. W., & Kuldau, J. M. (1986). Eating patterns in normal weight individuals: bulimia, restrained eating, and the night eating syndrome. *International Journal of Eating Disorders, 5,* 75–84.

Rodin, J., Silberstein, L. R., & Striegel-Moore, R. H. (1985). Women and weight: A normative discontent. In T. B. Sonderegger (Ed.), *Nebraska Symposium on Motivation* (pp. 267–308). Lincoln: University of Nebraska Press.

Rosen, J. C., Vara, L., Wendt, S., & Leitenberg, H. (1990). Validity studies of the Eating Disorder Examination. *International Journal of Eating Disorders, 9,* 519–528.

Rosenberg, M. (1979). *Conceiving the self.* New York: Basic Books.

Rossiter, E. M., & Agras, W. S. (1988). An empirical test of DSM-III–R definition of binge. *International Journal of Eating Disorders, 9,* 513–518.

Rossiter, E. M., Agras, W. S., & Losch, M. (1988). Changes in self–report food intake in bulimics as a consequence of antidepressant treatment. *International Journal of Eating Disorders, 7,* 779–783.

Rossiter, E. M., Agras, W. S., Losch, M., & Telch, C. (1988). Dietary restraint of bulimic subjects following cognitive–behavioral or pharmacological treatment. *Behavioral Research and Therapy, 26,* 495–498.

Rossiter, E. M., Agras, W. S., Telch, C. F., & Schneider, J. A. (1993). Cluster B personality disorder characteristics predict outcome in the treatment of bulimia nervosa. *International Journal of Eating Disorders, 13,* 349–357.

Ruderman, A. J. (1985). Dysphoric mood and overeating: A test of restraint theory's disinhibition hypothesis. *Journal of Abnormal Psychology, 9A,* 78–85.

Russell, G. (1979). Bulimia nervosa: An ominous variant of anorexia nervosa. *Psychological Medicine*, 9, 429–448.

Schotte, D. E., & Stunkard, A.J. (1987). Bulimia vs bulimic behaviors on a college campus. *Journal of Amercan Medical Association*, 258, 1213–1215.

Schwalberg, M. D. (1990). *A comparison of bulimics, obese binge eaters, social phobics, and individuals with panic disorder on anxiety, depression, chemical abuse, and borderline personality disorder.* Unpublished doctoral dissertation.

Schwalberg, M. D., Barlow, D. H., Alger, S. A., & Howard, L. J. (1992). Comparison of bulimics, obese binge eaters, social phobics, and individuals with panic disorder on comorbidity across DSM-III-R anxiety disorders. *Journal of Abnormal Psychology*, 101, 675–681.

Silberstein, L. R., Striegel–Moore, R. H., & Rodin, J. (1987). Feeling fat: A woman's shame. In H. B. Lewis (Ed.), *The role of shame in symptom formation* (pp. 89–108). Hillsdale, NJ: Erlbaum.

Sjostrom, L. V. (1992a). Morbidity of severely obese subjects. *American Journal of Clinical Nutrition*, 55, 508S–515S.

Sjostrom, L. V. (1992b). Mortality of severely obese subjects. *American Journal of Clinical Nutrition*, 55, 516S–523S.

Smith, D. E., Marcus, D. E., & Kaye, W. (1992). Cognitive behavioral treatment of obese binge eaters. *International Journal of Eating Disorders*, 12, 257–262.

Spiegel, D., Bloom, J. R., Kraemer, H. C., & Gottheil, E. (1989). The beneficial effect of psychosocial treatment on survival of metastatic breast cancer patients: A randomized prospective outcome study. *Lancet*, 12, 888–891.

Spira, J. L. , & Spiegel, D. (1993). Group psychotherapy for the medically ill. In A. Stoudemire & B. Fogel (Eds.), *Principles of medical psychiatry.* New York: American Psychiatric Press.

Spitzer, R. L., Devlin, M., Walsh, B. T., Hasin, D., Wing, R., Marcus, M. D., Stunkard, A. J., Wadden, T., Yanovski, S., Agras, W. S., Mitchell, J., & Nonas, C. (1991). Binge eating disorder: To be or not to be in DSM-IV. *International Journal of Eating Disorders*, 10, 627–629.

Spitzer, R. L., Devlin, M. J., Walsh, B. T., Hasin, D., Wing, R. R., Marcus, M. D., Stunkard, A., Wadden, T. A., Yanovski, S., Agras, W. S., Mitchell, J., & Nonas, C. (1992). Binge eating disorder: A multisite field trial for the diagnostic criteria. *International Journal of Eating Disorders*, 11, 191–203.

Spitzer, R. L., Williams, J. B. W., & Gibbon, M. (1987). *Structured Clinical Interview of DSM-III-R—Patient version (SCID-P).* New York: Biometrics Research Department, New York State Psychiatric Institute.

Spitzer, R. L., Yanovski, S., Wadden, T., Wing, R., Marcus, M. D., Stunkard, A., Devlin, M., Mitchell, J., & Hasin, D. (1993). Binge eating disorder: Its further validation in a multisite trial. *International Journal of Eating Disorders*, 12, 137–153.

Spurrell, E. B., Wilfley, D. E., Tanofsky, M. B., & Brownell, K. B. (in press). Age of onset for binge eating: Are there different pathways to binge eating? *International Journal of Eating Disorders*.

Striegel-Moore, R. H. (1993). Etiology of binge eating: A developmental perspective. In: C. G. Fairburn & G. T. Wilson (Eds.), *Binge eating: Nature, assessment and treatment* (pp. 144–172). New York: Guilford Press.

Striegel-Moore, R. H., Silberstein, L. R., & Rodin, J. (1986). Toward an understanding of risk factors for bulimia. *American Psychologist, 41*, 246–263.

Striegel–Moore, R. H., Silberstein, L. R., & Rodin, J. (1993). The social self in bulimia nervosa: Public self-consciousness, social anxiety, and perceived fraudulence. *Journal of Abnormal Psychology, 102*, 297-303.

Strober, M., & Humphrey, L. L. (1987). Familial contributions to the etiology and course of anorexia nervosa and bulimia. *Journal of Consulting and Clinical Psychology, 55*, 654–659.

Strober, M., & Katz, J. (1987) Do eating disorders and affective disorder share a common etiology? A dissenting opinion. *International Journal of Eating Disorders, 6*, 171–180.

Stunkard, A. J. (1959). Eating patterns and obesity. *Psychiatric Quarterly, 33*, 284–295.

Stunkard, A. J., & Messick, S. (1985). The three-factor eating questionnaire to measure dietary restraint, disinhibition and hunger. *Journal of Psychosomatic Research, 29*, 71–83.

Stunkard, A. J., & Wadden, T. A. (1992). Psychological aspects of severe obesity. *American Journal of Clinical Nutrition, 55*, 524S–532S.

Telch, C. F., & Agras, W. S. (1992). *Group cognitive-behavioral therapy for Binge Eating Disorder: Therapist manual.* Unpublished manuscript, Stanford University.

Telch, C. F., & Agras, W. S. (1993). The affects of a very low calorie diet on binge eating. *Behavior Therapy, 24*, 177–193.

Telch, C. F., & Agras, W. S. (1994). Obesity, binge eating, and psychopathology: Are they related? *International Journal of Eating disorders, 15*, 53–61.

Telch, C. F., Agras, W. S., & Rossiter, E. M. (1988). Binge eating increases with increasing adiposity. *International Journal of Eating Disorders, 7*, 115–119.

Telch, C. F., Agras, W. S., Rossiter, E. M., Wilfley, D., & Kenardy, J. (1990). Group cognitive-behavioral treatment for the nonpurging bulimic: An initial evaluation. *Journal of Consulting and Clinical Psychology, 58*, 629–635.

Thelen, M.H., Farmer, J., Wonderlich, S., & Smith, M. (1991). A revision of the bulimia test: The BULIT–R. *Psychological Assessment, 3*, 119–124.

Thompson, J. K. (Ed.). (1996). *Body image, eating disorders, and obesity: An integrative guide for assessment and treatment.* Washington, DC: American Psychological Association.

Thoresen, C. E., Friedman, M., Powell, L., Gill, J., & Ulmer, D. (1985). Altering the Type-A behavior pattern in postinfarction patients. *Journal of Cardiopulmonary Rehabilitation, 5*, 258–266.

Van Buren, D. J., & Williamson, D. A. (1988). Marital relationships and conflict resolution skills of bulimics. *International Journal of Eating Disorders, 7*, 735–741.

Vinogradov, S., & Yalom, I. D. (1989). *A concise guide to group psychotherapy.* New York: American Psychiatric Press.

Wadden, T. A., Foster, G. D., Letizia, K. A., & Wilk, J. E. (1993). Metabolic, anthropometric, and psychological characteristics of obese binge eater. *International Journal of Eating Disorders, 14*, 17–25.

Wadden, T. A., & Stunkard, A. J. (1985). The psychological and social complications of obesity. *Annals of Internal Medicine, 103*, 1062-1067.

Walsh, B. T., Hadigan, C. M., Devlin, M. J., Gladis, M., & Roose, S. P. (1991). Long–term outcome of antidepressant treatment for bulimia nervosa. *American Journal of Psychiatry, 148,* 1206–1212.

Weissman, M. M., & Bothwell, S. (1976). Assessment of social adjustment by patient self–report. *Archives of General Psychiatry, 33,* 1111–1115.

Weltzin, T. E., Fernstrom, M. H., Hansen, D., McConaha, C., & Kaye, W. H. (1991). Abnormal caloric requirements for weight maintenance in patients with anorexia and bulimia nervosa. *American Journal of Psychiatry, 148,* 1675–1682.

Wilfley, D. E. (1989). *Interpersonal analyses of bulimia: Normal-weight and obese.* Unpublished doctoral dissertation.

Wilfley, D. E., Agras, W. S., Telch, C. F., Rossiter, E. M., Schneider, J. A., Cole, A. G., Sifford, L., & Raeburn, S. D. (1993). Group cognitive-behavioral therapy and group interpersonal psychotherapy for the nonpurging bulimic: A controlled comparison. *Journal of Consulting and Clinical Psychology, 61,* 296–305.

Wilfley, D. E., Frank, M. A., Welch, R. R., Spurrell, E. B., & Rounsaville, B. J. (in press). Adapting interpersonal pyschotherapy to a group format (IPT-G) for binge eating disorder: A Model for adapting empirically validated treatments. *Psychotherapy Research.*

Wilfley, D. E., Kunce, J. T., & Welch, R. R. (1992). Psychological and interpersonal profiles of normal-weight and obese bulimic women in comparison to non-binge-eating normal-weight and obese women. Unpublished manuscript.

Wilson, G. T. (1984). Clinical issues and strategies in the practice of behavior therapy. In G.T. Wilson, C. M. Franks, K. D. Brownell, & P. C. Kendall (Eds.), *Annual review of behavior therapy: Theory and practice* (pp. 288–317). New York: Guilford Press.

Wilson, G. T. (1993). Binge eating and addictive disorders. In C.G. Fairburn & G.T. Wilson (Eds.), *Binge eating: Nature, assessment, and treatment* (pp. 97–120). New York: Guilford Press.

Wilson, G. T. (1996). Treatment of bulimia nervosa: When CBT fails. *Behaviour Research and Therapy, 34,* 197–212.

Wilson, G. T. (in press). Acceptance and change in the treatment of eating disorders and obesity. *Behavior Therapy.*

Wilson, G. T., & Fairburn, C. G. (1993). Cognitive treatments for eating disorders. *Journal of Consulting and Clinical Psychology, 61,* 261–269.

Wilson, G. T., Nonas, C. A., & Rosenblum, G. D. (1993). Assessment of binge-eating in obese patients. *International Journal of Eating Disorders, 13,* 23–33.

Wilson, G. T., & Pike, K. M. (1993). Eating disorders. In D. H. Barlow (Ed.), *Clinical handbook of psychological disorders* (2nd ed.). New York: Guilford Press.

Wilson, G. T., & Smith, D. (1989). Assessment of bulimia nervosa: An evaluation of the Eating Disorder Examination. *International Journal of Eating Disorders, 8,* 173–179.

Wilson, G. T., & Walsh, B. T. (1991). Eating disorders in the DSM-IV. *Journal of Abnormal Psychology, 100,* 362–365.

Wing, R. R. (1992). Weight cycling in humans: A review of the literature. *Annals of Internal Medicine, 14,* 113–119.

Yalom, I. D. (1985). *The theory and practice of group psychotherapy* (3rd ed.). New York: Basic Books.

Yanovski, S. Z. (1993). Binge eating disorder: Current knowledge and future directions. *Obesity Research, 1,* 305–324.

Yanovski, S. Z., Nelson, J. E., Dubbert, B. K., & Spitzer, R. L. (1993). Binge eating is associated with psychiatric co-morbidity in the obese. *American Journal of Psychiatry, 150,* 1472–1479.

Young, J. E., & Beck, A. T. (1982). Cognitive therapy: Clinical applications. In A. J. Rush (Ed.), *Short-term psychotherapies for depression: Behavioral, interpersonal, cognitive, psychodynamic* (pp. 182–214). New York: Guilford Press.

Zotter, D. L., & Crowther, J. H. (1991). The role of cognitions in bulimia nervosa. *Cognitive Therapy and Research, 15,* 413–426.

CHAPTER 7

Interactive Group Therapy for Substance Abusers

ROBERT A. MATANO
IRVIN D. YALOM
KIM SCHWARTZ

Substance abuse in the United States has continued unabated through the last several decades, giving rise to a host of political, social, and health problems (Winick, 1992). The abuse of drugs and alcohol affects every sector of the population, regardless of race, gender, age, income, or educational level. Although drug an alcohol abuse exist throughout the world, the use of mood-modifying substances in the United States is higher than in any other industrialized country (Winick, 1992).

Reports of the extent to which Americans use drugs vary widely. Research conducted by the National Institute on Drug Abuse (NIDA) and the National Institute of Mental Health (NIMH) report that substance abuse effects approximately 6% of the population (Reiger et al., 1984). Other epidemiological surveys place this figure much higher. NIDA indicates that 14.5 million Americans had used marijuana, cocaine, or another illicit drug within the 30 days preceding the interview. Of these, 8 million persons had used cocaine in the last month (NIDA, 1990). Although alcohol consumption in the United States has been declining since 1981, there are still approximately 19 million individuals exhibiting dependence and loss of control, features contributing to the definition of an alcohol (Clark & Midanik, 1982; Reiger et al., 1984).

Epidemiological studies offer a demographic perspective of the abusing population. Gender makes a difference, with males using more drugs, especially, cigarettes, alcohol, marijuana, and cocaine (Winick, 1992). The elderly are unequivocally the largest users of legal drugs in the United States, and this trend is expected to continue to grow (Widner & Zeichner, 1991). Not only do elderly users have a propensity to use multiple drugs, but their sensitivity to drug toxicity is especially high, thus accentuating the problem. There is an alarmingly high rate of substance abuse among the poor, especially within the homeless population. Studies conducted in several cities indicate that nearly 30% of the homeless population have alcohol problems, and as many as 40% may have problems with other drugs (Ropers & Boyer, 1987).

Ethnic background also is a risk factor. According to Weissman et al. (1980), the NIMH multisite study found lifetime prevalence rates for alcoholism to be nearly 20% for nonwhites compared to 5% for whites. Alcohol abuse has been found to be consistently higher for men in all Hispanic groups except Cuban-Americans (Lex, 1987). Alcohol-related arrests and mortality are also greater among Hispanics than in the general adult population (Winick, 1992). The proportion of drinkers among adult Native Americans is about the same as the general population, with the exception of Native American youth. Native American youths use more marijuana and other inhalants than youths in any other ethnic background (Winick, 1992). Drug use, other than alcohol, occurs in African Americans at a rate similar to the general population. However, African Americans tend to use alcohol at greater rates than the general population.

EFFECT ON HEALTH

Alcohol and drug abuse lead to numerous psychological and physiological dysfunctions. Ross, Glaser, and Germanson (1988) found that nearly 50% of 501 male and female Canadians seeking treatment at an alcohol and drug treatment facility met the criteria for a lifetime psychiatric disorder as well as a substance abuse disorder. A study of 133 narcotic users concluded that more than 75% met an Axis I diagnosis according to the *Diagnostic and Statistical Manual of Mental Disorders*, third edition, revised (American Psychiatric Association, 1987). Moreover, 93% of the subjects met the criteria for either an Axis I or an Axis II diagnosis, and nearly 50% had diagnosis on both axes (Khantzian & Treece, 1985).

Although these rates appear to be very high, one should keep in mind the extraordinary complexity surrounding the diagnosis of a psychiatric disorder in a substance abuser (Weissman & Myers, 1980). Clinicians attempting to diagnose depression in substance abusers are confronted with an especially difficult task. For instance, various studies have reported a prevalence rate of depression in alcoholics ranging from 3% to nearly 100%. This enormous disparity among researchers may be caused by several factors, including widely varying definitions of depression and the use of different diagnostic assessments (Weiss & Mirin, 1989; Weissman & Myers, 1980). Further, the causal relationship between psychiatric disorders and substance abuse is unclear. Determining whether psychiatric disorders lead to or result from substance abuse may need to be taken into account in the overall management of the patient (Ross et al., 1988). Moreover, with detoxification and continued abstinence, psychiatric disorders may tend to dissipate for some individuals.

Alcohol and drug abuse frequently result in medical complications and are highly correlated with excess mortality (Romelsjo, 1993; Ashley, 1989). For instance, a Norweigan study concluded that the increase in alcohol consumption has produced a substantial increase in mortality rates from a specific group of diseases. However, the effects on general mortality for other diseases are less clear (Skog, 1987). It is also well-known that cessation of such abuse can improve both health and survival.

One problem with assessment of comorbid conditions concomitant with substance abuse is that physicians frequently fail to interview patients regarding their substance use. In one hospital study examining intervention for alcoholism, only 58% of patients with at least one alcohol-related illness were asked about their consumption of alcohol (Mehler, McClellan, Lezotte, Casper, & Gabrow, 1995). Almost twice as many alcohol-related illnesses were found in those asked about their drinking than in those who were not asked. Promotion of physician awareness was found to be among the major factors determining whether patients were asked about their substance use.

Heart disease has been found to be the leading cause of death among male alcoholics, with traumatic injury second and liver cirrhosis third (Schmidt & Popham, 1981). Liver damage is an inevitable result of heavy drinking, often resulting in serious illness or death if left untreated or if drinking continues. However, it is often reversable with the cessation of alcohol ingestion.

Several studies have set out to determine the correlation between alcohol consumption and cancer. According to Tuyns (1979), epidemiological studies indicate that alcohol consumption is a cancer hazard. Cancer rates are higher among alcoholics than in the general population. In addition, several behaviors common among alcoholics, such as smoking, contribute to this population's elevated risk in cancer (Blott et al., 1988).

Pregnant women who abuse drugs and alcohol are afflicting both their own life and the future life of their unborn babies. A substance-abusing mother is creating an extremely tenuous environment for the developing fetus. Neurological damage that was suffered in the womb, as a result of the substance abuse, can be permanent and devastating (Chasnoff, 1989). More than 15% of newborn infants born in certain regions of the country already have cocaine in their system (Bateman & Heagarty, 1992).

Intravenous (IV) drug use is the second most common risk behavior among cases of acquired immune deficiency syndrome (AIDS) in the United States and Europe. AIDS case statistics show that IV drug use is associated with a substantial and growing percentage of AIDS cases in many countries. Mortality rates among drug users has increased drastically as a result of this disease (Des Jarlais, Friedman, Woods, & Milliken, 1992).

INTERVENTION

The past decade has seen a major expansion in the treatment of addictive disorders. It is estimated that more than $2 billion per year is spent on alcohol and drug inpatient and outpatient treatment programs (Frances, 1988). Programs have proven to be effective not only in reducing addiction (U.S. Preventive Services Task Force, 1989) but also in reducing concomitant illnesses. In a long-term study of 3,729 persons with alcoholism, health care costs after treatment (including the cost of treatment) declined by up to 55% of pretreatment levels, while health care costs for a matched group of untreated alcoholics increased by 202% (Genetello, Donovan, Dunn, & Rivara, 1995).

Intervention programs may use therapies ranging from pharmocotherapies to behavioral approaches either singly or in combination. Pharmacotherapies are often the initial treatment of choice for persons addicted to certain substance. For instance, opiate antagonists, partial agonists, and mixed agonist/antagonists are the substances used in treating the opiate abuser. Opiate receptor sites are occupied by the antagonist, such that the effects of agonists at the cellular level are blocked, helping to keep addicts from relapsing (Jaffe, 1992). Of considerable recent interest in the treatment of alcoholism has been the trial of naltrexone—an opiate antagonist—as a pharmacological adjunct. Several studies have demonstrated significant reductions in the number and intensity of relapses in those patients taking naltrexone as an adjunct to their treatment (Volpicelli, Alterman, Hayashida, & O'Brien, 1992; O'Malley et al., 1992).

An appropriate psychosocial treatment is clearly one of the most widely employed and effective aspects of a substance abuser's path to recovery (Daley & Raskin, 1991; Brown, 1995; Genetello et al., 1995). An alcoholic is likely to experience some type of relapse during his or her recovery process. However, several factors play an integral role in facilitating the recovery process, including a satisfactory living environment, a stable work situation, and compliance with follow-up treatment, all of which are highly correlated with successful recovery (Svanum & McAdoo, 1989).

Common treatment options for the substance abuser include the following:

1. Therapeutic communities.
2. Multimodal rehabilitation programs.
3. Alcoholics anonymous.
4. Individual psychotherapy.
5. Structured outpatient group therapy.
6. Family therapy.
7. Methadone maintenance and pharmacotherapies.

The therapeutic community is established as having a firm and unique position among the array of drug treatment modalities. Therapeutic communities are characterized by the following basic standards: drug-free supervised abstinence, emphasis on peer self-help model, active participation of residents, role modeling accountability and socially responsible behavior, and feedback and confrontation of behavior (O'Brien & Biase, 1992).

The rehabilitation model was developed in Minnesota approximately 40 years ago with the primary intention of treating alcoholics. Over the past four decades the emphasis has changed to treating substance abusers, regardless of their drug of choice. Rehabilitation programs utilize five key ingredients:

1. Psychological testing and evaluation.
2. Strong group support orientation.
3. Skilled substance abuse counselors as primary therapists.
4. Medical and psychiatric support for coexisting problems.
5. Therapists trained in systemized methods of treatment (Geller, 1992).

Alcoholics Anonymous (AA) has universally influenced the treatment of alcoholism. A recovery from alcoholism is achieved through various types of meetings employing psychosocial support. It would be difficult today to find a substance abuse treatment program that does not espouse the principles of AA (Nace, 1992). The primary purpose of AA members is to stay sober and help other alcoholics achieve sobriety through the philosophy that AA is a fellowship of men and women who share a common experience, strength, and hope to solve their common problem. Participants of AA are guided by the "Twelve Steps" and the "Serenity Prayer," which offer the alcoholic a satisfying way of life without alcohol. The Twelve Steps and the Serenity Prayer are as follows[1]:

[1]The Twelve Steps are reprinted with permission of Alcoholics Anonymous World Services, Inc. Anonymous World Services, Inc. Permission to reprint the Twelve Steps does not mean that AA has reviewed or approved the contents of this publication, nor that AA agrees with the views expressed herein. AA is a program of recovery from alcoholism *only*—use of the Twelve Steps in connection with programs and activities which are patterned after AA, but which address other problems, or in any other non-AA context, does not imply otherwise.

1. We admitted that we were powerless over alcohol—that our lives had become unmanageable.
2. Came to believe that a Power greater than ourselves could restore us to sanity.
3. Made a decision to turn our will and our lives over to the care of God *as we understood Him.*
4. Made a searching and fearless moral inventory of ourselves.
5. Admitted to God, to ourselves, and to another human being the exact nature of our wrongs.
6. Were entirely ready to have God remove all these defects of character.
7. Humbly asked Him to remove our shortcomings.
8. Made a list of all persons we had harmed and became willing to make amends to them all.
9. Made direct amends to such people wherever possible, except when to do so would injure them or others.
10. Continued to take personal inventory and when we were wrong promptly admitted it.
11. Sought through prayer and meditation to improve our conscious contact with God, *as we understood Him,* praying only for knowledge of His will for us and the power to carry that out.
12. Having had a spiritual awakening as a result of these steps, we tried to carry this message to alcoholics and to practice these principles in all our affairs.

The AA Serenity Prayer in many ways encapsulates these steps: "God grant me the serenity to accept the things I cannot change, courage to change the things we can and the wisdom to know the difference."

Cocaine Anonymous (CA) and Narcotics Anonymous (NA) have emerged as a result of AA's enormous effectiveness, utilizing the same format. CA and NA members also employ the sense of "powerlessness" over their abusing chemical and become submissive to a "power greater than ourselves." AA (1976) claims that cocaine addicts have consistently been able to reduce their feelings of inferiority and isolation and, hence, remain abstinent. However, the AA format is not without controversy. Adversaries to the Twelve Step program emphasize the level of dependency that the addict assumes with the program as being unhealthy and a substitute for the drug dependency. Therefore, educating the drug abuser with the process of recovery may need to be stressed (Millman, 1986).

The family of the drug-dependent individual has recently received a great deal of attention, with increased focus on therapy including the family. Some researchers contend that family therapy with substance abusers has been the most successful of approaches studied in the past decade (Kaufman, 1986). At the very least, the social context within which a drug abuser lives must be considered an integral part of the problem as well as the solution.

Substance abusers' reactions to treatment depend on several factors. According to Watson, Brown, Tilleskjor, Jacobs, and Pucel (1988), alcoholics who were coerced into treatment had a lower rate of recovery than alcoholics who entered willingly. Jarvis (1992) found that female alcoholics had better outcomes in programs that focused on the medical and educational aspects of recovery and emphasized moderation of usage. Male alcoholics responded better to inpatient treatment programs that emphasized a group or "peer" orientation. Possibly, the fear of stigmatization make women more receptive to nongroup treatments. However, both men and women tended to do better when more females were present in their treatment groups. Although women were able to be more self-revealing with an all-female treatment group, men also discussed their feelings more frequently with the increase of female group members. Clearly, the interactive nature of group therapy is beneficial in recovery from substance abuse. The remaining portion of this chapter focuses on the principles and practice of interactive group therapy for substance abusers.

GROUP THERAPY INTERVENTIONS [2]

Group therapy has in recent years become the treatment of choice for chemical dependency. This preference is, no doubt, because of the influence of AA, which demonstrated the power of groups—the power to counter prevailing cultural pressures to drink, to provide effective support to those suffering from the alienation of addiction, to offer role modeling, and to harness the power of peer pressure—an important force against denial and resistance.

Groups are used for alcoholic patients in nearly all the therapeutic contexts, including acute-care inpatient units and outpatient settings. The models for conducting these groups vary widely, ranging from social skills training to cognitive-behavioral models.

Despite this widespread use, most contemporary group therapy with alcoholics fails to take advantage of a very powerful therapeutic element: the interactive group process. This chapter focuses on methods for adapting interactive group therapy to the unique needs of the chemically dependent.

Interactive Group Therapy

The primary feature distinguishing the interactive method from other types of group therapy is its focus on the interpersonal realm. Based on the funda-

---

[2]This section is adapted from Matano and Yalom (1991). Copyright 1991 by the American Group Psychotherapy Association, Inc. Adapted by permission.

mental assumptions that interpersonal relationships play a crucial role in the development of the individual and that maladaptive interpersonal patterns result in psychiatric symptomology, the interactive group process focuses on the dynamic interplay of individuals within the "here and now" of the group meeting. Interpersonal learning—insight that results from the examination of this dynamic interaction—is considered a primary vehicle of therapeutic change (Yalom, 1985).

The process of interpersonal learning in interactive group therapy rests on two basic factors: (1) the importance of interpersonal relationships as manifested in the here and now and (2) a view of the group as a social microcosm.

The interactional approach calls for primary attention to the here and now, on the transactions occurring in the immediate present in the course of the group meeting. This is basically an ahistoric approach, yet it should not be seen as a denial of the importance of each person's past history or of the importance of relationships outside the group. Focusing on the immediate interpersonal events within the group is simply a way of maximizing the effectiveness of therapy.

The effective use of the here and now occurs in two stages. First, the group must plunge into its own interaction. Second, the group has to step outside itself and begin to understand what has just transpired. This means that the therapist has two different functions, each requiring a different set of techniques. For the first function, the therapist requires *activating* techniques to plunge the group into its own interaction, that is, to help group members take risks, express feelings, disclose fears, and become fully engaged with one another. For the second function, the therapist requires a set of *clarifying and interpretive techniques* to help group members make sense of what has just transpired and ultimately develop a cognitive map to guide them in future interpersonal situations.

An interactive approach assumes that patients will, sooner or later, within the group, tend to display the same maladaptive thoughts and behaviors they exhibit outside therapy. Thus, the group develops into a social microcosm in which individual pathology is reproduced and is clearly observable in the here-and-now interactions among group members. Through the reactions and feedback of other group members, patients become acutely aware of the their maladaptive behavior and alternate approaches within the safe confines of the psychotherapy group.

TRADITIONAL APPROACHES TO
CHEMICAL DEPENDENCY TREATMENT

Although interactional groups have been successful in treating a wide variety of psychological symptoms, traditional group treatments for chemical dependency generally have not incorporated an interactional focus into their therapeutic orientation. The most likely explanation for this omission is that most chemical dependency treatments are based on the disease model, which views substance addiction as an incurable, progressive, life-threatening illness in which an individual loses control over the ability to regulate use. The disease model holds that the key etiological determinants of addictions are genetic and physiological factors for which the addict is not motivationally responsible. Moreover, the addict's psychological and interpersonal problems are usually viewed as a consequence, not the cause, of the chemical dependency. According to this view, the interpersonal problems of an addict will for the most part resolve spontaneously following sobriety.

Treating interpersonal problems is, therefore, not considered a central component of existing models of group therapy for the chemically dependent. Rather, the emphasis is on maintaining abstinence through behavioral and cognitive change. The first step in the recovery process is clearly the elimination of drinking behavior. Attention is also given to the development of social networks supportive of sobriety. From a cognitive point of view, the desired goal is to alter beliefs about drug use, to help the patient become more aware of behavioral antecedents of relapse, and to develop strategies that will aid in the recovery process.

These goals are addressed therapeutically by providing a highly structured group atmosphere in which any potential threat to sobriety, including anxiety and conflict, is avoided. Patients are encouraged by the therapist, and through peer pressure, to subscribe unconditionally to group beliefs about the disease concept of addiction, the individual's inability to control drinking, and the cognitive and behavioral process of recovery. Therapists promote this view with an authoritative, confrontational stance: They stress identification as an addict, deemphasize differences among patients, and posit abstinence as the primary topic of discussion.

Limitations of Traditional Treatments

Although the disease model is extremely useful in explaining the physiological aspects of addiction, many clinicians and researchers acknowledge its limitations in explaining the psychological and social experience of the addict (Pattison & Kaupman, 1982). Recently, efforts have been made to expand the disease-based model of addiction to include cultural, familial, and psychological variables (Levin, 1990). There is growing recognition that many addicts continue to suffer from a variety of interpersonal and psychological problems following sobriety—problems that, left unchecked, can contribute to relapse. In some cases, these difficulties precede substance abuse, but even those addicts who appeared, prior to addiction, to have relatively intact psychological makeup and social-support systems cannot assume that these assets will easily reemerge following sobriety. Their behavior while using drugs or alcohol is likely to have significantly damaged their interpersonal relationships, self-esteem, and ability to rebuild friendships and family ties. These developments in turn can lead to such persisting feelings of alienation and despondency that successful recovery is unlikely.

INTEGRATING AN INTERACTIONAL APPROACH WITH A TRADITIONAL CHEMICAL DEPENDENCY APPROACH

Traditional chemical dependency approaches and interactive group therapy represent very different conceptions of chemical dependency. The disease concept stresses the physiological and genetic variables; the interactive process stresses the role of interpersonal relationships in the genesis and perpetuation of addiction. Our view is that both models have validity and, in practice, may enrich and complement one another. The challenge in integrating and applying these models in clinical practice lies in knowing when to emphasize which approach.

Five principles provide guidelines for the clinician attempting to integrate the two approaches: (1) priority of recovery, (2) identification as an alcoholic/addict, (3) careful modulation of anxiety levels, (4) a therapeutic approach to responsibility, and (5) modification of the group process to incorporate into therapy the language and belief systems of AA.

Priority of Recovery

Patients in the earliest stages of recovery often lack the ability to cope with even low levels of anxiety or frustration. To end this, treatment in the earliest phase of recovery must provide needed support and alleviate dysphoria: all available resources must be channeled into sobriety. Nothing takes precedence over recovery—it is a life-or-death issue.

This priority raises a potential challenge to integrating an interactive approach. The process of resolving maladaptive patterns of interpersonal relationships does not seem to the alcoholic patient relevant to effecting abstinence. Although patients may understand on some level that this more indirect approach ultimately leads to a lasting foundation for future sobriety, they are unlikely to grasp its immediate importance for recovery. Further, there is a strong behavioral emphasis in early recovery (the AA slogan, "Don't analyze, utilize"). This emphasis is often necessary to combat the addict's defenses of intellectualization—rationalizing, minimizing, and generalizing to deny the consequences of addiction. Unfortunately, patients often interpret this emphasis to mean that they should engage in no form of insight-oriented therapy.

In our interactional groups we support the absolute priority of recovery and suspend the analysis of the interpersonal realm long enough for sober supports to consolidate and behavioral change to become entrenched. Without such supports, the interactive focus in the group may raise anxiety levels and possibly induce a relapse.

However, even in this earliest stage of recovery, an interpersonal approach may facilitate the achievement of sobriety. For example, abrasive and distrustful interpersonal relationships with others threaten recovery by impeding the development of the supportive network so necessary for sobriety. In these instances it is absolutely necessary for the leaders to explore interpersonal issues that interfere with the patient establishing the group as a supportive network. Thus, we might address the patient's abrasiveness, expectation of negative judgments from others, or projected self-hatred. The interpersonal approach at this point must be gentle, supportive, and directly supportive of sobriety.

When it becomes evident that a group member is in danger of relapse and demonstrates reckless or "slippery" behaviors, attention should shift from the interpersonal focus to refortifying the patient's basic behavioral and social supports. Thus, the therapist must analyze interpersonal dynamics in the group while maintaining a vigilant eye for threats to the recovery process. In fact, changes in the interpersonal style of group members can often be the first signal of impending relapse, as the following example illustrates:

A typically serious college professor came to group one day in an unusually rebellious mood and lamented the flaws of therapists and the entire psychotherapy enterprise. Normally somewhat deferential to the leader, on this occasion the patient immediately challenged all the leader's interventions. Alarmed by this behavior, the leader did not attempt to explore the interaction between the patient and himself but rather asked the patient if he had been drinking. Other group members, also noticing the patient's unusual bravado, followed the leader's approach and confronted the patient, citing the change in his interactive style as evidence of relapse. The group member finally admitted to drinking, and the group then focused on whether it provided enough support for this member. The other group members soon decided that he needed more structure and recommended that he leave the group to receive intensive inpatient care.

As soon as this was accomplished, the remaining group members explored this event. They discovered that many group members sensed that the patient had been drinking for quite some time, but they were reluctant to comment upon it. Group discussion focused on their reluctance and their reliance on the group leader to confront the patient. This then led to a productive exploration of the members' urges to drink, their dependency, and their shifting the entire responsibility for therapy to the therapist.

Identification as Alcoholic/Addict

Traditional approaches to chemical dependency always require group members to identify themselves as alcoholics/addicts. There are two compelling reasons. One is to break down the denial commonly seen in addiction which so often acts as a resistance to therapy. Another is to encourage a sense of common purpose among members.

Identification as an alcoholic has a number of implications in interactive group therapy. A continual tension exists in groups between uniformity and differentiation. An emphasis on sameness among the members increases cohesion, trust, safety, and the belief that others can help. These feelings can be vitally important to members in early recovery who generally experience profound isolation, distrust, and shame. Although members of the group are encouraged to identify with one another in one very important respect—their addiction—they are also clearly different in many other aspects. Ultimately, differentiation is necessary for growth though it may decrease the feeling of connectedness and produce anxiety for some.

Even during the early phases, an interactional approach can enrich the group sessions. For example, in an interpersonal context, group members can explore the problems that they experience in admitting or accepting their addiction. Leaders may inquire: What does it mean to admit that one is similar to others? What does it mean to admit vulnerability? To ask for help? To acknowledge helplessness?

Many alcoholics familiar with self-help groups find even this process of discussing their similarities with other group members somewhat strange. "Cross-talk"—or talking about how one feels about another—is discouraged in AA meetings. Nonetheless, asking members to identify themselves as alcoholics and encouraging them to explore their similarities to others may reinforce the process of recovery, as this clinical example reveals:

> A young physician who joined an ongoing group immediately differentiated herself from other members. She felt the group was too intellectualized, that members were "conning" each other, and, in a condescending manner, she expressed disbelief that members with years of sobriety were still struggling with issues of who they were. It was clear to the members that she believed her identity as a physician made her better than others in the group. The leaders began by asking whether she was an alcoholic. She replied that it was hard to accept this definition of herself. She felt that identifying herself both as a physician and as an alcoholic presented an essential conflict. She was then asked whether she felt like anyone else in the group. Initially, she identified with another group member, who also rebelled against accepting this label and, later, the "stronger" group members, who did not reveal weaknesses. She was unable to accept her identity as an alcoholic until the focus turned to her need to be perfect, which made it difficult

for her to express any limitation or vulnerability. Only after these interpersonal aspects were explicitly addressed could this woman be a fully participating member of the group.

Modulating Anxiety Levels

People always experience anxiety in the process of personal growth. However, many alcoholics may have a low tolerance for anxiety and attempt to handle it by acting out, especially through drinking. Therefore, the modulation of the level of anxiety is vital to the success of the recovery group. The group therapist needs to make certain that anxiety levels do not overwhelm the members' coping resources.

Therapy group members are often asked to engage in activities that temporarily extend them beyond their personal comfort zone. Anxiety typically accompanies many necessary group activities: self-disclosure, receiving feedback about blindspots, expressing feelings, experiencing conflict or intimacy.

The alcoholic brings other specific sources of anxiety into the group setting. First, many alcoholics are fearful of therapy: They are grateful to AA and believe AA to be hostile to therapy, and they may have heard of the failures or even dangers of psychotherapy. The relatively fluid structure of the interactional group also generates a high degrees of anxiety for the alcoholic whose experience with most treatment and self-help is highly ritualized and structured.

A number of therapeutic techniques can help reduce the patients' anxiety. Generally speaking, the more structure and support provided, the lower the anxiety. This can be best accomplished if the therapist is active and supportive and explicitly teaches about the process of group therapy and addiction., If here-and-now interactions become emotionally charged, the therapist can titrate the level of anxiety by steering the group into a stage of objective reflection about the interaction.

Thus, the therapist does not aim to eradicate anxiety from the group but to manage it carefully according to the patients' tolerance levels. By successfully navigating anxiety-producing situations, a patient can develop confidence about performing adequately in similar interactions outside the group and may also learn that such negative emotional states can be tolerated without recourse to drugs or alcohol.

A THERAPEUTIC APPROACH TO RESPONSIBILITY

Every psychotherapeutic approach that is ambitious and hopes to precipitate extensive change in the individual has to presume that patients have some responsibility for the genesis and alteration of their condition. Yet the disease concept holds that alcoholics are not responsible for their illness; the disease is the culprit.

How to resolve this dilemma? The first step is to delineate the boundaries of responsibility and to clarify our meaning of the term.

What Are Patients Not Responsible For?

Patients are not to be held responsible for the addiction itself. Much research has demonstrated an organic substrate to alcoholism:

1. Genetic studies have demonstrated predisposing factors to alcoholism as evidenced by biological marker, family, and twin studies (Cloninger, Bohman, & Sigvardsson, 1981; Schuckit, 1980).
2. Metabolic studies have demonstrated alterations in alcohol metabolism that minimize the negative effects of intoxication (Schuckit & Rayes, 1979).
3. Psychophysiological studies demonstrate differences in autonomic reactivity (e.g., P3 waves are less pronounced in sons of alcoholics) (Begleiter, Porjescz, & Kissin, 1984; Tarter, Alterman, & Edwards, 1985).

In addition, alcoholics experience a psychological loss of control, for which they similarly should not be held accountable. They are unable to stop drinking after the first drink and lack the ability to predict the consequences of their drinking. Though their judgment becomes impaired, the massive defensive system inextricably linked with the disease prevents awareness of this impairment. Heavy drinkers often literally lose conscious control via blackouts.

Alcoholics should not be considered responsible for beliefs and values about drinking—these are deeply ingrained in our culture and transmitted pervasively through the media and families. Finally, alcoholics inevitably experience psychological sequelae to their loss of drinking control (anxiety, depression, shame, guilt) that call forth a series of restorative or compensatory defenses (denial, intellectualization, projection, grandiosity, and defiance).

In summary, alcoholics experience these powerful forces as being out of control (prompting them to take the first AA step). We advocate validating their experience through the concepts of the disease model, which maintains that they are not responsible for the addictive process. At the same time, however, we demand that patients assume responsibility for their recovery.

What Are Patients Responsible For?

Patients are responsible for many things:

1. *Patients are responsible for the first drink.* Once the patient has made it through detoxification and entered treatment in a state of abstinence, the physiological craving for alcohol has diminished. The first drink reactivates a powerful process over which the patient has no control. However, patients do make a conscious choice to take the first drink; not to hold them responsible for this would undermine the goal of sobriety and make treatment untenable.
2. *Patients are responsible for the series of behaviors outlined in AA's Twelve Steps.* For example, the patient is responsible for self-examination and understanding, for making amends to others, for carrying the AA message to others, and so forth. AA and psychotherapy can provide structure, support, and encouragement, but ultimately it is the responsibility of individual patients to take the active steps.
3. *Patients are responsible for how they choose to relate to others in the immediate here and now.* In the group psychotherapy session, interactional therapists must view patients as free and responsible for the innumerable decisions they make and behaviors they display (e.g., whether patients choose to engage with others or recede into silence, to support other members or attack them, or to be helpful to others or to exploit them).

MODIFICATION OF GROUP PROCESS TO INCORPORATE THE LANGUAGE AND BELIEF SYSTEMS OF AA AND OTHER SELF-HELP GROUPS

AA is an extremely powerful force in the treatment program of alcoholics. Not only is it intrinsically valuable—many decades have led to an accretion of valuable knowledge about the recovery process—but AA has an extraordinary influence over the thinking of a substantial number of recovering alcoholics. Therefore, if therapists, are to be effective with the alcoholic population, it behooves them to be thoroughly familiar with the AA traditions. There are two reasons for this: (1) to draw on the knowledge of AA and incorporate that knowledge into the therapy process and (2) to spot and prevent the misuse of AA concepts (i.e., their distortion and utilization in therapy resistance) (Vannicelli, 1988).

Relationship between AA and Psychotherapy:
Sources and Perceived Conflict

Interactive group therapy is in no way meant to replace AA's important role in the recovery program; in fact, the group therapist often actively enlists the aid of AA. Yet many recovering alcoholics view the process of psychotherapy (and in particular group therapy) as antithetical to AA. Why does this misunderstanding arise? We have identified five perceived conflicts between AA and psychotherapy.

1. Traditional psychotherapy has had a long tradition of failing to help alcoholics.
2. Psychotherapy is seen as rationalistic whereas AA places a heavy emphasis on spirituality.
3. Group therapy emphasizes interpersonal interaction and analysis whereas AA eschews that and relies on other therapeutic mechanisms.
4. AA insists on nonprofessional leaders who have recovered from alcoholism, as opposed to the traditional professional leadership of group psychotherapy.
5. Traditional psychotherapy is viewed as not placing a heavy emphasis on abstinence and lacking the methodology to prevent drinking.

These are serious "charges." They suggest fundamental and irreconcilable differences between AA and psychotherapy, and we must, if we wish to recruit alcoholics into psychotherapy programs, respond effectively to these concerns.

It is our position that these statements are based on inaccuracies or misunderstandings of either AA or psychotherapy and that there are no fundamental inconsistencies. In this section we first address these five charges and then translate some of the basic principles of AA into an interpersonal point of view.

1. *Traditional psychotherapy has had a long tradition of failing to help alcoholics.* The early psychotherapists, for the most part psychoanalytically oriented, viewed addiction solely as a function of underlying psychological disturbance and ignored biochemical and social etiological factors (Levin, 1990). Therapy, often nondirective and psychoanalytical, placed a heavy emphasis on insight and failed to provide the structure and support so necessary for containing anxiety and maintaining sobriety.

Because these early, now outmoded methods did not work, many traditional therapists became pessimistic, even nihilistic, about the effectiveness of psychotherapy for alcoholic patients. AA emerged, in effect, to fill this void and to help those deemed untreatable by contemporary psychotherapeutic methods.

2. *Psychotherapy is seen as rationalistic whereas AA heavily emphasizes spirituality.* Perhaps as a reaction to the overemphasis of psychological etiological theories, advocates of the disease model stressed the biochemical and sociocultural aspects of addiction (Vaillant, 1983). This viewpoint deemphasizes personal responsibility and considers that psychological forces are overwhelmed by the power of the addictive experience. This deemphasis on personal responsibility created the need for an alternate theory of mastery and change and has resulted in a heavy emphasis on the spiritual component of AA as the driving force behind recovery.

This opposition between spiritual and psychological approaches is inconsistent with the basic tenets of AA, which does indeed invoke a spiritual component in its recovery approach but also insists on self-understanding as a basis of recovery. (See the discussion of the fourth and tenth steps of AA.)

As for religious faith, psychotherapy is no more a threat to the alcoholics' belief in a higher power than therapy is a threat to adherence to any religious system. The responsible psychotherapist never attempts to question or remove a patient's working, satisfying religious belief system. The polemics around psychotherapy and antireligiosity dwell almost entirely in the professional theoretical literature, not in the clinician's office.

3. *Group therapy emphasizes interpersonal interaction and analysis whereas AA eschews that and relies on other therapeutic mechanisms.* The format of AA meetings is highly structured: Roles are assigned, topics for discussion are suggested, and literature is assigned and read. Interactions with other members during the meetings are nearly always discouraged; AA members address topics (e.g., the need for honesty in recovery) by speaking to the group as a whole about their experiences. This format is in striking contrast to the relatively unstructured approach in group psychotherapy, where here-and-now interpersonal exchanges are not only discouraged but seen as an essential ingredient in therapy.

AA has adopted a uniform structure for several reasons. Because many alcoholics suffer from serious interpersonal difficulties, the prohibition against interaction between members in AA meetings prevents conflict and anxiety. AA also discourages interpersonal exchanges in the meetings because of the fear that an unhealthy dependency on a person may serve as a substitute for a drug. AA slogans, such as, "Principles, not personalities" and "Don't rely on people, places, or things," guide the members away from potentially unhealthy dependencies. Finally, the absence of formal, professional leaders makes the use of interpersonal interaction inadvisable. Considerable skill and training are required for the effective therapeutic use of the interpersonal approach.

Nonetheless, the interpersonal realm is both formally and informally addressed in AA (specifically, as we discuss shortly, in the second, fifth, eighth, ninth, and twelfth steps). The importance of interpersonal relationships in the recovery process is also acknowledged in the role of the sponsor and in the encouragement to perform roles within the AA organization, such as chairing a meeting, serving as a secretary, or, more generally, carrying the message to other alcoholics. In fact, we have heard alcoholics joke that the most important parts of AA meetings are the pre- and postmeeting social encounters.

4. *AA insists on nonprofessional leaders who have recovered from alcoholism, as opposed to the traditional professional leadership of group psychotherapy.* Several related factors are responsible for the leaderless nature and the nonprofessional tradition of AA. Consider traditions Two and Eight in AA's *Twelve Steps and Twelve Traditions* (1996). (Note that the Twelve Steps in AA are guides for individual members, whereas the 12 traditions are guidelines for AA group interactions.)

> *Tradition Two*—For our purpose there is but one ultimate authority—a loving God as He may express himself in our group conscience. Our leaders are but trusted servants; they do not govern. (p. 132)
> *Tradition Eight*—Alcoholics Anonymous should remain forever non-professional, but our service centers may employ special workers. (Alcoholics Anonymous World Services, Inc., 1996, p. 166)

One of the primary therapeutic factors in AA is the sense of fellowship that it creates. Any methodological approach that would alter this sense of equality of its members is therefore discouraged. Furthermore, one of the most consistent characteristics of alcoholics is their deep difficulty with authority, manifested by rebelliousness; AA is responsive to this trait by deemphasizing human authority.

AA believes that help can only be offered by other alcoholics—that only people who have gone through the same turmoil and struggles have the same requisite empathy and knowledge to offer help. AA augments this belief by fostering a dichotomy between the "we" (AA members) and the "they" (the noncomprehending, nonsympathetic outside world, a world where it is abnormal not to drink).

AA clearly serves many important functions that cannot be realistically provided by a professional therapist. The AA culture serves as a counterculture that normalizes sobriety. AA provides role models and inspiration to those who are newly recovering: Other recovering alcoholics provide both hope for recovery and support and advice for staying sober. It is vital for the recovering alcoholic to be immersed in a culture of recovering people.

314 TREATING BEHAVIORS THAT INTERFERE WITH HEALTH

But the fact that alcoholics can reap great benefits from a supportive social network of other recovering individuals does not also mean that *only* alcoholics can help each other. Although a well-trained psychotherapist who is also a recovering alcoholic might have some additional insight into the experience, by no means does the recovery experience substitute for extensive clinical training.

Even though therapists need not be recovering alcoholics, it is imperative that they be thoroughly familiar with AA steps and traditions and with the AA experience: It permits them to harness the wisdom of AA in the service of therapy, to undermine the use of AA as resistance, and to disarm patients' negativity toward psychotherapy.

5. *Traditional psychotherapy is viewed as not placing a heavy emphasis on abstinence and as lacking the methodology to prevent drinking.* We believe that the need for a supportive social network is at the heart of the perception that therapy is in and of itself insufficient to help a person stop drinking. Social pressure to drink is massive: advertisements, movies, books, television, and day-to-day social settings abound with overt and covert messages about the positive functions to alcohol. Therapy can help strengthen an awareness of these cues and develop alternative coping strategies, but it, in itself, is rarely capable of helping the patient achieve and maintain abstinence. Most patients need the additional support of AA or other self-help groups.

There is another component of the negative perception about therapy. In nearly all cases therapy seeks to increase a person's sense of mastery; this coupled with recent scholarly debate about the possibility of controlled drinking for recovering alcoholics may have increased the suspicion that traditional psychotherapy is ambivalent about the goal of abstinence. To work effectively with this population, therapists must clarify their own attitudes about drinking and abstinence. Therapists uncomfortable with the notion of abstinence unwittingly reinforce a patient's difficulty in accepting this position. On this issue, our position is unequivocal—drinking is life-threatening for the alcoholic.

It is important to resolve these perceived areas of incompatibility between AA and psychotherapy. AA and psychotherapy are not competing forces that threaten the survival or efficacy of the other but are mutually augmentative. Their goals are similar, and they share more common methods than generally thought. It must be remembered, however, that both psychotherapy and AA are diverse entities, containing a wide range of practices and interpretations of theory and traditions. There will, unfortunately, always be AA "hard liners," openly antagonistic to the idea of therapy, as well as psychotherapists who scorn AA.

THE TWELVE STEPS OF AA: AN INTERPERSONAL VIEW

The twelve steps have proven their value in the AA recovery process, and an interpersonal interpretation of these steps proves useful for the group therapist. However, therapists should keep in mind that each step may be viewed in a psychological context and may have different meanings for different individuals, even for the same individual over time (Brown, 1985).

Therapists frequently experience some confusion about how to handle the use of "God" in these steps. This discussion translates religious concepts into interpersonal symbolic equivalents. Alcohol and drugs fulfill many psychological functions for addicts, eventually assuming the significance of primary relationships in their lives. Recovering individuals who relinquish this pathological relationship need something to replace it. They urgently seek a new source of soothing, nurturance, and hope. A higher power may be one such source; a significant, rewarding interpersonal relationship may be another.

Let us now examine the Twelve Steps for this perspective.

1. We admitted that we were powerless over alcohol—that our lives had become unmanageable.
2. Came to believe that a Power greater than ourselves could restore us to sanity.
3. Made a decision to turn our will and our lives over to the care of God as we understood Him.

In the first step, individuals must acknowledge that they are in pain, powerless to help themselves, and, therefore, in need of assistance. This step requires the alcoholic to relinquish two common defenses: grandiosity and counterdependency. In the second step, the alcoholic understands that the restorative process takes place through relationships. The first step emphasizes that the addict has reached the point of being unable to solve problems in isolation; the second step teaches that redemption is possible only through the establishment of important human connections.

The third step asks the individual to make a "leap into trust"—that is, to temporarily put aside customary defenses against social intimacy and instead to place faith and trust in the larger group. This step sharply differentiates treatment of the alcoholic versus a more traditional treatment of other neurotic conditions. Most patients are expected to develop trust gradually, but alcoholic patients in early stages of recovery cannot afford to wait: they must be exhorted to take an immediate leap into trust, which then provides the human relatedness and sustenance that make abstinence possible. In this phase of therapy the alcoholic often becomes strongly merged with the group or recovery program.

4. Made a searching and fearless moral inventory of ourselves.
5. Admitted to God, to ourselves, and to another human the being, the exact nature of our wrongs.

Steps 4 and 5 constitute a sequence of self-discovery and self-disclosure. Because of the AA tradition and the prior exposure of alcoholic group members to steps 4 and 5 in their AA experience, the alcoholic group is often able to engage in these processes at a fast pace—provided the group therapist is familiar with and draws upon the AA Twelve Step procedure.

6. Were entirely ready to have God remove all these defects of character.

In many AA chapters, members approach this sixth step by considering their character defects. Alcoholics will only be willing to give up their defects when they can clearly see the effects of the ensuing negative consequences on their relationships with others. Behaviors such as aggressiveness and seclusiveness may insulate the alcoholic from the pain and problems of intimacy, but they also result in the alcoholic not receiving the type of nurture or support he or she desires. Part of the group work consists in demonstrating to alcoholic patients the self-defeating nature of their behavior.

7. Humbly asked Him to remove our shortcomings.

Steps 6 and 7 together constitute a sequence beginning with awareness and resulting in change. Step 6, as we have discussed, involves the awareness that the defective character no longer serves any positive function; step 7 consists of the actual step of removal and correction of interpersonal patterns. Thus, in the context of the therapy group, these two steps include learning as much as possible about one's behavior via self-exploration and assimilation of feedback from other members, and, finally, making active attempts to experiment with new behaviors. Group therapists must urge and support such experimentation.

8. Made a list of all persons we had harmed and became willing to make amends to them all.
9. Made direct amends to such people wherever possible, except when to do so would injure them or others.

Steps 8 and 9 also constitute a sequence leading from awareness to willingness to making amends to actual respirations. In the AA program, members are expected to examine all dimensions of their life to determine whom they have harmed and to take responsibility for making appropriate amends.

These steps are an attempt to ameliorate the alcoholic's ubiquitous guilt and shame, which so often cripple satisfactory interpersonal interactions. Alcoholics are asked to be more empathic in their relationships—a process in which therapy groups play an important role. The group therapist encourages members to progress through these steps in the here-and-now context of the group: Members examine those group members against whom they have, in some minor but representative way, transgressed and make appropriate amends. This is both a real experience (with real people, in real time) and a rehearsal for the work that must be done in their outside life.

10. Continued to take personal inventory and when we were wrong promptly admitted it.

This is a "maintenance" step, calling for an ongoing process of self-reflection and self-disclosure. The therapist supports this process by urging members to self-disclose, to express feelings about other members, and to study their here-and-now interactions within the group.

11. Sought through prayer and meditation to improve our conscious contact with God as we understand Him, praying only for knowledge of His will for us and the power to carry that out.

This is obviously an explicitly religious step that has no direct counterpart in the interactional group process. Note, however, that many AA programs use this eleventh step to encourage meditative practice—a practice that does not necessarily have religious overtones. Therapists working with alcoholic patients in either individual or group should be familiar with and sympathetic to such meditative practices; such practices may offer an effective mode of anxiety control that may play an important role in the recovery process.

12. Having had a spiritual awakening as the result of these steps, we tried to carry this message to alcoholics and to practice these principles in all our affairs.

Within the framework of AA, this step can be understood on a number of levels. In its simplest interpretation, it refers to the idea of carrying the message to other alcoholics by personal example. This step promotes a sense of family, which serves as an antidote to the alcoholics' deep sense of alienation. For the self-absorbed alcoholic, the development of an active concern for others is an important ingredient in recovery.

The ramifications of step 12 for the interactional group are several. Patients, once they have established a modicum of equilibrium and moved past the survival stage in recovery, can be useful guides to other members in early recovery. The fact that others have struggled with the same issues and transcended them provides hope for newer members and results in continuous renewal in the alcohol group. Furthermore, there is persuasive research indicating that altruism not only increases the cohesiveness of the group but elevates the self-esteem of the individual offering the help.

COMMON CLINICAL THEMES IN GROUP THERAPY WITH ALCOHOLICS

Idealization and Devaluation

Addicts' tendency to idealize or devalue others is particularly evident in their attitudes toward the group leaders. This process is particularly threatening to the recovery process because disappointment in and devaluation of the leadership often increase the likelihood of turning to drugs and alcohol to combat negative emotional states.

Therapists must be prepared for rapid fluctuations in group members' evaluation of them. The more that therapists are imbued with extreme wisdom, insight, and power, the more likely they are ultimately to disappoint their group members. Alcoholics frequently have strong unmet dependency needs. To protect themselves from disappointment they frequently withdraw or assume a strong counterdependent posture. Leaders are advised to call attention to these trends early in therapy and not to allow themselves to be seduced by the idealization or become threatened by the inevitable devaluation. A firm, reliable, benevolent therapist is essential to the recovering alcoholic.

Tendency to Externalize

Alcoholics often see themselves as being influenced or controlled primarily by external events. Research with prealcoholics also indicates a projective predisposition, that is, tendencies toward high levels of external locus of control and field dependency rather than an internal locus of control and field independence (O'Leary, Donovan, & Hague, 1974).

The defining characteristic of alcoholics—their pathological relationship with alcohol—is clearly symptomatic of their externalizing tendency. They look to alcohol to provide soothing, support, or power rather than considering internal sources of need gratification. Indeed, addiction is driven by the belief that one cannot function without the all-powerful addictive substance.

Alcoholics experience guilt from a number of sources: from the loss of control and mastery over their drinking and the damage they have done to themselves, to their physical health, to their families, to their relationships with their spouses, and to their careers. They frequently attempt to ameliorate intolerable levels of guilt by externalization, by blaming others for their failures. In the course of a therapy group, it is not unusual for alcoholics to blame the group for a drinking slip. They may say, for example, that the group's criticism of them the previous week created such discomfort that they were forced to drink.

This tendency to externalize exists at such a fundamental level that it is unlikely that it can be substantially altered or uprooted; instead, the therapy process has to utilize it. AA routinely makes use of this tendency by encouraging reliance on some higher power outside the individual. Therapy groups may make use of it by permitting, even encouraging, high levels of dependency on the therapist and the group.

Experiencing others as having the power and resources to help them often leaves alcoholics feeling empty, passive, and dependent on some external event to solve their difficulties. Thus, a major issue in treatment of the alcoholic patient is to help patients differentiate between what they *are* and *are not* responsible for and to help them assume responsibility for changing those things they can change. The AA Serenity Prayer, "God grant me the serenity to accept the things I cannot change, courage to change the things we can and the wisdom to know the difference," is particularly potent in this regard. Therapists should know this slogan well and be able to exploit its therapeutic leverage.

Compensatory Tendencies

One of the chief psychological tasks of actively abusing addicts is to deal with loss of personal control. They commonly employ the defenses of defiance, grandiosity, and counterdependency as a way of compensating for loss of control.

Defiance

The loss of control often results in alcoholics being infantilized and parented by others. Yet this response by others often makes alcoholics bristle, and they respond in a defiant manner with the clear message, "Don't tell me what to do." This typical dynamic has considerable implications for group therapy technique. Patients resist therapists who rely excessively on the authority inherent in their role. Chairpersons of AA meetings "quality" for their position by virtue of "experience, strength and hope." Therapists, too, must be expected to qualify for their position of leadership not through *ex cathedra* authority but by virtue of their expertise.

Alcoholics often deny any dependent feelings—including their dependence on alcohol. In therapy, this often takes the form of patients suddenly deciding to leave the group just when they seem to be more fully engaged: Their growing awareness of their dependency needs becomes threatening to them and precipitates a flight from therapy. Therapists must be sensitive to alcoholics' reluctance to acknowledge their dependency needs and help them to accept and express these needs gradually.

Grandiosity

Another method of defending against loss of control (and low self-esteem) is through grandiosity. This defense should not be challenged too suddenly in psychotherapy or severe depression may result. Proper timing and support are necessary to help alcoholics develop substitute defenses and coping skills. AA posits that recovery entails "ego deflation." Alcoholics need to deflate their false egos and instill a true sense of pride. There is no better source of self-confidence and esteem than continued sobriety.

Tendency to Con or Avoid

It is well-known that alcoholics tend to lie, con, and engage in avoidant behavior. Therapists working with alcoholic groups repeatedly observe examples of this: Patients lie, engage in passive–aggressive behaviors, drop out of therapy, are silent or passive, or pretend to agree rather than face up to conflicts.

AA has long recognized these tendencies and has always insisted that the alcoholic bring the attitudes of "willingness" and "rigorous honesty" into the recovery process. An alcoholic's unwillingness to begin from this stance indicates that he or she is not yet ready for a recovery endeavor.

These tendencies present a continuing problem in the psychotherapy of alcoholic patients and have rendered nondirective therapy approaches ineffective. However, we believe that traditional chemical dependency programs have erred in the opposite direction by assuming an overly confrontative therapy stance. This confrontative style was designed to break down denial or resistance but often causes the alcoholic to leave the treatment program or to dissemble compliance while inwardly retreating.

Psychotherapy, like AA, must find a way to encourage "willingness" (i.e., high motivation) and rigorous honesty. Therapists must be ready to confront and challenge behaviors that are not consistent with recovery, yet they must also recognize the limits and consequences of a confrontational approach and, when appropriate, be ready to adopt a more supportive posture.

Ultimately it is the individual's responsibility to be honest and seriously committed to recovery—no amount of exhortation from family or therapists can replace this. Alcoholics are similar to any other psychotherapy patients in that they display resistance to change; it is only that their defenses tend to be more rigid and manipulative. There are times when massive confrontation is absolutely essential: in life-threatening situations, when abstinence is jeopardized, or when it is exceedingly evident that patients are lying or being evasive.

But when recovery is not at issue, confrontative techniques may be counterproductive, and therapists need to treat alcoholics in the same way they work with other patients—that is, by relating to them in an empathic, supportive, and understanding manner. Sheer confrontation alone will not result in substantial personal growth.

On a practical level, at times the therapist may be required to be more active than in clinical situations. Silence and avoidant behavior in the alcoholic group should be challenged more rapidly and actively than in other psychotherapy situations. If, for example, a patient misses group, it is generally indicated for the therapist to call and immediately confront the patient.

Therapists must find a way to be both empathic and distrustful with this population. If the therapist is suspicious, for example, that a patient is drinking or using drugs, it is important to voice these suspicions. If these concerns are well grounded yet meet with denial by the patient, the therapist may well wish to employ other validating methods, including the use of breath analyzers and urine screening.

Often the task of confrontation is effectively carried out by other group members—a positive development in the group because the patients themselves may be particularly able to spot using in their peers. It is also important that therapists have access to information about patients that comes form other sources: treatment programs of codependents, other family members, employers, physicians. It must be made clear, at the onset of therapy, that the therapist has the right, even the mandate, to reveal in the group any available information that patients are drinking or engaging in other forms of behavior detrimental to recovery.

To summarize, we believe that group approaches to alcoholism can be made more effective if the therapist takes advantage of a powerful group therapeutic factor—interpersonal learning. However, special factors associated with alcohol addiction may mandate a modification of the standard interactional approach. Group therapists must always be aware of the absolute primacy of recovery, they must insist that patients accept identity as an alcoholic; they must modulate anxiety to prevent acting out and relapse, they must understand the concept of responsibility, and they must create a powerful working liaison with AA. Finally, they must be prepared to deal in the therapy group with themes that are often specific to work with alcoholic patients.

REFERENCES

Alcoholics Anonymous World Services, Inc. (1996). *Twelve steps and traditions*. New York: AA Grapevine.

American Psychiatric Association. (1987). *Diagnostic and statistical manual of mental disorders* (3rd ed., rev.). Washington, DC: Author.

Ashley, M. J. (1989). How extensive is the problem of alcoholism? *Alcohol and Research World, 13*(4), 305–309.

Bateman, D. A., & Heagarty, M. C. (1992). Passive freebase cocaine ("crack") inhalation by infants and toddlers. *American Journal of Diseases of Children, 143*, 25–27.

Beardsley, S., Gardocki, G. J., Larson, D. B., & Hidalgo, J. (1988). Prescribing of psychotropic medication by primary care physicians and psychiatrists. *Archives of General Psychiatry, 45*, 1117–1119.

Begleiter, H., Porjesz, B., & Kissin, B. (1984). Event-related brain potentials in children at risk for alcoholism. *Science, 255*, 1493–1496.

Blott, W. J., McLaughlin, J. K., Winn, D. M., Austin, D. F., Greenberg, R. S., Preston-Martin, S., Bernstein, L., Schoeberg, J. B., Stemhagen, A., & Fraumeni, J. F. (1988). Smoking and drinking in relation to oral and pharyngeal cancer. *Cancer Research, 48*, 3282–3287.

Brown, S. (1985). *Treating the alcoholic: A developmental model of recovery*. New York: Wiley.

Brown, S. (1995). *Treating alcoholism*. San Francisco: Jossey-Bass.

Chasnoff, R. (1989). Cocaine, pregnancy, and the neonate. *Women and Health, 15*(3), 23–35.

Clark, W., & Midanik, L. (1982). Alcohol use and alcohol problems among United States adults. In *NIAAA: Alcohol consumption and related problems* (pp. 3–52). Washington, DC: U.S. Government Printing Office.

Cloninger, C. R., Bohman, M., & Sigvardsson, S. (1981). Inheritance of alcohol abuse: Cross fostering analysis of adopted men. *Archives of General Psychiatry, 38*, 861–868.

Daley, D. C., & Raskin, M. S. (1991). Relapse prevention and treatment effectiveness studies. In D. C. Daley & M. S. Raskin (Eds.), *Treating the chemically dependent and their families* (pp. 129–171). Newbury Park, CA: Sage.

Des Jarlais, D. C., Friedman, S. R., Woods, J., & Milliken, J. (1992). HIV infection among intravenous drug users: Epidemiology and emerging public health perspectives. In J. H. Lowinson, P. Ruiz, R. B. Millman, & J. G. Langrod (Eds.), *Substance abuse: A comprehensive textbook* (pp. 734–743). Baltimore: Williams & Wilkins.

Frances, F. J. (1988). Update on alcohol and drug disorder treatment. *Journal of Clinical Psychiatry, 49*(9, Suppl.), 13–17.

Geller, A. (1992). Rehabilitation programs and halfway houses. In J. H. Lowinson, P. Ruiz, R. B. Millman, & J. G. Langrod (Eds.), *Substance abuse: A comprehensive textbook* (pp. 458–466). Baltimore: Williams & Wilkins.

Genetello, L. M., Donovan, D. M., Dunn, C. W., & Rivara, F. P. (1995). Alcohol interventions in trauma centers: Current practice and future directions. *Journal of the American Medical Association, 274*, 1043–1048.

Gottheil, E., Druly, K. A., Skoloda, T. E., & Waxman, H. M. (1983). *Etiologic aspects of alcohol and drug abuse.* Springfield, IL: Charles C. Thomas.

Ishak, K. G., Zimmerman, H. J., & Mukunda, R. B. (1991). Alcoholic liver disease: Pathologic, pathogenetic and clinical aspects. *Alcoholism: Clinical and Experimental Research, 15*(1), 45–66.

Ito, J. R., Donovan, D. M., & Hall, J. J. (1988). Relapse prevention in alcohol aftercare: Effects on drinking outcome, change, process, and aftercare attendance. *British Journal of Addiction, 83,* 171–181.

Jaffe, J. H. (1992). Opiates: Clinical aspects. In J. H. Lowison, P. Ruiz, R. B. Millman, & J. G. Langrod (Eds.), *Substance abuse: A comprehensive textbook* (2nd ed., pp. 186–194). Baltimore: Williams and Wilkins.

Jarvis, T. J. (1992). Implications of gender for alcohol treatment research: A quantitative and qualitative review. *British Journal of Addiction, 87,* 1249–1261.

Kaufman, E. (1986). A workable system of family therapy for drug dependence. *Journal of Psychoactive Drugs, 18*(1), 43–50.

Khantzian, E. J., & Treece, C. (1985). DSM-III psychiatric diagnosis of narcotic addicts. *Archives of General Psychiatry, 42,* 1067–1071.

Levin, J. D. (1990). *Treatment of Alcoholism and other addictions: A self-psychology approach.* Northvale, NJ: Jason Aronson.

Lex, B. W. (1987). Review of alcohol problems in ethnic minority groups. *Journal of Consulting and Clinical Psychology, 55*(3), 293–300.

Matano, R., & Yalom, I. (1991). Approaches to chemical dependency and interactive group therapy—A synthesis. *International Journal of Group Psychotherapy, 41*(3), 269–293.

Mehler, P. S., McClellan, M. D., Lezotte, D., Casper, E., & Gabrow, P. A. (1995). Improving identification of and intervention for alcoholism. *Western Journal of Medicine, 163,* 335–340.

Miller, N. S., Belkin, B. M., & Gold, M. S. (1991). Alcohol and drug dependence among the elderly: Epidemiology, diagnosis, and treatment. *Comprehensive Psychiatry, 32*(2), 153–165.

Millman, R. B. (1986). Considerations on the psychotherapy of the substance abuser. *Journal of Substance Abuse Treatment, 3*(2), 103–109.

Nace, E. P. (1992). Alcoholics Anonymous. In J. H. Lowinson, P. Ruiz, R. B. Millman, & J. G. Langrod (Eds.), *Substance abuse: A comprehensive textbook* (pp. 486–495). Baltimore: Williams & Wilkins.

National Institute on Drug Abuse. (1990). *National household survey on drug abuse—Main findings, 1988.* Rockville, MD: National Institute on Drug Abuse.

O'Brien, W. B., & Biase, D. V. (1992). Therapeutic community (TC): A coming of age. In J. H. Lowinson, P. Ruiz, R. B. Millman, & J. G. Langrod (Eds.), *Substance abuse: A comprehensive textbook* (pp. 446–457). Baltimore: Williams & Wilkins.

O'Leary, M. R., Donovan, D. M., & Hague, W. H. (1974). Relationships between locus of control and MMPI scales among alcoholics: A replication and extension. *Journal of Clinical Psychology, 30,* 312–314.

O'Malley, S. S., Jaffe, A., Chang, G., Schottenfeld, R. S., Meyer, R. E., & Rounsaville, B. (1992). Naltrexone and coping skills therapy for alcohol dependence: A controlled study. *Archives of General Psychiatry, 49,* 881–887.

Pattison, M., & Kaupman, E. (1982). The alcoholism syndrome: Definitions and models. In M. Pattison & E. Kaupman (Eds.), *Encyclopedic handbook of alcoholism* (pp. 3–30). New York: Garner Press.

Reiger, D. A., Myers, J. K., Kramer, M., Robins, L. N., Blazer, D. G., Hough, R. L., Eaton, W. W., & Locke, B. Z. (1984). The NIMH epidemiologic catchment area program. *Archives of General Psychiatry, 41,* 934–941.

Romelsjo, A. (1993). The prevalence of alcohol-related mortality in both sexes: Variations between indicators. *American Journal of Public Health, 83*(6), 838–844.

Ropers, R. H., & Boyer, R. (1987). Homelessness as a health risk. *Alcohol Health and Research World, 11,* 38–41.

Ross, H. E., Glaser, F. B., & Germanson, T. (1988). The prevalence of psychiatric disorders in patients with alcohol and other drug problems. *Archives of General Psychiatry, 45,* 1023–1031.

Rutan, J. S., & Sonte, W. N. (1984). *Psychodynamic group therapy.* Lexington, MA: Collamore Press.

Schmidt, W., & Popham, R. E. (1975). Heavy alcohol consumption and physical health problems: A review of the epidemiological evidence. *Drug and Alcohol Dependence, 1,* 27–50.

Schmidt, W., & Popham, R. E. (1981). The role of drinking and smoking in mortality from cancer and other causes in male alcoholics. *Cancer, 47,* 1031–1041.

Schuckit, M. A. (1980). Biological markers: Metabolism and acute reactions to alcohol in sons of alcoholics. *Pharmacology, Biochemistry, and Behavior, 13,* 9–16.

Schuckit, M. A., & Rayes, V. (1979). Ethanol ingestion: Differences in blood acetaldehyde concentrations in relatives of alcoholics and controls. *Science, 203,* 54–55.

Skog, O. J. (1987). Trends in alcohol consumption and deaths from diseases. *British Journal of Addiction, 82,* 1033–1041.

Solomon, S. D. (1983). *Evaluation of drug treatment programs.* Haworth Press.

Svanum, S., & McAdoo, W. G. (1989). Predicting rapid relapse following treatment for chemical dependence: A matched subjects design. *Journal of Consulting and Clinical Psychology, 57*(2), 222–226.

Tarter, R. E., Alterman, A. I., & Edwards, K. L. (1985). Vulnerability to alcoholism in men: A behavior–genetic perspective. *Journal of Studies on Alcohol, 46,* 329–356.

Tuyns, A. J. (1979). Epidemiology of alcohol and cancer. *Cancer Research, 39,* 2840–2843.

U.S. Preventive Services Task Force. (1989). *Guide to clinical preventive services: An assessment of effectiveness of 169 interventions* (M. Fisher, Ed.). Baltimore: Williams & Wilkins.

Vaillant, G. E. (1983). *The national history of alcoholism: Causes, patterns and paths to recovery.* Cambridge, MA: Harvard University Press.

Vanicelli, M. (1988). Group therapy after care for alcoholic patients. *International Journal of Group Psychotherapy, 38,* 337–353.

Volpicelli, J. R., Alterman, A. I., Hayashida, M., & O'Brien, C. P. (1992). Naltrexone in the treatment of alcohol dependence. *Archives of General Psychiatry, 49,* 876–880.

Watson, C. G., Brown, K., Tilleskjor, Jacobs, L., & Pucel, J. (1988). The comparative recidivism rates of voluntary- and coerced-admission male alcoholics. *Journal of Clinical Psychology, 44*(4), 573–581.

Weiss, R. D., & Mirin, S. M. (1989). Tricyclic antidepressants in the treatment of alcoholism and drug abuse. *Journal of Clinical Psychiatry, 50*(7 Suppl.), 4–9.

Weissman, M. M., & Myers, J. K. (1980). Clinical depression in alcoholism. *American Journal of Psychiatry, 137*(3), 372–373.

Weissman, M. M., Myers, J. K., & Harding, P. S. (1980). Prevalence and psychiatric heterogeneity of alcoholism in a United States urban community. *Journal of Studies on Alcohol, 41*(7), 672–681.

Widner, S., & Zeichner, A. (1991). Alcohol abuse in the elderly: Review of epidemiology research and treatment. *Clinical Gerontologist, 11*(1), 3–18.

Winick, C. (1992). Epidemiology of alcohol and drug abuse. In J. H. Lowinson, P. Ruiz, R. B. Millman, & J. G. Langrod (Eds.), *Substance abuse: A comprehensive textbook* (pp. 15–29). Baltimore: Williams & Wilkins.

Yalom, I. D. (1985). *The theory and practice of group psychotherapy.* New York: Basic Books.

Index

327

hostility in, 96
intervention studies, 104–107
modification in Recurrent Coronary
    Prevention Project, 97–104
narcissism in, 121–122
social and cultural factors affecting,
    107–108
in women, 103
Type of disease, and format of groups, 43

U

Unusual patients, 39–40

Z

Zen Buddhism, and existentialism,
    174–175, 186–190